# The Illustrated Encyclopedia of
# NATURAL REMEDIES

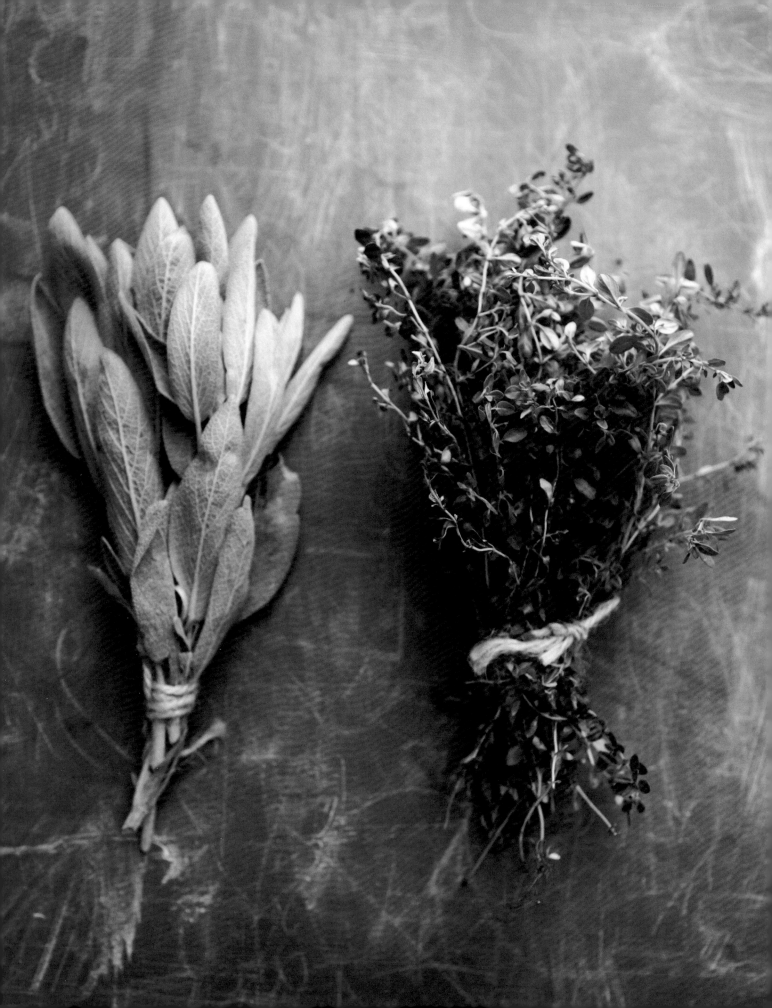

# The Illustrated Encyclopedia of
# NATURAL REMEDIES

## Edited by Abigail R. Gehring
### Foreword by Alyssa Holmes

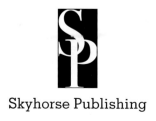
Skyhorse Publishing

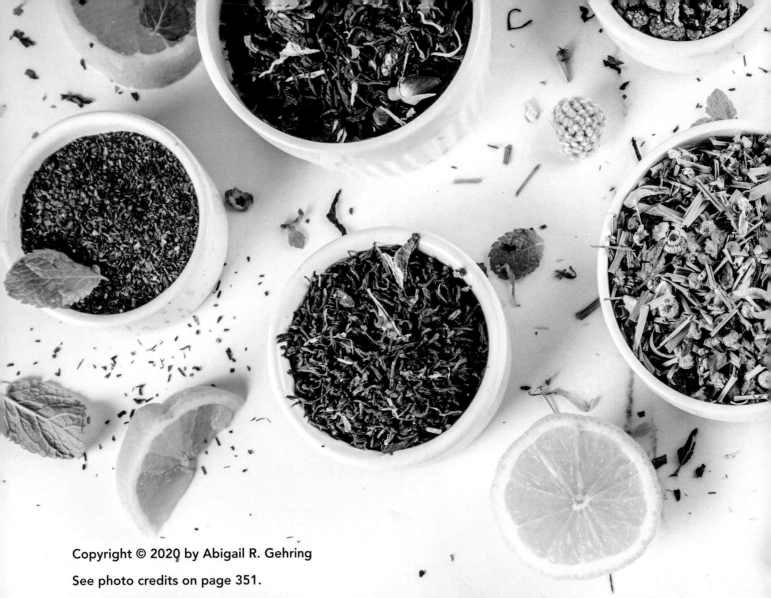

Skyhorse Publishing books may be purchased in bulk at special discounts for sales promotion, corporate gifts, fund-raising, or educational purposes. Special editions can also be created to specifications. For details, contact the Special Sales Department, Skyhorse Publishing, 307 West 36th Street, 11th Floor, New York, NY 10018 or info@skyhorsepublishing.com.

Skyhorse® and Skyhorse Publishing® are registered trademarks of Skyhorse Publishing, Inc.®, a Delaware corporation.

Visit our website at www.skyhorsepublishing.com.

10 9 8 7 6

Library of Congress Cataloging-in-Publication Data is available on file.

Cover design by Daniel Brount
Cover images by Getty Images

Print ISBN: 978-1-5107-4999-3
Ebook ISBN: 978-1-5107-5002-9

Printed in China

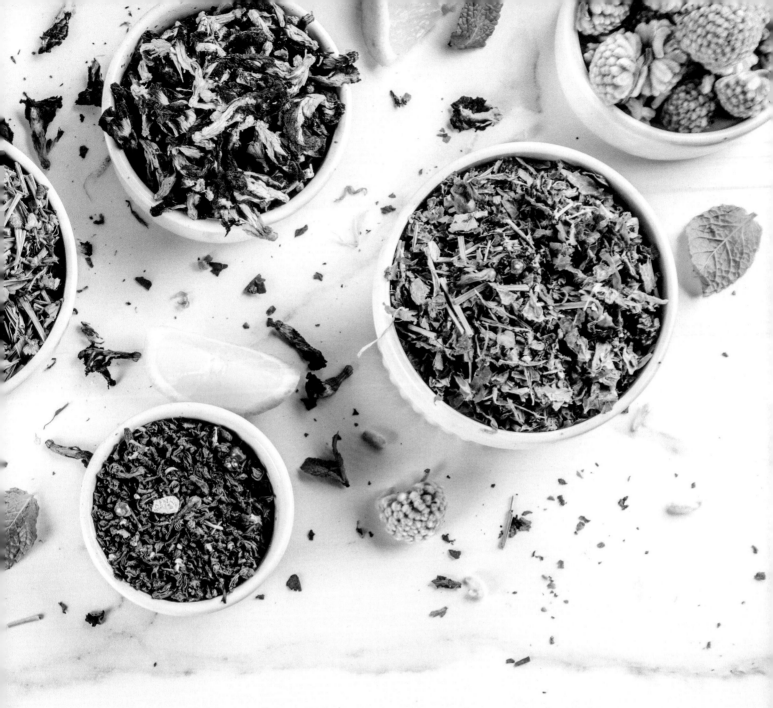

"The part can never be well unless the whole is well." —Plato

"A cheerful heart is a good medicine . . ." —Proverbs 17:22

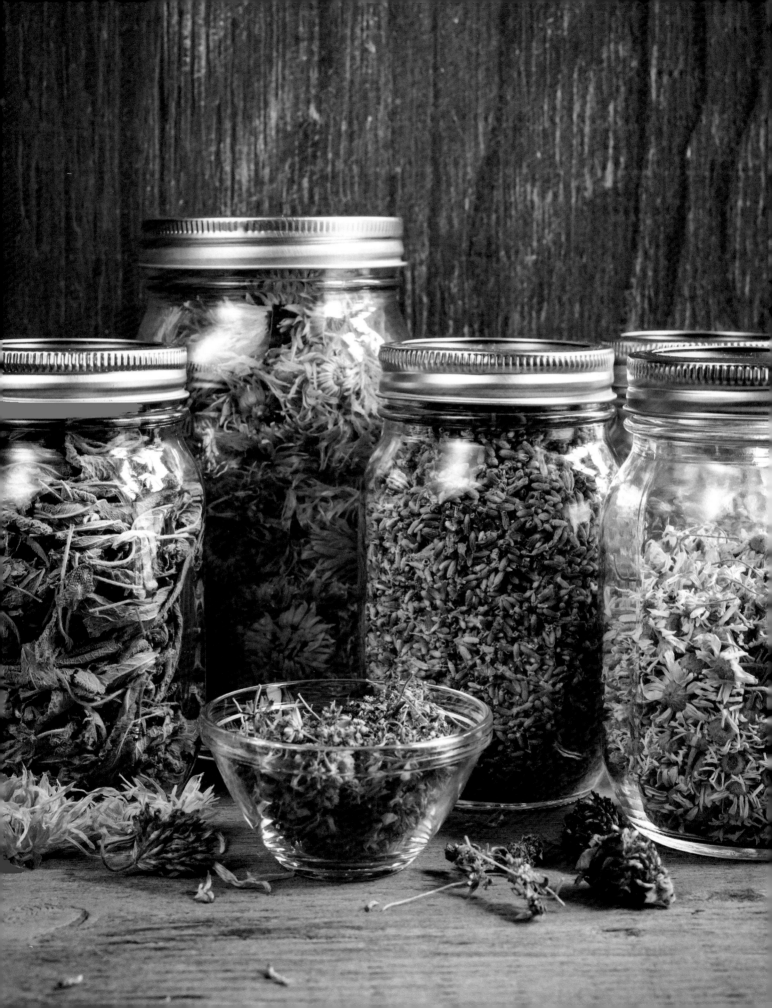

# CONTENTS

Foreword.................................................. xi
Introduction........................................... xiii
- How to Use This Book.......................xiii
- Pantry Tips.....................................xiii
- Choosing Herbs and Essential Oils .....xiv
- Safety Concerns............................xiv

## Part One: Natural Remedies for Common Ailments ............................ I

Mind and Emotions..................................... 3
- Anxiety ............................................ 4
- Depression ...................................... 6
- Insomnia........................................ 7
- Memory Loss ................................. 8
- Stress............................................. 10

Nervous System.................................... 13
- Alzheimer's Disease ......................... 14
- Headache ...................................... 16
- Migraine ........................................ 19
- Multiple Sclerosis............................. 20

Digestive System ................................. 23
- Constipation ................................... 24
- Crohn's Disease ............................. 26
- Diarrhea......................................... 28
- Flatulence ...................................... 29
- Irritable Bowel Syndrome.................. 30
- Heartburn and Acid Reflux............... 32
- Nausea and Vomiting....................... 33

Respiratory System .............................. 35
- Asthma .......................................... 36
- Common Cold ................................ 38
- Coughs .......................................... 42
- Flu ................................................. 44
- Hay Fever ...................................... 46
- Pneumonia and Bronchitis ............... 48
- Sinusitis ......................................... 50

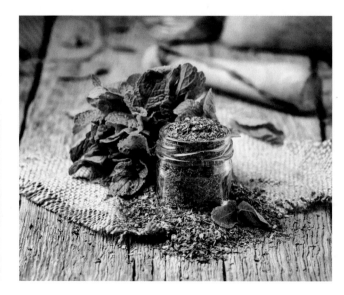

**Skin** ............................................... **52**

- Acne .......................................... 54
- Athlete's Foot ........................... 56
- Cold Sores ................................ 57
- Corns ......................................... 58
- Cuts and Sores ......................... 59
- Dandruff .................................... 60
- Eczema ...................................... 61
- Hemorrhoids ............................. 62
- Insect Bites .............................. 63
- Poison Ivy ................................. 64
- Psoriasis .................................... 65
- Rashes ....................................... 66
- Sunburn ..................................... 67

**Heart and Blood Health** ........................ **69**

- Anemia ....................................... 70
- Cholesterol ............................... 71
- High Blood Pressure ................ 72
- Varicose Veins ........................... 74

**Bones, Muscles, and Joints** ..................... **77**

- Arthritis ..................................... 78
- General Pain .............................. 80
- Osteoporosis ............................ 81
- Sprains and Pulled Muscles .............. 82

**Eyes and Ears** ................................... **85**

- Ear Wax Buildup ......................... 86
- Eyestrain ..................................... 87

**Women's Health** .............................. **89**

- Breastfeeding ............................ 90
- Infertility ................................... 92
- Menstrual Cycle and PMS ......... 94
- Morning Sickness ...................... 96
- Urinary Tract Infection ............. 98
- Yeast Infection .......................... 100

**Men's Health** ................................. **103**

- Baldness .................................... 104
- Infertility .................................. 105
- Shaving Care ............................ 107

**Babies and Children** ....................... **109**

- Diaper Rash .............................. 110
- Earache ..................................... 111
- Head Lice ................................. 113
- Sore Throat .............................. 114
- Teething .................................... 116

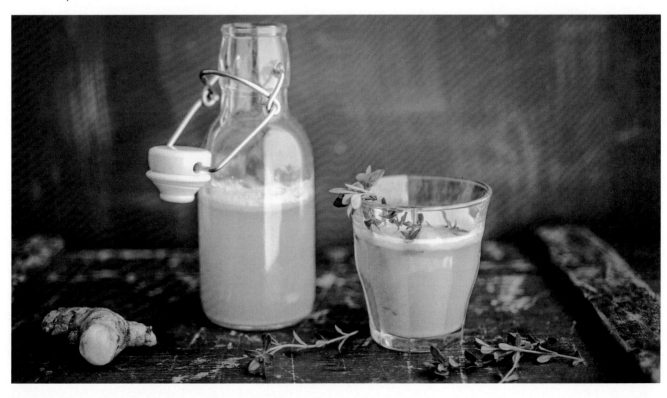

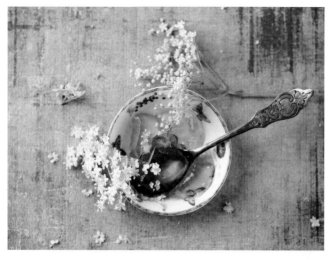

## Part Two: Healing Herbs, Spices, and Superfoods .....................119

**Herbs** ........................................ 121
- Planning an Herb Garden ............... 122
- Herbs to Avoid During Pregnancy.... 124
- Properties and Actions of Herbs ...... 126
- Aloe Vera ................................... 130
- Calendula ................................... 132
- Chamomile ................................. 134
- Chickweed.................................. 136
- Daisy ........................................ 138
- Lavender .................................... 140
- Lemon Balm................................ 143
- Mint.......................................... 144
- Oregano .................................... 146
- Parsley...................................... 148
- Rosemary ................................... 150
- Sage ......................................... 154
- Sunflower .................................. 156
- Thyme ...................................... 158
- Watercress ................................. 160
- Edible Wild Plants ........................ 163

**Juices and Cleanses** ..................... 167
- The Truth about Toxins ................... 168
- The Power of Juicing ..................... 170
- Detox Juicing 101......................... 174
- Juice Recipes.............................. 177

**Smoothies**................................. 185
- Benefits of Smoothies.................... 186

**Teas & Elixirs** ............................. 193
- Tea ........................................... 194
- Elixirs........................................ 199

**Tinctures**.................................. 203
**Tonics and Shots** ........................ 207
- Cool Tonics................................. 210
- Health Shots ............................... 216
**Broths**.................................... 219
**Medicinal Cooking** ...................... 233
**Natural Baby and Toddler Treats** ............ 253
- Baby Food.................................. 254
- Bigger Bites................................ 256

## Part Three: Homemade Cosmetics and Natural Cleaning Products ............. 261

**Natural Cosmetics and Beauty Rituals** ..... 263
- Body Butters................................ 265
- Body Oiling ................................. 266
- Dry Brushing................................ 268
- Facial Oiling ................................ 270
- Facial Steams............................... 271
- Hair Treatments ........................... 274
- Hand and Foot Treatments ............. 278
- Makeup Remover........................... 280
- Masks ....................................... 281
- Natural Deodorant......................... 284
- Scrubs ...................................... 287

**Natural Remedies for the Bedroom** ........ 295
- Aphrodisiacs/Stimulation ............... 296

**Natural Cleansers for the Home** ............ 305
- Houseplants for Clean Air ............... 306
- Kitchen and Bathroom Cleaning ...... 314
- Laundry Room ............................. 323
- Pet Care .................................... 325
- Soaps ....................................... 329
- Toothpaste and Mouthwash ............ 341

**Acknowledgments** ...................... 345
**Resources** ............................... 347
**Photo Credits** ........................... 351
**About the Editor**........................ 353
**Conversion Charts**....................... 355
**Index** ..................................... 357

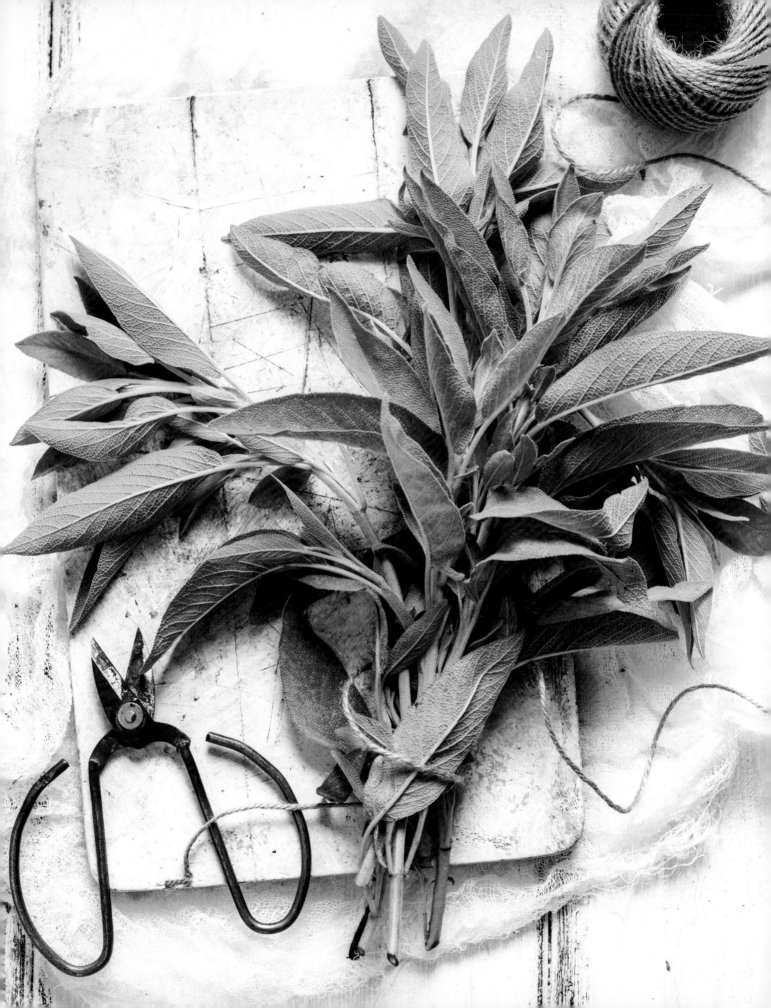

# FOREWORD

This book is truly like no other! I have been practicing herbalism, nutrition, and holistic health in general for two decades, and have collected quite a library of books. There are so many wonderful books covering all topics health related, but this book offers something unique—something we have been waiting for. This book has it all! As much as one book can, it includes everything you would want to know about herbal medicine, nutritious foods, rituals for whole health, and general well-being. The way it is organized is very comprehensible, and the pages are filled with articulate information from knowledgeable health practitioners, medicine makers, nutritionists, and specialists. I love that I can look up a body system and find remedies and rituals that correspond. Then, I can take it further, and find recipes to add to my cooking repertoire as well!

There is so much information out there in the world, of value, from the hearts and minds of amazing people, and this book does the best job of any book I have ever read of putting so much of it together. You can find out how to treat everything naturally, from anxiety, to digestive issues, to acne, to varicose veins!

I believe this book is very needed and of high value for our world today, and my hope is that it will travel far and wide and help to empower people to take their health into their own hands as much as possible. I believe it will support the movement toward taking better care of ourselves, and in turn others in our families and communities. I will be utilizing this book in my own practice, and be recommending it to many. It is guaranteed to make a great addition to any library, for anyone who has the desire to learn and grow and heal. Thank you to everyone who has been part of this book—for the healing of our families, communities, and the world!

—Alysssa Holmes, herbalist,
coauthor of *Healing Herbs* and
*Medicinal Gardening Handbook*

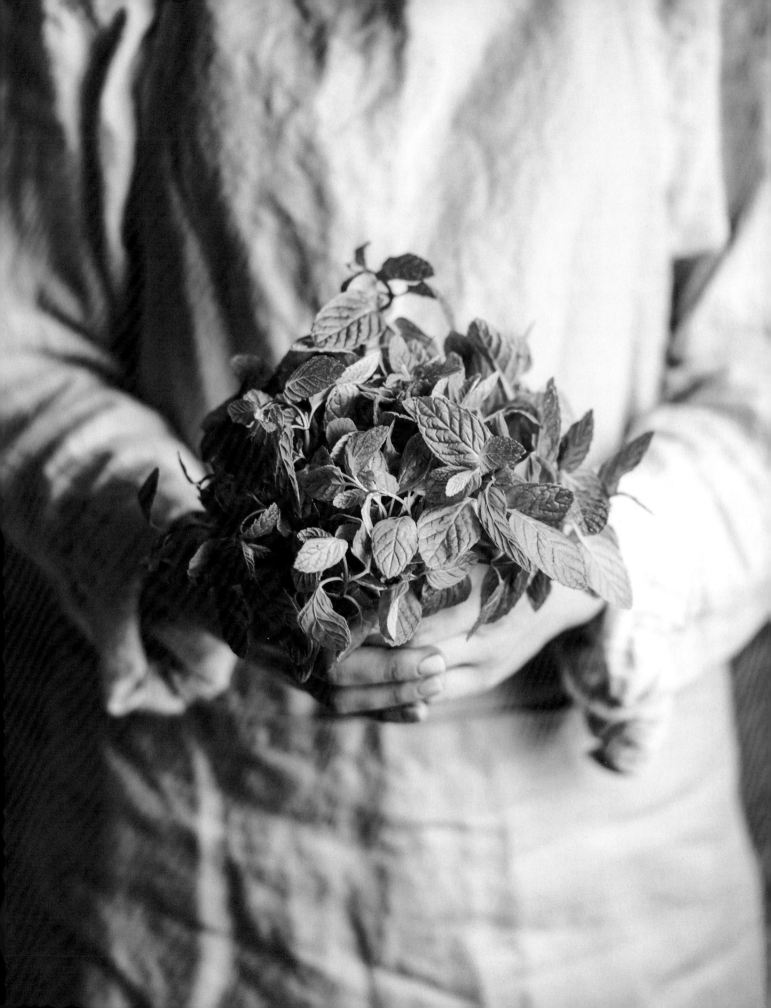

# INTRODUCTION

Once you begin discovering all the good medicine that God has gifted us in the form of herbs, spices, fruits, and vegetables, you may find yourself thirsty for more knowledge—and, perhaps, a little overwhelmed. Not only is there a whole world of healing plants, but there are myriad ways to tap the benefits of each plant: essential oils, tinctures, teas, elixirs, scrubs, poultices, sprays . . . and the list goes on! This book, though hefty and chockfull of recipes, tips, and information, is merely an introduction to the world of natural remedies. The material here has been selected and compiled from a wealth of literature authored by knowledgeable and experienced herbalists and healers of many kinds, and then peppered with my own research. My goal is not necessarily to be exhaustive (as if that would even be possible in one lifetime or one book), but rather to include the most useful information and recipes so that you and your loved ones can dive into the world of natural healing with curiosity, creativity, and confidence.

## How to Use This Book

As you can see in the table of contents, this book is split into three sections. If you are experiencing a particular ailment or condition, **Part One** will be the best place to start. Flip to the bodily system that is affected (such as, "Digestive System") and you'll find that the specific conditions (such as, "Constipation" and "Crohn's Disease") are in alphabetical order. There you'll find recipes to immediately begin your healing journey.

To learn more about specific plants and herbs and their properties, as well as how to grow them in a garden or in your home, flip to **Part Two**. In that section you'll also find recipes for healing food and drinks, including juices, teas, broths, superfood meals, and even baby and toddler treats.

In **Part Three**, you'll find inspiring beauty rituals and instructions for making natural cosmetics and cleaning solutions for your home, because wellness is impacted by much more than just what we consume. The substances we put on our skin and the environment in which we live can have a major impact on our health and well-being, too.

Be sure to check out the Resources section in the back to see the list of books that much of this material is compiled from. Also note that because the research and experience of many authors are represented in this book, if you come across text written in the first person, don't assume I'm the one writing. See pages 347–349 to find the author and his or her book. Credit where credit's due!

## Pantry Tips

Apart from specific herbs and spices, which have unique healing properties, there are certain ingredients you'll see show up again and again throughout this book. There's a good chance you already have them in your pantry, but if not, you may want to stock up.

- Apple cider vinegar (choose organic, raw, unfiltered)
- Baking soda
- Beeswax
- Coconut oil
- Epsom salt
- Garlic (always use fresh cloves, not powdered)
- Ginger (fresh ginger root is best)
- Honey (raw, local is best)
- Olive oil

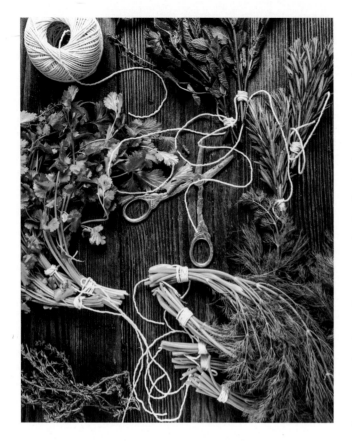

# Choosing Herbs and Essential Oils

Not all herbs and essential oils are created equal, and, since most natural products you can buy are not regulated by the FDA, you can't always trust the labels. For herbs, either grow and harvest your own (using organic methods), or ask around to find an herbalist you can trust. For essential oils, it will be tempting to buy the cheapest ones you can find online. But you should know that doing so will likely lead to poor results. Many essential oils are diluted with carrier oils, and some may not even be safe. It takes a lot of plants to get a small amount of essential oil, so there's a pretty good chance that a very cheap oil is not pure. Look for essential oils that are organic or wildcrafted (you want concentrated plant essence, but you don't want concentrated levels of pesticides and herbicides). Also look for brands that do gas chromatography and mass spectrometry tests (GC/MS testing) on all their oils. You can find that information by looking on their website or asking a representative.

- Shea butter
- Sweet almond oil
- Vodka (or other high-proof alcohol)
- Witch hazel

You'll also find these tools helpful:

- Mortar and pestle
- Blender
- Glass bottles with tight-fitting lids (various sizes)
- Glass bottles with spray tops
- Teakettle
- Glass bowls in various sizes
- Measuring cups
- Cheesecloth
- Glass tincture vials with droppers

# Safety Concerns

Not all herbs and essential oils are safe for pregnant women, nursing women, babies, children, and pets. Also, any natural remedy may interfere with other medications you are taking or conditions that you have. Check with your doctor and do your own research! Some herbs should only be taken short term. Consult with an herbalist or naturopath for the safest, most effective use of any herb or natural remedy. Remember, each body is unique; this book is not meant to take the place of professionals who can customize a health plan to the specific needs of you and your loved ones.

Always keep herbs and essential oils locked up and out of reach of children and pets. Babies or children who ingest essential oils could be at risk of seizures, choking, pneumonia, liver failure, brain swelling, and other serious conditions. Essential oils splashed directly on the skin can cause burns and, if gotten in the eyes, can cause eye damage. Never use essential oils directly on skin or undiluted in baths—always dilute in a carrier oil. Don't diffuse essential oils around children 6 months or younger. Some recommend not using essential oils at all around children under 6 years. Essential oils can be deadly for dogs, cats, birds, and other pets, even when diffused. Research any particular oils you wish to use and consider their safety for children and pets prior to use.

For more information on herbs and essential oils to use or avoid during pregnancy, see pages 96 and 124.

Natural remedies are a powerful way to support your own health. That doesn't mean that the recipes and instructions in this book should take the place of your doctor's advice or the tools, medicine, and techniques offered by Western medicine. For most of us, taking our health seriously means employing a combination of modern healthcare practices and ancient healing remedies, of modern medicine and plant medicine.

## Ask Your Doctor and Independently Research Regarding...

- Any medications you are taking and how they might interact with herbs
- Whether certain herbs or essential oils are safe for pregnancy, nursing, or babies or young children
- Specific remedies and how they may affect other conditions you're experiencing

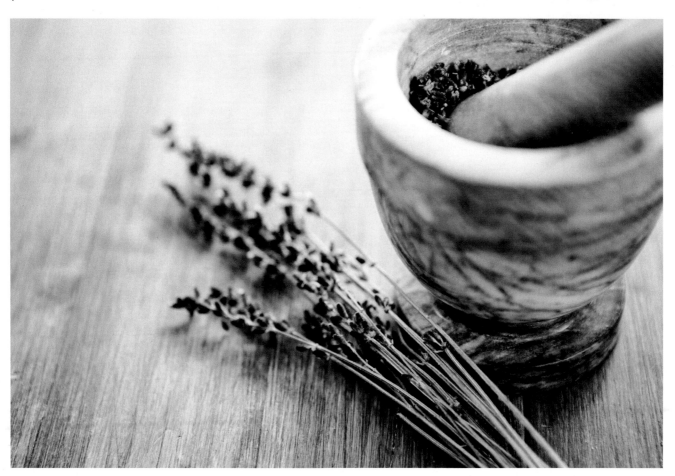

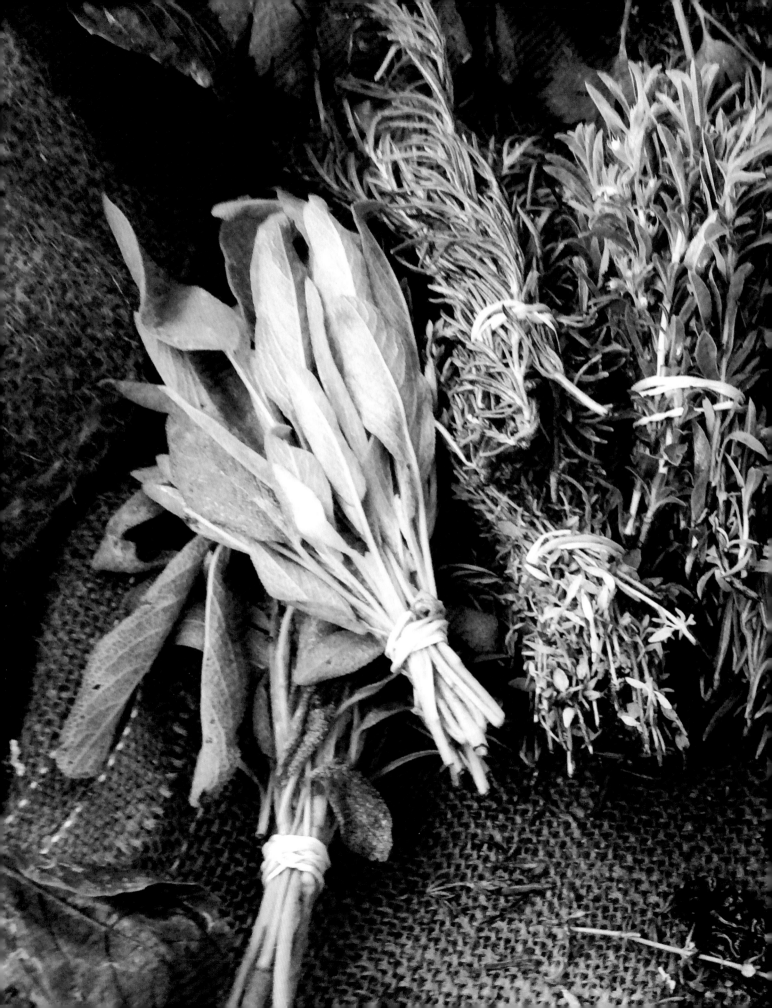

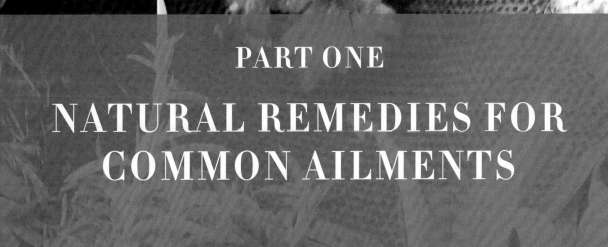

# PART ONE
# NATURAL REMEDIES FOR COMMON AILMENTS

Mind and Emotions    3

Nervous System    13

Digestive System    23

Respiratory System    35

Skin    52

Heart and Blood Health    69

Bones, Muscles, and Joints    77

Eyes and Ears    85

Women's Health    89

Men's Health    103

Babies and Children    109

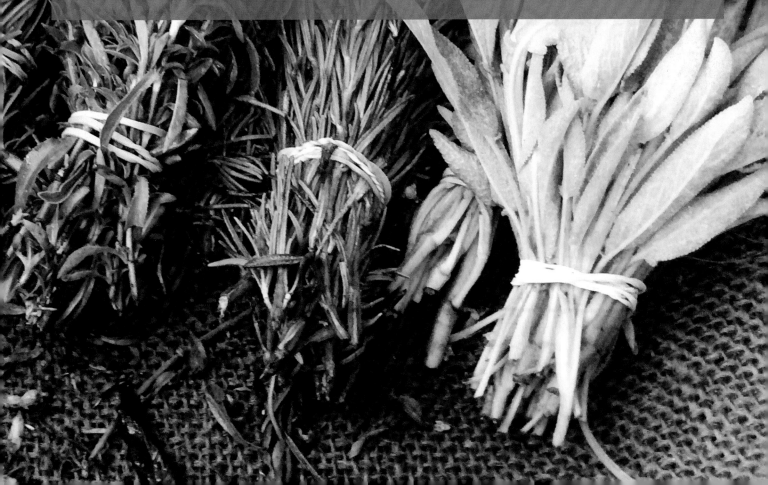

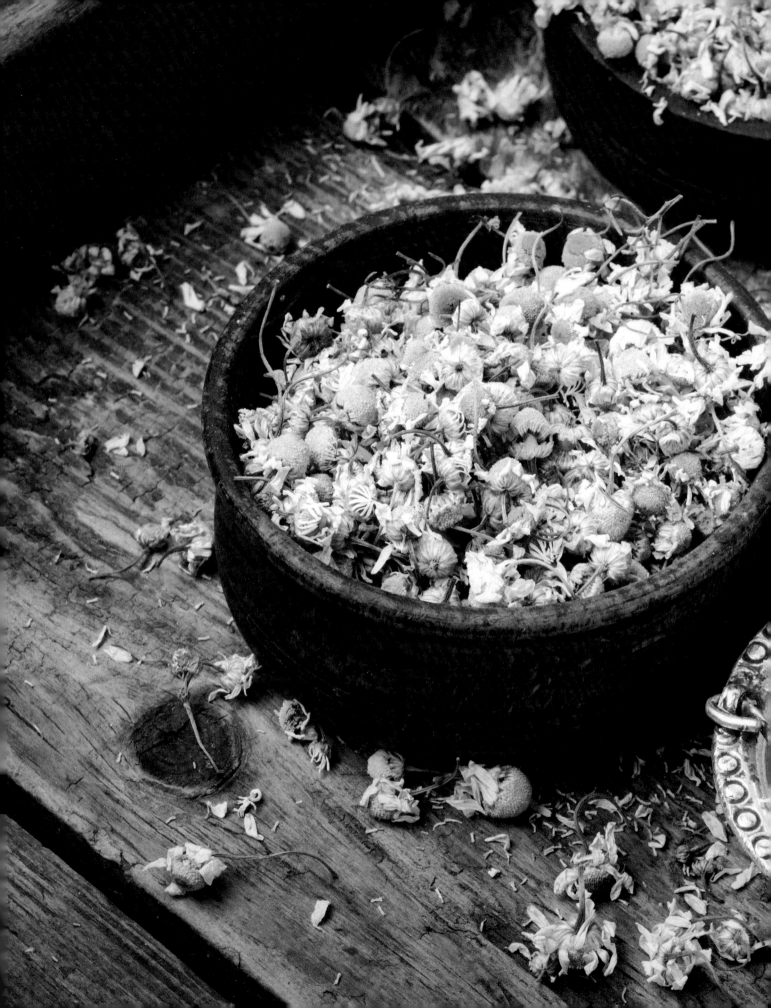

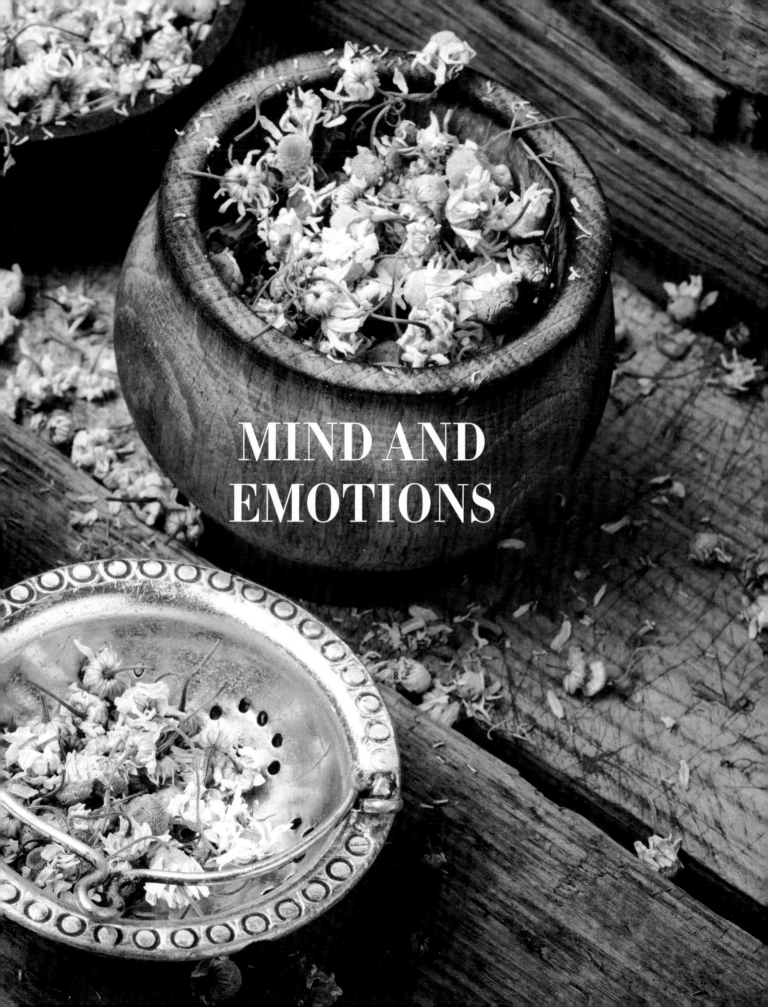

# MIND AND
# EMOTIONS

# Anxiety

## DIY Chamomile Flower Tea for Anxiety and Stress

Drinking three cups of chamomile tea per day can help you relieve some anxiety and stress, while also reducing your inflammation and pain! This one-stop shop of herbal goodness is an easy way to incorporate herbal medicine, and it tastes good! Chamomile is unique in its sweet and fruity taste. Using an infuser pot to brew your tea is an easy way to make fresh tea using loose leaves. If you don't have an infuser teapot, find a strainer or cheesecloth in order to make a makeshift tea bag.

### Ingredients:
3–4 tablespoons fresh chamomile flowers
1 sprig fresh mint
8 ounces boiling water

### Directions:
1. Harvest your chamomile flowers the same day you plan to use them for tea. Pop the heads of the flowers off the stems, and mix together with fresh mint sprig.
2. Boil your 8 ounces of water and place it in your teapot with the herbs, or over the cheesecloth. Steep your flowers and mint in the water for five minutes.

### Tips for Reducing Anxiety
- Exercise regularly
- Quit or reduce smoking, alcohol consumption, and caffeine consumption
- Practice deep breathing
- Try eating foods that have been shown to help reduce anxiety, including Brazil nuts, almonds, salmon, eggs (including yolks), dark chocolate, turmeric, asparagus, blueberries, and yogurt

## Beam Me Up Melissa Balm Tea

### Ingredients:
1 teaspoon lemon balm leaves
1 teaspoon pineapple weed herb
1 teaspoon lavender flowers
1 teaspoon California poppy herb

### Directions:
1. Prepare as an infusion (see page 194).
2. Use as an uplifting subtle tea blend for raising the spirits and a gentle relaxant for condition of anxiety and stress.

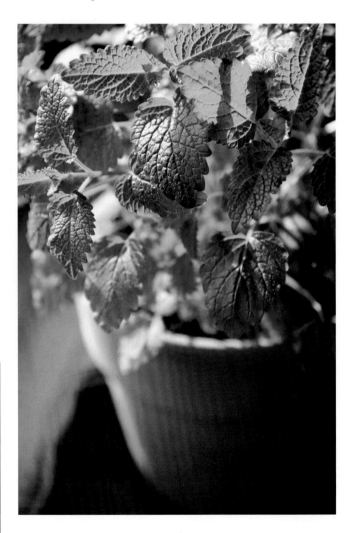

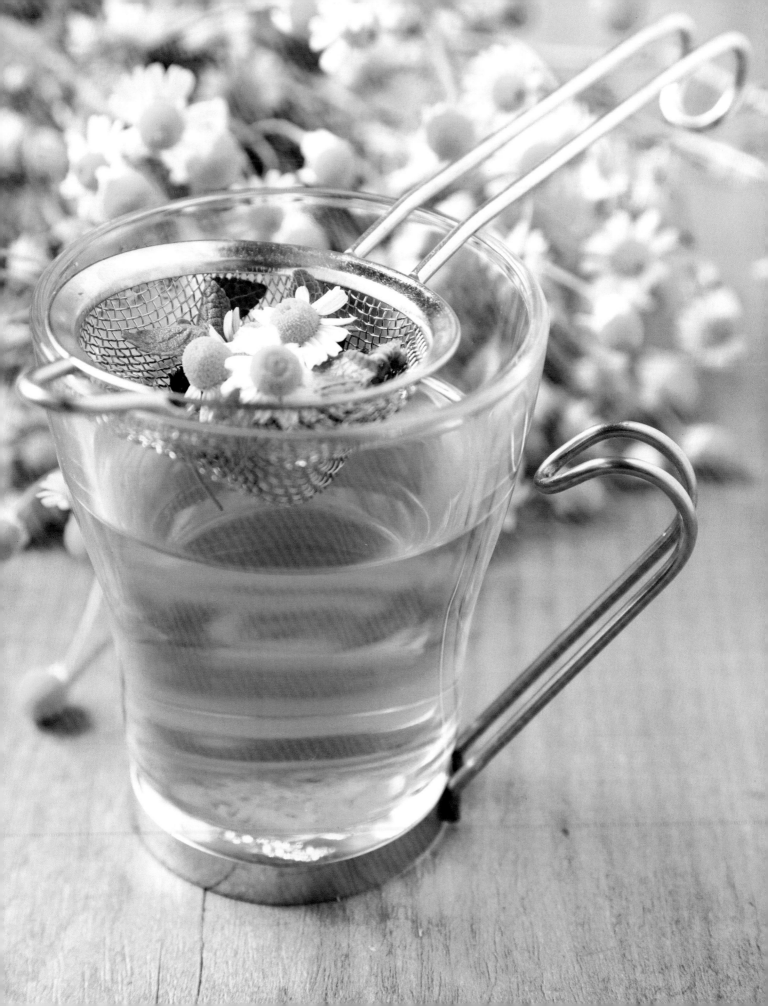

# Depression

## Apple Cider Vinegar

Depression can range from serious metabolic disorders to occasional mood problems. The severity and causes can vary widely from individual to individual. Serotonin levels have been found to greatly influence moods. Apple cider vinegar is also believed to help with serotonin levels in the brain. Some Eastern medicine practices subscribe to the belief that depression is caused by having a stagnant liver. Taking a daily dose of apple cider vinegar works as a liver-cleansing tonic. This is promoted by the amino acids that it contains.

## Antidepressant Tea

### Ingredients:

1 part lemon balm leaf
1 part hawthorn leaf, flower, or berry
2 parts St. John's wort flower and leaf
8 oz. hot water

### Directions:

1. Combine dried herbs and steep in water, covered, for 10–15 minutes. Remove herbs from water, and sip tea slowly.
2. Feel free to sweeten with honey.

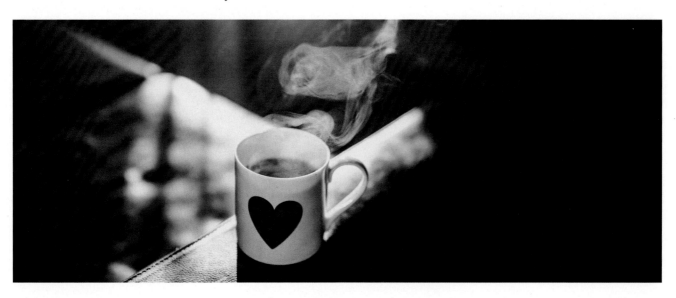

# Insomnia

## Sleepy Time Chamomile Tincture

This easy-to-make chamomile tincture is a safe and simple way to help your body relax and fall asleep naturally. A dose right before bedtime will relax the mind and body and help you drift off smoothly. Chamomile tinctures can be found widely online or in stores, but if you're looking for a cheaper and homemade option, this is a wonderful recipe. For adults, take up to one teaspoon, one to three times a day or as needed.

### Ingredients:
½ cup dried chamomile flowers
Glass jar with airtight lid, quart size
1¾ cups boiling water
1¾ cups vodka
Cheesecloth
Tincture vial with droppers

### Directions:
1. Place your dried chamomile flowers in your clean and sterile glass jar.
2. Pour boiling water over the flowers, making sure you just cover them.
3. Fill the rest of the jar with the vodka of your choice. Cover the jar with an airtight lid.
4. Store the jar in a cool and dark place for four to six weeks. I like placing the jars in my kitchen cabinets.
5. After four to six weeks, take your jar and strain the liquid out into a cheesecloth or strainer. Once the liquid is separated out from the flowers, you have your tincture. Place the liquid in a tincture vial with dropper.

## Apple Cider Vinegar

Apple cider vinegar can be used as a natural treatment for insomnia. Try making a mixture of apple cider vinegar and honey mixed with a glass of water. Keep a second glass ready for if you wake during the night. Both apple cider vinegar and honey are known to activate serotonin production in the brain, which promotes relaxation and induces sleepiness.

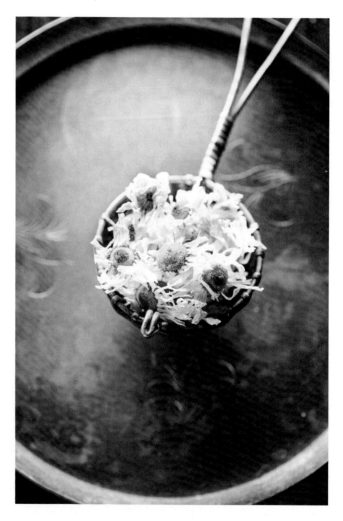

# Memory Loss

## Forget-Me-Not Tea

### Ingredients:
1 part parsley leaf and stem
1 part ginseng root
2 parts ginkgo leaf
8 oz. hot water

### Directions:
1. Combine dried herbs and steep in water, covered, for 10–15 minutes.
2. Remove herbs from water, and sip tea slowly. Feel free to sweeten with a pinch of stevia.

*See Sage section, page 154*

## Herbs to Improve Memory, Mental Clarity, and Overall Brain Health

- Ashwagandha
- Ginseng
- Ginko biloba
- Gotu kola
- Hawthorn
- Lemon balm
- Peppermint
- Rosemary
- Sage
- Turmeric

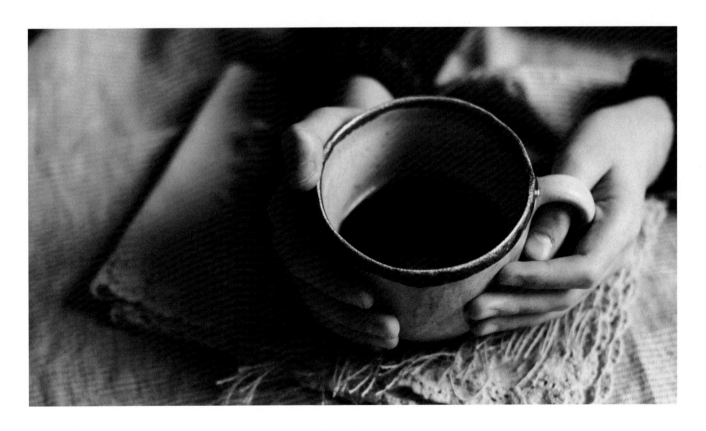

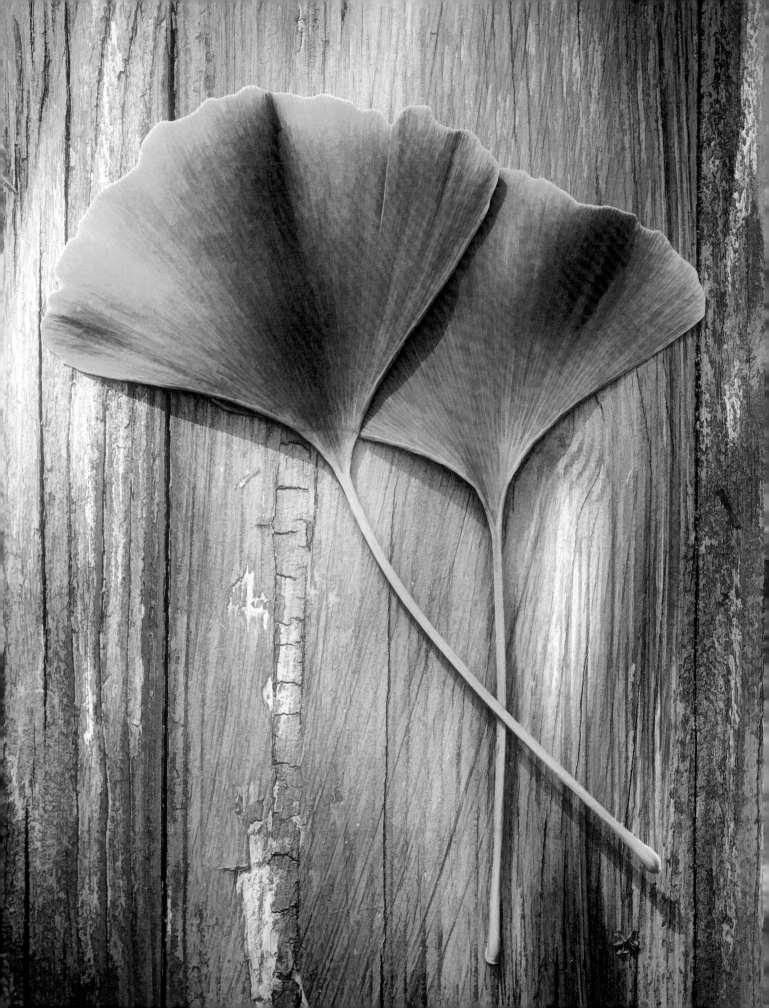

# Stress

## Stress-Relieving Diffuser Blend

Stress is a part of life, but too much stress has serious consequences for our health and well-being. Continuously high stress levels are leading causes of heart disease, stroke, inflammatory diseases, premature aging, and getting sick in general. Stress can come in many forms—including work, family, and emotional and financial distress—but no matter the cause, there are ways to deal with stress in a healthy manner. The Stress-Relieving Diffuser Blend helps your body mitigate the effects of stress and your mind feel at peace.

### Ingredients:

½ cup water
4 drops lavender essential oil
3 drops bergamot essential oil
2 drops lemon essential oil

### Preparation:

1. Add ½ cup of water (or the amount recommended by your diffuser) to the well of your diffuser.
2. Add 4 drops of lavender essential oil, 3 drops of bergamot essential oil, and 2 drops lemon essential oil to the water.

### Administration:

1. Place your diffuser on your desk at work or in the bathroom when you are taking a stress-relieving bath or shower—or wherever you are when you need some stress relief
2. Turn on your diffuser and let the room fill with the relaxing aroma.
3. Take several deep breaths and then continue to breath normally.

## Stress and Anxiety Support Syrup

Make a decoction (see box) with the following:

- 1 part eleuthero
- 1 part astragalus

At the end, add the following herbs to steep in the decoction mixture, before straining:

- ½ part lemon balm
- ½ part oat tops

Let steep for an hour, strain, and add equal part honey, mix well, let cool, bottle, label, and store in the fridge.

---

### Herbal Decoctions

To make an herbal decoction, add 2–3 teaspoons of herbs per one cup of water. Add herbs and cold water in a pan and bring to a gentle boil. Simmer with a lid on for about half an hour. Remove from heat, cool to room temperature, and then strain out the herbs. Decoctions are best consumed right away or refrigerated for up to one day.

---

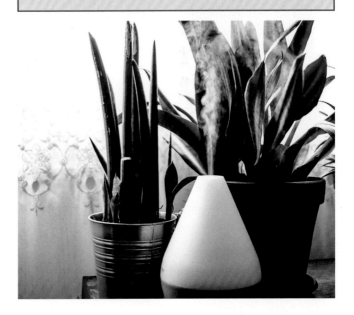

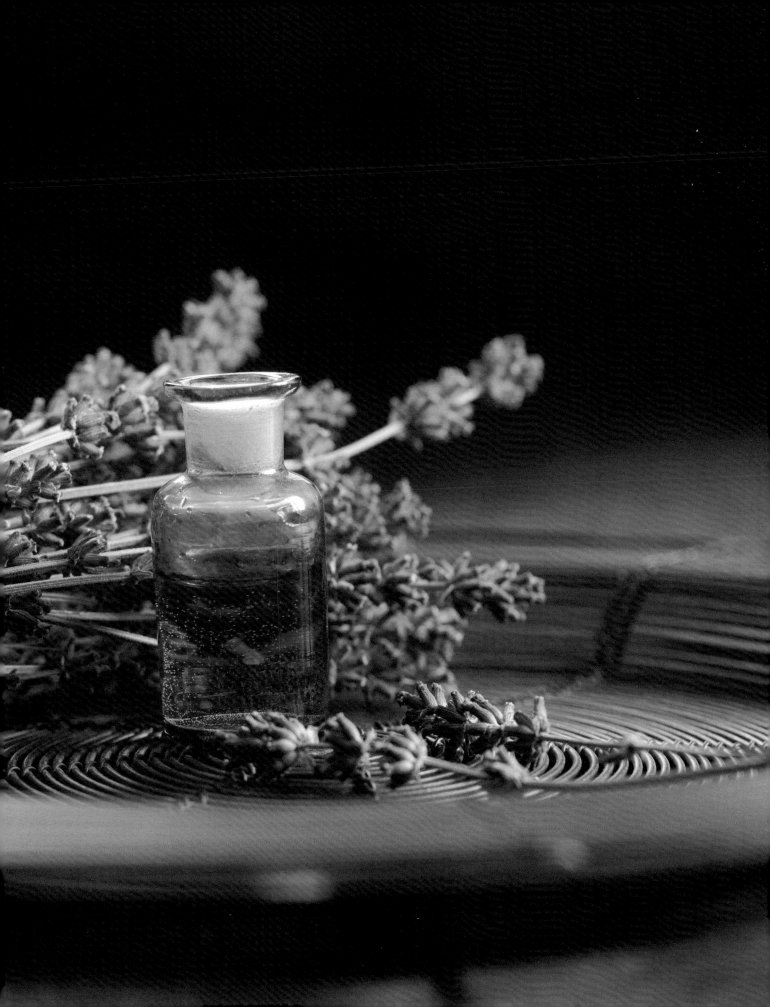

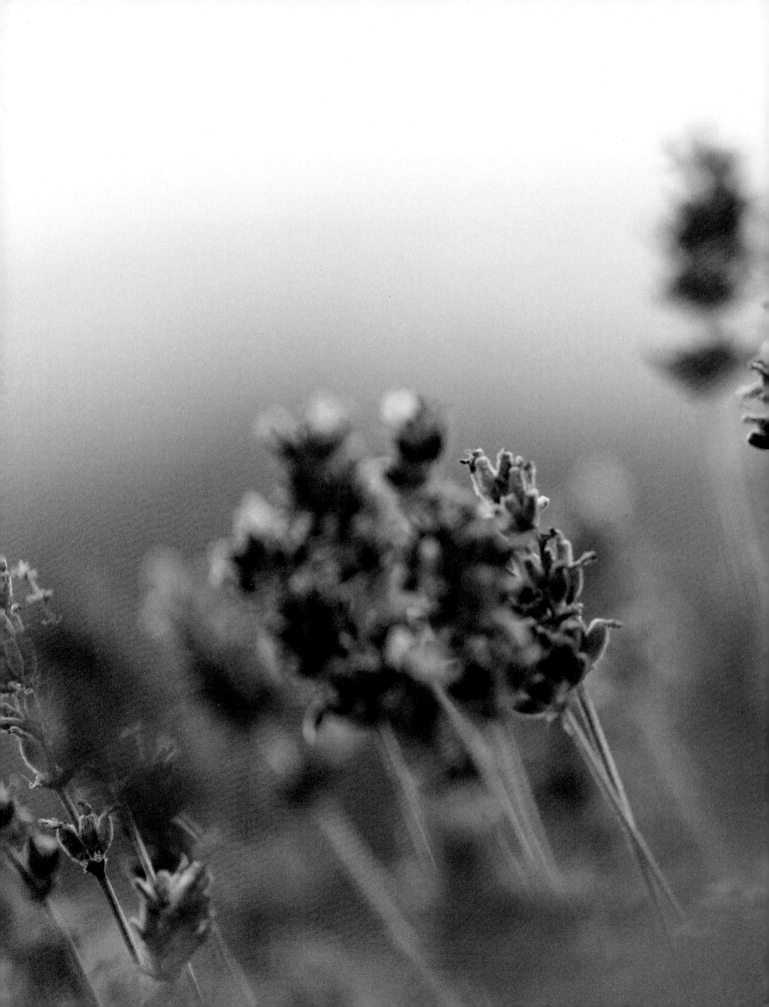

# NERVOUS SYSTEM

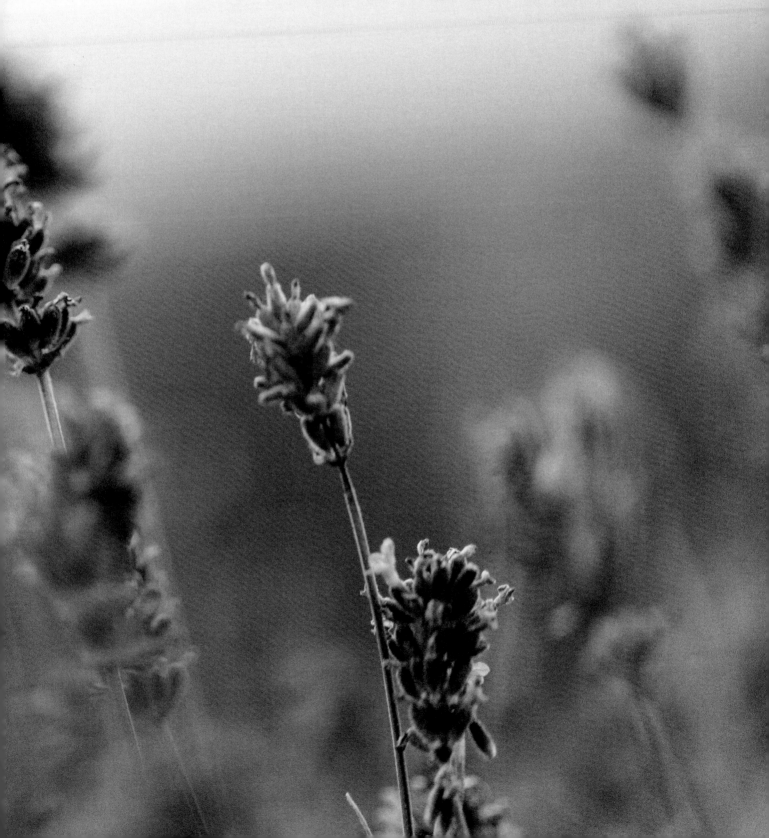

# Alzheimer's Disease

## Coconut Oil

One of the indications of Alzheimer's disease is that some sections of the brain stop processing glucose. For this reason, people with diabetes have a higher risk of developing Alzheimer's disease, as they already have problems processing sugars. Researchers have figured out that, by supplying more energy to the brain, they could find a solution to the downward spiral of Alzheimer's.

The brain uses an energy source called ketones. The liver converts medium-chain triglycerides into ketones, and coconut oil is rich in medium-chain triglycerides. Many researchers of small-scale studies have found that daily doses of coconut oil have helped slow the development of Alzheimer's and it is believed this is because the medium-chain triglycerides are providing the necessary energy to keep the brain cells from deteriorating.

## Omega-3 Fatty Acids

Eating foods rich in omega-3 fatty acids may help prevent or repair cognitive impairment. Good food sources of omega-3 include fish, seaweed, chia or hemp seeds, walnuts, and edamame. You can also take it in supplement form.

## Acupuncture

Some have found that acupuncture can improve mood and cognitive function including verbal and motor skills in individuals with Alzheimer's.

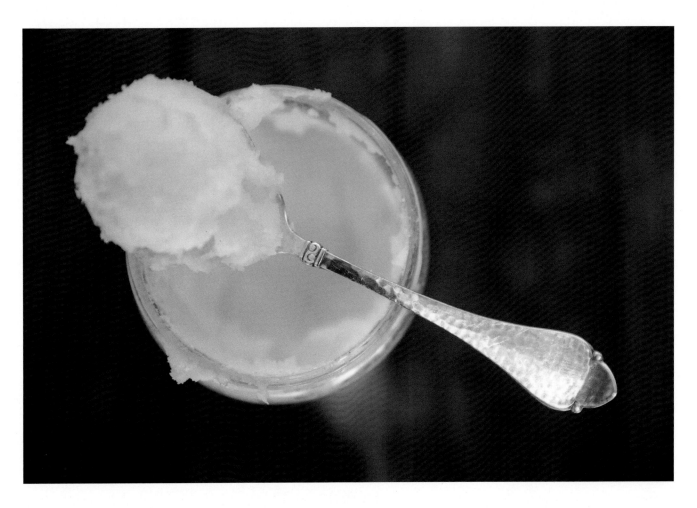

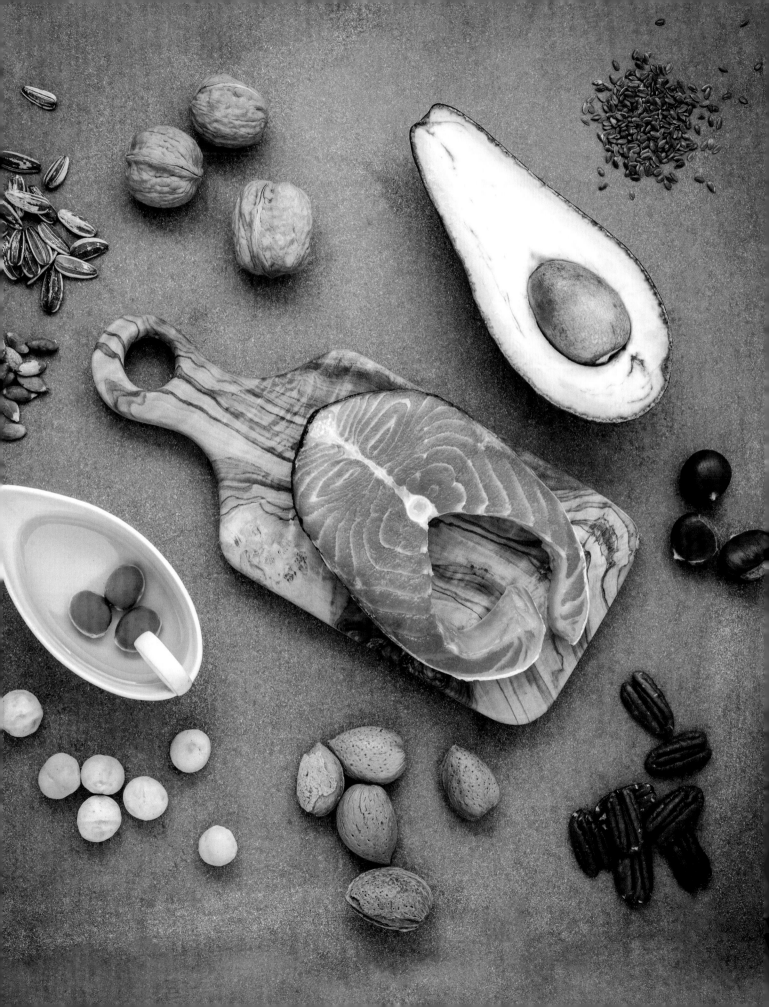

# Headache

## Headache Be Gone

### Ingredients:

2 parts lavender flowers
1 part peppermint leaf
2 parts rosemary herb

### Directions:

1. Prepare as a strong infusion (see page 194) using 1 heaping teaspoon of herb mixture or prepare a tincture.
2. Drink 3–4 cups of tea daily for prevention and treatment of headaches, or take the tincture: 1 teaspoon 3 times daily.

## Headache Tincture

### Ingredients:

2 parts feverfew
1 part rosemary
1 part lemon balm
½ part lavender menstruum

*See instructions for making a tincture on page 204.*

See page 194; page 204.

### Essential Oils for Headaches

Smelling certain essential oils may help to relieve headaches. Dilute a few drops in several drops of a carrier oil (such as jojoba or sweet almond) and massage into your shoulders or temples. Try these:

- Chamomile
- Eucalyptus
- Frankincense
- Lavender
- Peppermint
- Rosemary

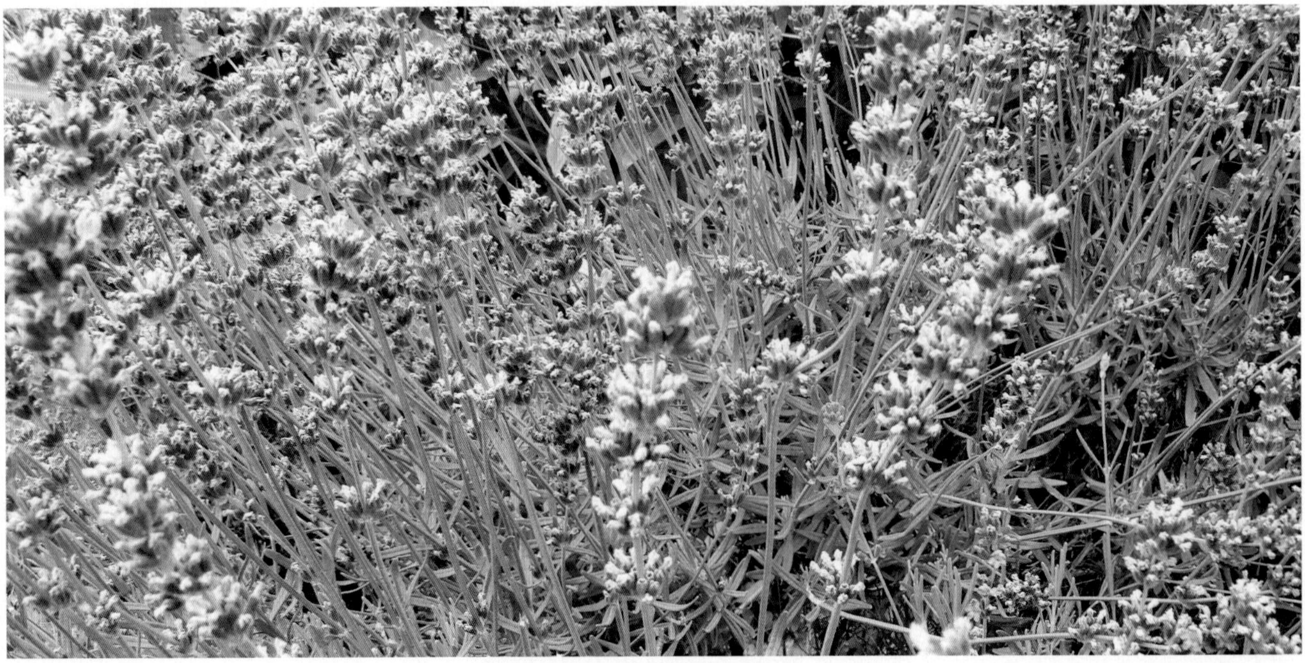

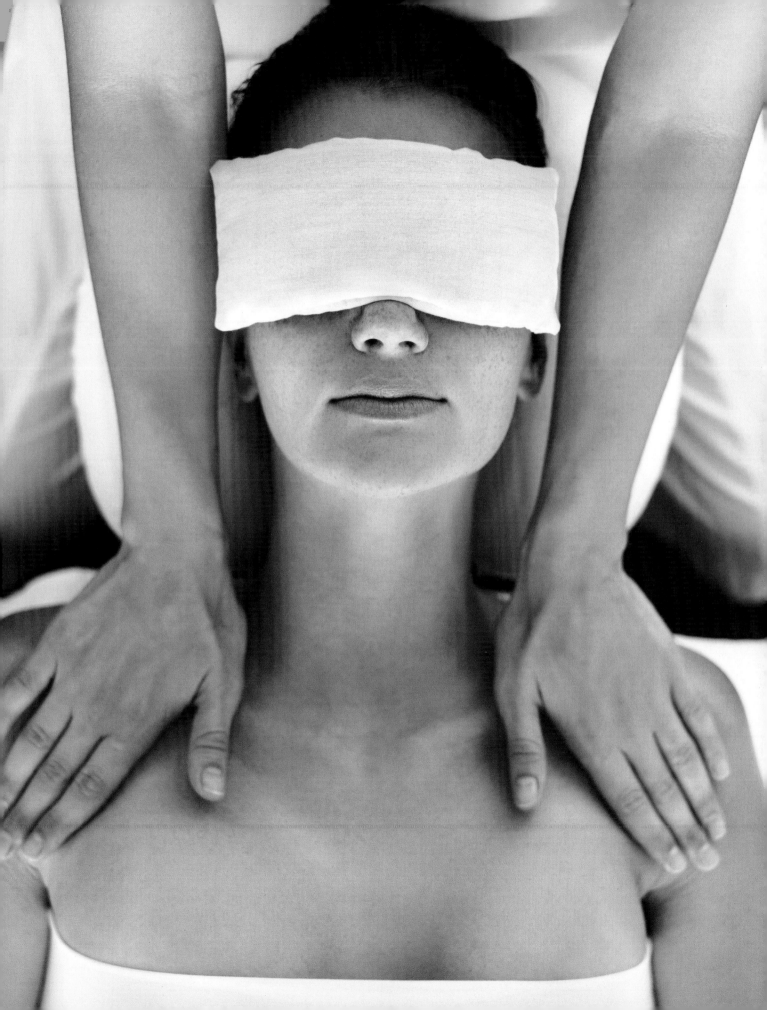

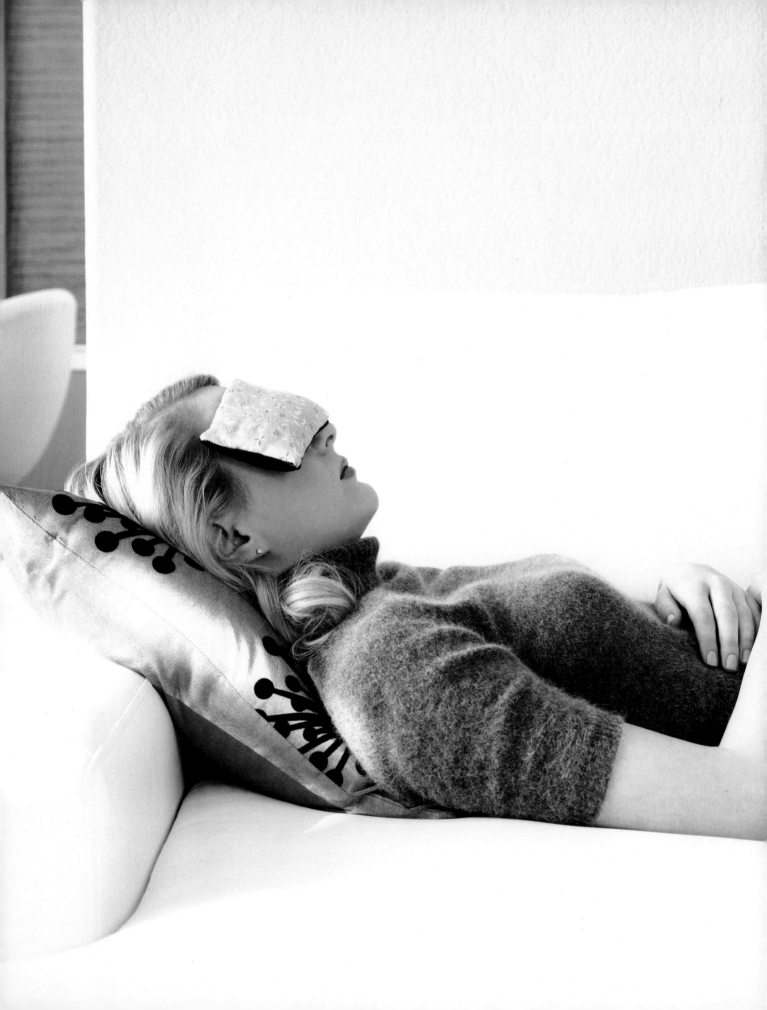

# Migraine

## Tea for Migraines

**Ingredients:**

1 part peppermint leaf
1 part lavender flower
2 parts dong quai root and leaf
8 oz. hot water

**Directions:**

1. Combine dried herbs and steep in water, covered, for 10–15 minutes.
2. Remove herbs from water, and sip tea slowly.

## Healing Plants for Migraine Relief

- Betony
- Butterbur
- Coriander seed
- Dong quai
- Evodia
- Feverfew
- Ginger
- Hops
- Horseradish
- Honeysuckle
- Lavender
- Linden
- Mullein
- Peppermint
- Rosemary
- Teaberry
- Valerian
- Willow

## Migraine Triggers

As with any ailment, it's a good idea to consult with your doctor to make sure your migraines are not your body's way of telling you there's something more serious going on. Be sure to mention any other symptoms and any recent lifestyle or dietary changes. A visit to your eye doctor may be wise, too, as vision problems are a common cause of migraines.

You may also wish to keep to keep a food diary to help determine if the migraines are stemming from something you're eating or drinking.

Some common migraine triggers include:

- Alcohol
- Caffeine (although, in some cases, caffeine may help relieve a migraine)
- Chocolate
- Hormonal shifts
- Muscle tension
- Red wine
- Stress
- Sudden changes in weather

## Soothing Eye Pillow

This herbal eye pillow can be kept in the freezer or warmed in the microwave and then placed over your eyes while you lay on your back. Cut a 9-inch x 10-inch piece of cotton fabric or two 9-inch x 5-inch pieces. Fold in half (if using the larger piece of fabric) or place together so that right sides are facing each other. Sew along three sides, keeping one short side open. Turn right side out, so that seams are now on the inside of the bag. Add ¾ cup flaxseeds and ½ cup of dried herbs (lavender, rosemary, and peppermint are great options). If desired, add essential oils for a stronger scent. Fold the fabric on the open end over to create a seam and sew up.

For an even simpler version, fill a clean sock with flaxseeds and herbs and knot the open end.

# Multiple Sclerosis

## Coconut Oil

Coconut oil improves the absorption of magnesium, an essential mineral for neurological health. The medium-chain fatty acids create ketones, the energy source required by the brain, so that damaged brain cells can be repaired. This in turn can improve the communication between the brain and the rest of the body.

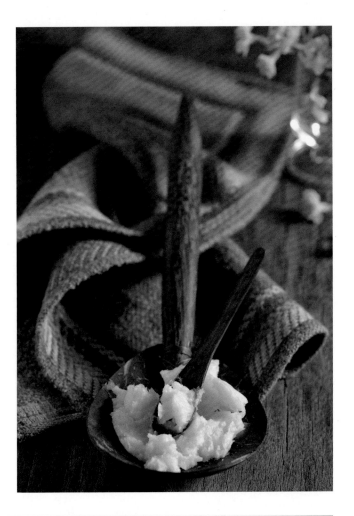

### Ways to Enjoy Coconut Oil

- Spread on toast
- Use in baking (instead of butter or other oils)
- Sauté vegetables in a tablespoon of melted coconut oil
- Pour coffee into a blender and add a small scoop of coconut oil. Blend for 10–20 seconds. If desired, add honey, maple syrup, or a dash of cinnamon.

### Herbs and Supplements for MS

There are many herbs and supplements that may reduce the symptoms and/or slow the progression of MS. Note that MS is thought by many to be an autoimmune disease or disorder, so herbs that are known to boost the immune system may not be a good choice. Be sure to check with your doctor before trying anything new, as herbs may interfere with other medications or not be right for you for a variety of other reasons. Speak with an herbalist or naturopath about proper dosage; more is not always better when it comes to supplements!

- Ashwagandha
- Chamomile
- Cranberry
- Dandelion root and leaf
- DHA
- Echinacea
- Ginger

- Ginko biloba
- Omega-3 and omega-6 essential fatty acids
- Peppermint
- Sage
- St. John's wort
- Turmeric
- Vitamin B1 (thiamine)

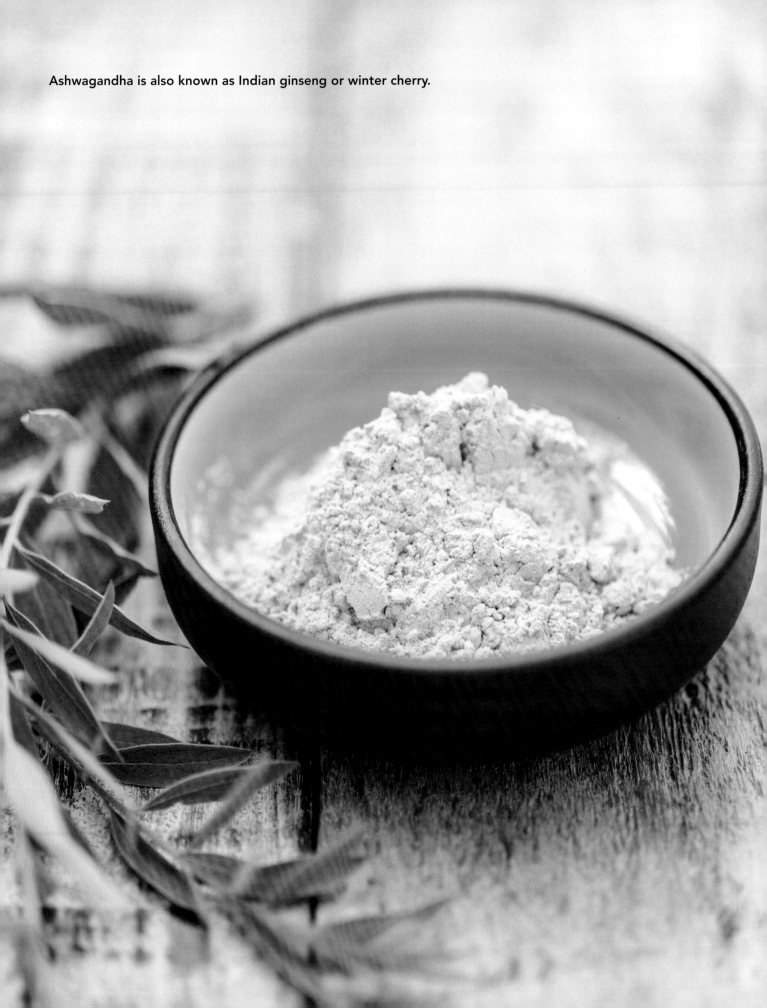

Ashwagandha is also known as Indian ginseng or winter cherry.

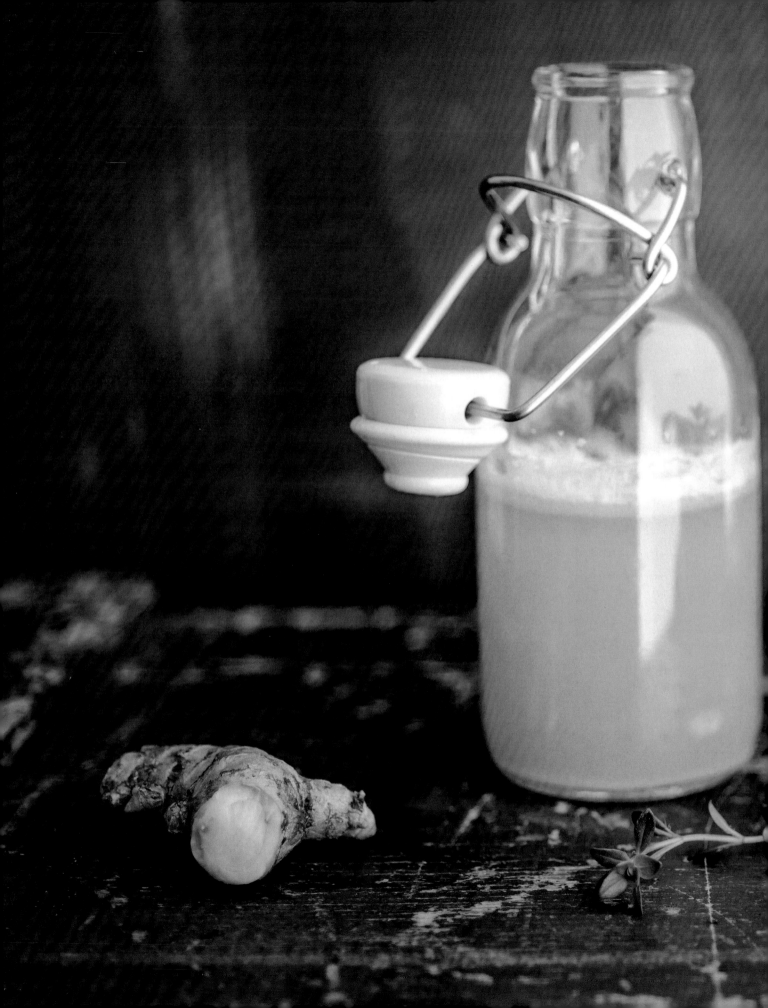

# DIGESTIVE SYSTEM

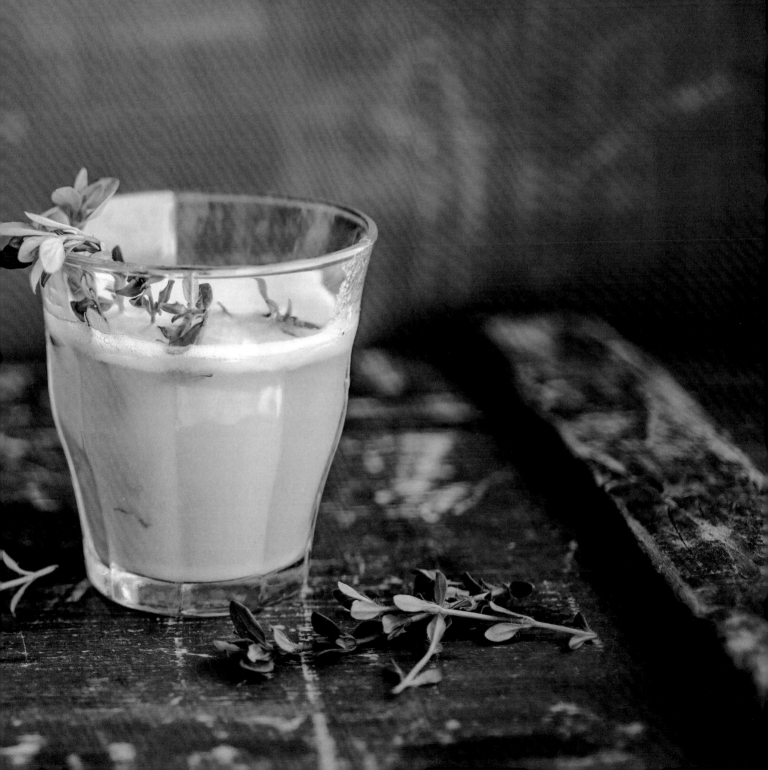

# Constipation

## Coconut Oil

Coconut oil is both fibrous and easily absorbed, so it is an excellent remedy for constipation. It also works as a cleansing and balancing agent for your entire digestive tract, so regular doses will have a positive effect on your digestion.

## Apple Cider Vinegar

Constipation is usually caused by eating a poor diet too low in fiber. It is also a normal sign of aging as the volume of digestive acids reduces as we age. Constipation can lead to serious health problems because of the increased amount of time digested food remains in the colon. This leads to a greater number of toxins being reabsorbed into the body, leading to damage caused by free radicals and a host of secondary illnesses. Eating a diet with a high fiber content is the most effective and natural way of combating and alleviating constipation. Apple cider vinegar is a good source of pectin, a water soluble fiber. You can supplement your diet with a daily tonic of apple cider vinegar or you can try a well-known recipe from Patricia Bragg. You need to boil two cups of distilled water and a quarter cup of flaxseed for ten minutes. Then remove it from the heat. The mixture will become gelatinous as it cools. You then take a teaspoon of apple cider vinegar and mix it with two tablespoons of the flaxseed gel. Take this mixture every morning and again one hour after dinner.

## Foods to Get Things Moving

- Apple cider vinegar
- Apples
- Artichokes
- Avocados
- Bananas
- Berries
- Chia seeds
- Figs
- Flaxseeds
- Ginger
- Kefir
- Kiwi
- Lentils
- Oat bran
- Pears
- Prunes
- Raw seeds and nuts
- Rhubarb
- Spinach
- Sweet potatoes
- Tomatoes
- Turmeric

## Five Super Simple Ways to Relieve Constipation

1. Exercise. Move your body to get things moving (if you know what I mean). Take a walk, do some yoga, dance around the kitchen.
2. Eat more fiber. Especially soluble fibers, such as avocados, bananas, and oatmeal.
3. Drink more water. Dehydration can contribute to constipation.
4. Consume probiotics. Try lactofermented sauerkraut or pickles, kombucha, yogurt, or a quality probiotic supplement.
5. Have a cup of coffee. Caffeine is a stimulant, which can get the muscles in your digestive system working.

*See Watercress section, page 160*

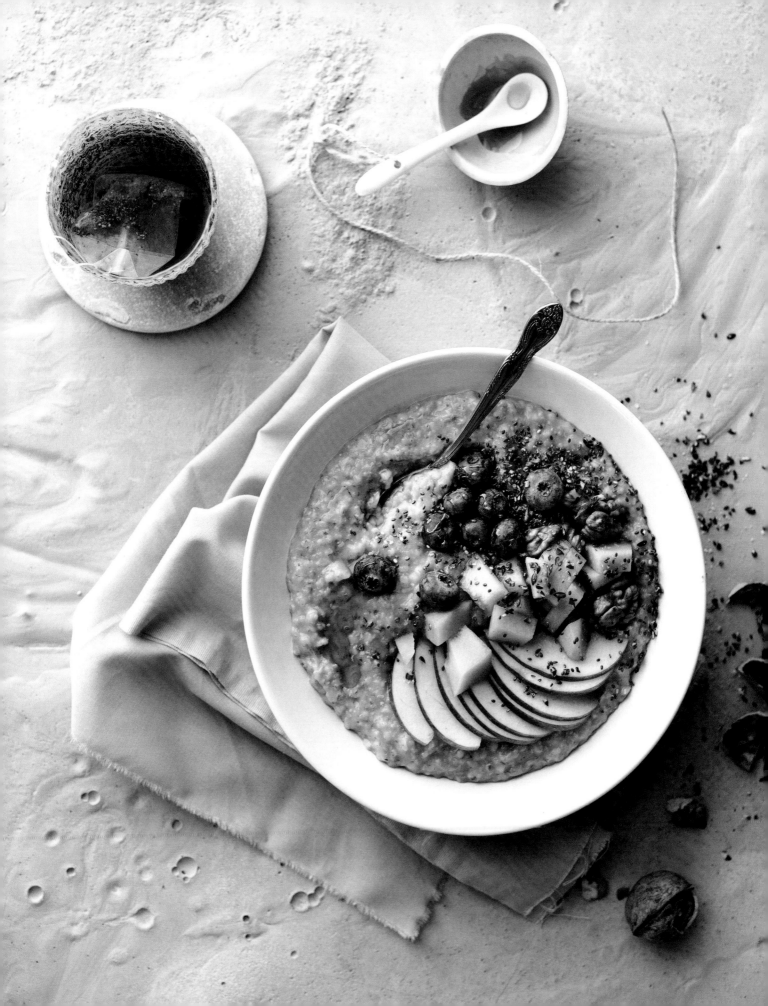

# Crohn's Disease

## Coconut Oil and Crohn's Disease

Crohn's disease causes major ulcerations along the digestive system, preventing patients from absorbing nutrients and fluids, so they become dehydrated and/or malnourished. Coconut oil works in two ways to ease the symptoms and aftereffects of Crohn's disease. First, it helps to heal the ulcerated sections of the digestive tract, and second, it works to increase the absorption of essential nutrients such as calcium and magnesium. Crohn's patients can also benefit from drinking coconut water, as it is rich in electrolytes, which are lost through malabsorption.

### Gentle Ways to Alleviate Crohn's Symptoms

- Eat foods rich in probiotics and prebiotics, or take a quality supplement
- Turmeric helps to reduce inflammation. Use it in cooking, drinks, or teas, or purchase supplements. Fresh turmeric is more easily absorbed by the body than powdered.
- Try yoga or other forms of gentle exercise
- Find ways to relax, as stress can trigger flare-ups. Try journaling, taking a walk, deep breathing, and cutting back on unnecessary responsibilities.

### Probiotic Foods

- Kefir
- Kimchi
- Kombucha
- Lactofermented pickles
- Lactofermented sauerkraut
- Miso
- Yogurt

### Prebiotic Foods

- Apples
- Asparagus
- Bananas
- Barley
- Burdock root
- Chicory root
- Chickpeas
- Cocoa
- Dandelion greens
- Flaxseeds
- Garlic
- Leeks
- Oats
- Onions
- Savoy cabbage
- Seaweed

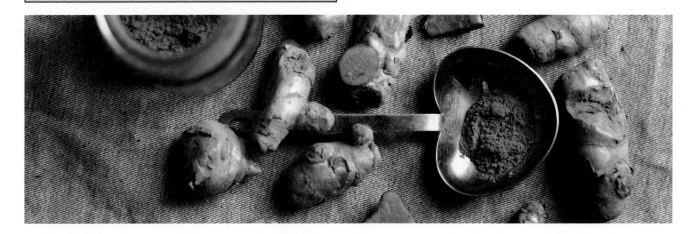

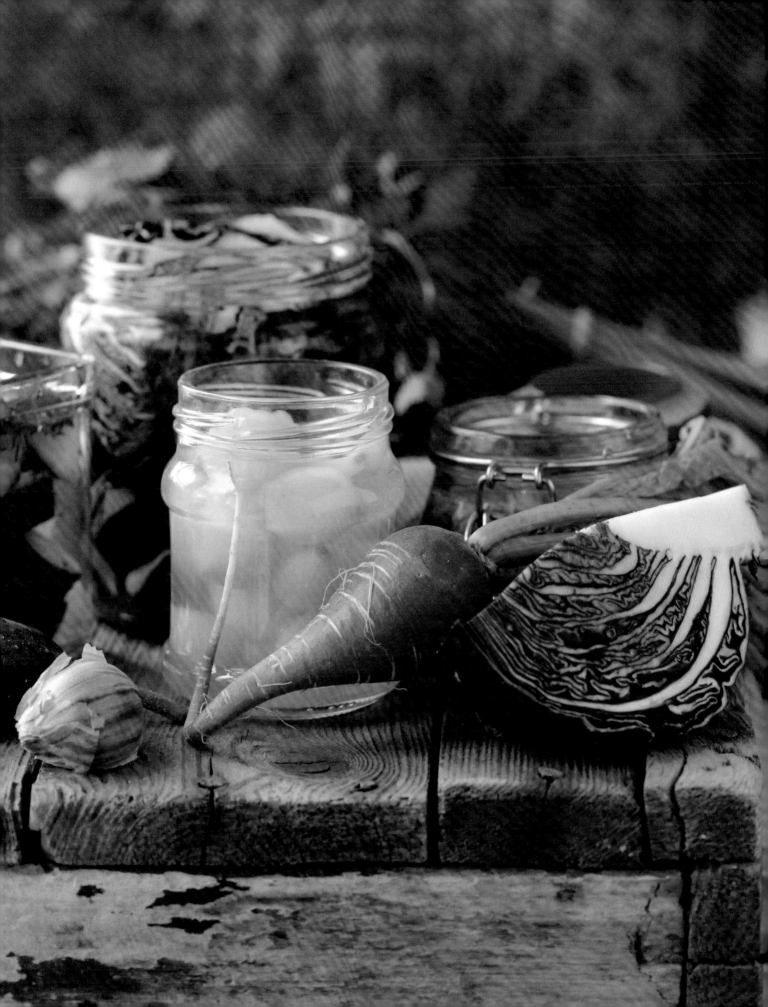

# Diarrhea

## Diarrhea Calming Capsule

### Ingredients:
vegetable capsule
6 drops black pepper essential oil
2 drops peppermint essential oil
2 drops chamomile essential oil
2 drops fennel essential oil
coconut oil

### Preparation and administration:
1. Open vegetable capsule.
2. Add 6 drops black pepper essential oil and 2 drops each of peppermint, chamomile, and fennel essential oils.
3. Top with coconut oil.
4. Close capsule.
5. Take capsule with water, coconut water, or coconut milk.

## Diarrhea Calming Massage Blend

### Ingredients:
1 teaspoon sweet almond oil (or other carrier oil)
3 drops chamomile essential oil
2 drops orange essential oil
1 drop ginger essential oil

### Preparation and administration:
1. Remove caps from essential oils.
2. Pour 1 teaspoon sweet almond essential oil into the palm of your hand.
3. Add 3 drops chamomile, 2 drops orange, and 1 drop ginger essential oils to your palm.
4. Rub the blend of oils over your entire abdomen.
5. Recap essential oils.

**Benefits:**
- Diarrhea is often accompanied by feelings of nausea. Ginger essential oil soothes this nausea and is in and of itself antidiarrhetic.
- Peppermint essential oil is particularly helpful with irritable bowel syndrome, which often results in spasmodic diarrhea. By reducing the spasms in the intestines, peppermint essential oil regulates the flow of digestion, allowing time for the proper absorption of fluid from the stools.
- Chamomile is also antispasmodic, calming the stomach and intestines.
- Black pepper contains constituents including piperine, which have both spasmodic and antispasmodic properties. This allows black pepper essential oil to aid the intestines in the appropriate speed of digestion.
- Orange essential oil reduces the perception of feelings of pain associated with diarrhea, but most importantly it relieves stress, which can contribute to gastrointestinal distress.
- Lemon balm is great for reducing stress.
- Fennel has been historically used—from ancient India, Greece, and Rome to colonial America—to aid in digestive health.

## NOTES AND TIPS:
The Diarrhea Calming Massage Blend is safe for children over the age of two. For children under the age of two, simply use chamomile essential oil diluted to a 0.5 percent dilution.

Peppermint essential oil can cause acid reflux when ingested directly (as opposed to in a capsule), but the lemon essential oil reduces acid reflux due to its gastroprotective qualities.

# Flatulence

## Apple Cider Vinegar

Flatulence occurs naturally in our bodies and is usually caused by swallowing air and gases produced by food that has not been digested properly. We swallow small amounts of air when we swallow our food and when we swallow our saliva. We either burp this air out through our mouths or it follows our digestive tract and is expelled from our back passage. Some foods like beans and cabbage are more likely to cause gas than others, but our individual food tolerances also play a role in what food gives us the most gas. Sipping a tablespoon of apple cider vinegar mixed with water before meals is known to aid digestion and reduce the volume and frequency of flatulence.

## Rosemary Digestive Tea

A great way to use your homegrown rosemary is to make your own tea! Additionally, this is the perfect way to aid your digestion before and after meals.

### Ingredients:

1–2 fresh sprigs of rosemary, or 1–1½ teaspoons of dried rosemary
2 cups boiling water
Honey (optional)

### Directions:

1. Break up your rosemary into small pieces and boil them in a pan with water and honey.
2. Reduce the heat when it is fully at a boil, and let sit for five minutes.
3. After the time is up, strain out the water from the mixture.

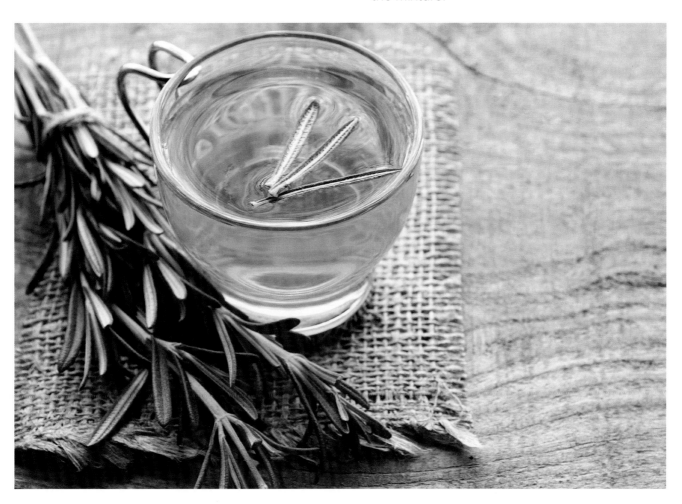

# Irritable Bowel Syndrome

## Peppermint Oil

If you're one of the twenty-five to forty-four million people in the United States suffering from IBS, it might be a good time to start growing peppermint in your backyard. Peppermint oil has been found to be an effective remedy for those who have abdominal pain and discomfort associated with IBS. One study found that those who took enteric-coated peppermint oil capsules twice a day for four weeks had a 50 percent reduction in total IBS symptoms.

## Tummy Tamer Tea

### Ingredients:

1 part lemon balm leaf
1 part ginger root
2 parts cramp bark
8 oz. hot water

### Directions:

1. Combine dried herbs and steep in water, covered, for 10–15 minutes.
2. Remove herbs from water, and sip tea slowly.

## Digestion Tincture

### Ingredients:

2 parts ginger
1 part dandelion root
1 part chamomile menstruum

*See instructions for making a tincture on page 204.*

## Kombucha

Kombucha is a medicinal drink full of healthy probiotics that aid digestion and the immune system. It is brewed by fermenting tea using a mass of yeast and bacteria that forms the kombucha culture, called the SCOBY (symbiotic colony of bacteria and yeast). Every batch of kombucha will create a new layer on the SCOBY, which can be peeled off and shared or discarded. So the best way to get started is to ask someone who is already brewing kombucha if you can have a layer of their SCOBY and a couple cups of kombucha to use as a starter. Alternately, you can purchase SCOBYs online. Don't skip the sugar in this recipe—it's essential to the fermenting process. However, the bacteria eat the sugar, so the end result is a tea that is fizzy and just barely sweet.

### Ingredients:

1½ quarts water
½ cup granulated sugar
4 bags green or black tea
1 SCOBY
1 cup already brewed kombucha

### Directions:

1. Bring the water to a boil, remove from heat, stir in the sugar, and add the tea bags. Allow the tea to brew until water is lukewarm and then remove the tea bags.
2. Add the brewed kombucha and pour into a clean 2-quart glass jar. Place the SCOBY into the jar with the tea, cover with cheesecloth or a paper towel, and secure with a rubber band.
3. Leave the jar at room temperature in a cupboard or somewhere where there's little direct light. Try not to disturb the jar while it's brewing. In about a week you should start to see bubbles floating around the SCOBY. Pour a little of the tea into a glass and taste it. If it's fizzy, it's ready to drink. Pour into a new jar and refrigerate, leaving a couple of inches of

kombucha in the jar with the SCOBY to keep it healthy until you brew another batch. If you'd like it fizzier, let it ferment a few more days.

## NOTE:

Check your SCOBY for any signs of mold. Any green spots mean that it has been compromised. Discard both the kombucha and SCOBY, and begin again.

### IBS and Stress

Stress and anxiety can aggravate IBS symptoms. Be sure to get adequate sleep and exercise, both of which help to reduce mental and emotional distress. Other self-care practices that may help include deep breathing, massage, acupuncture, and talk therapy to address underlying emotional concerns.

### Herbs to Relieve IBS Symptoms

- Bilberry (for intestinal spasms, inflammation, and diarrhea)
- Chamomile (to soothe and calm the digestive tract)
- Cramp bark (for abdominal and back pain relief, as well as for its antispasmodic values)
- Fennel
- Ginger
- Lemon balm
- Licorice (to reduce inflammation in the gut)
- Peppermint
- Slippery elm
- Wild yam (for general treatment of IBS symptoms)

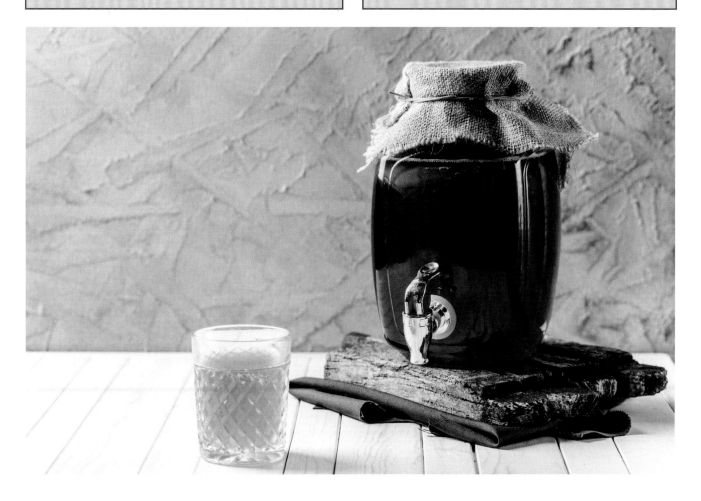

# Heartburn and Acid Reflux

## Heartburn Relief

**Ingredients:**

1 part spearmint leaf
1 part fennel seed
1 part pineapple weed
1 part organic orange peel
1 part hops strobiles

**Directions:**

1. Use for relief from indigestion and heartburn, a nervous stomach with gas, or for cramping and bloating. Prepare as a tea infusion (see page 194) using 1 heaping tablespoon tea mixture for 1½ cups of water.
2. Steep covered for 15 minutes.
3. Strain and drink 3 cups sipped after meals. Or for variety, prepare a larger amount and pour into Popsicle molds. Freeze. Enjoy as a cold pop.

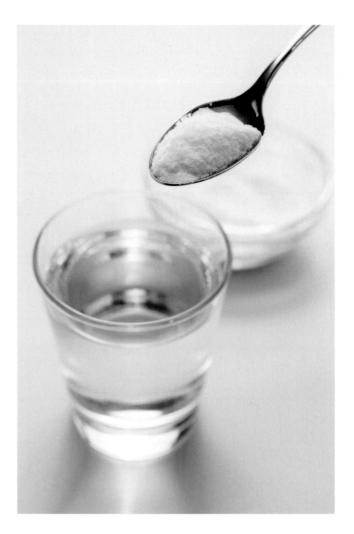

## Simple Ways to Relieve Heartburn or Acid Reflux

- Wear loose clothing.
- Avoid laying flat. Stand up, sit up straight, or prop up your upper body with pillows while reclining.
- Add a teaspoon of baking soda to a glass of water, stir until dissolved, and drink slowly.
- Don't stuff yourself. Overeating can contribute to heartburn.
- Avoid eating just before bed.
- Try a low-carb diet.
- Avoid alcohol.
- Reduce caffeine intake.

# Nausea and Vomiting

## Stomach-Stabilizing Tea

### Ingredients:
1 part ginger root
2 parts peppermint leaf
8 oz. hot water

### Directions:
1. Combine dried herbs and steep in water, covered, for 10–15 minutes.
2. Remove herbs from water, and sip tea slowly.

### Simple Ways to Relieve Nausea
- Consume ginger. Fresh ginger root can be used in cooking or steeped in hot water for tea.
- Drink bone broth.
- Eat crackers, toast, or bananas.
- Eat small portions frequently.
- Avoid very fatty, sweet, or spicy foods.
- Diffuse peppermint or citrus essential oil

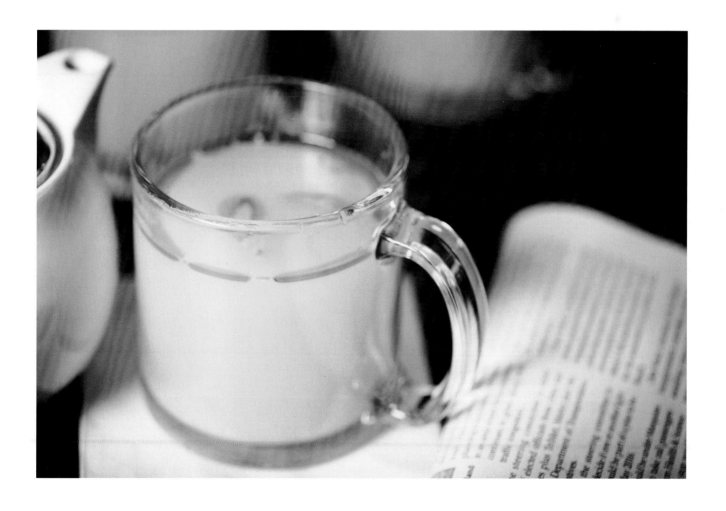

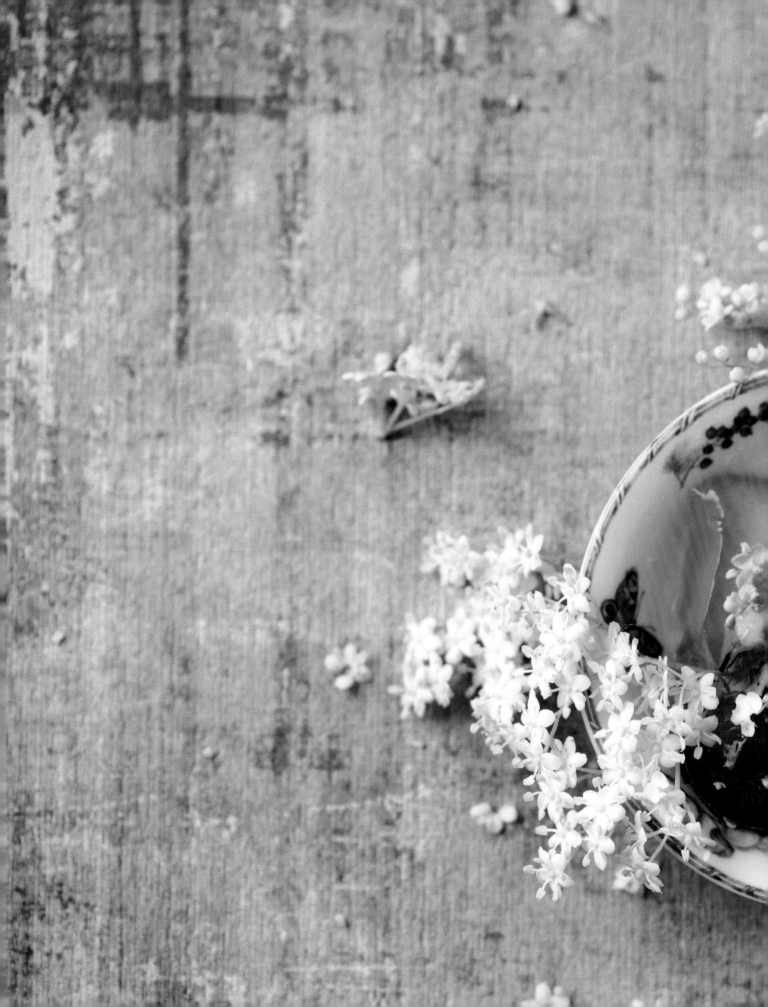

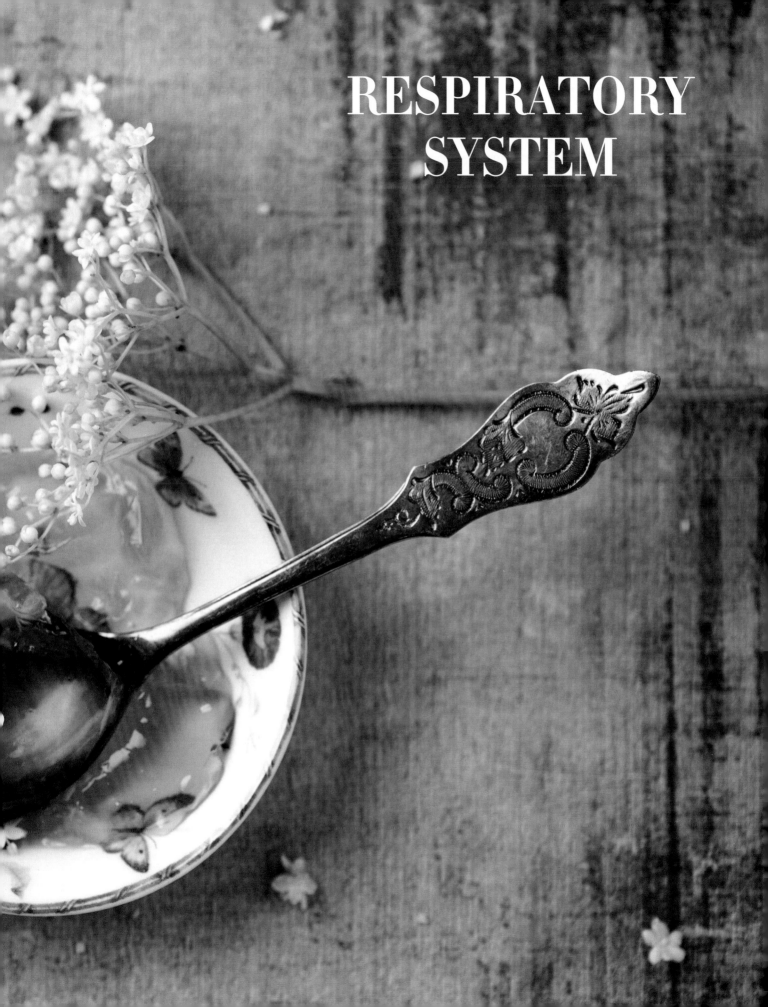

# RESPIRATORY SYSTEM

# Asthma

## Coconut Oil

Asthma is triggered by inflammation, which usually also limits the absorption of nutrients from food. Coconut oil not only works as an anti-inflammatory but also helps increase your ability to absorb nutrients, so you are generally stronger and fitter. The fatty acids in coconut oil are essential for the repair and maintenance of healthy lung tissue. Take a daily dose to counteract asthma symptoms.

## Apple Cider Vinegar

Apple cider vinegar has been found to strengthen the lungs and immune system, both of which are imperative for asthma sufferers. Combining apple cider vinegar with honey helps restore the acid/alkaline balance in the body, which helps stop the wheezing that generally accompanies an asthma attack. Sipping a tincture of 1 tablespoon of apple cider vinegar and 1 teaspoon of honey in half a cup of warm water over the course of thirty minutes will provide relief when you are in distress. If wheezing persists half an hour after finishing the drink, then try another dose, although you are not likely to need one as breathing difficulties should have subsided by then. If the first dose of apple cider vinegar and honey does not work, another tried-and-tested remedy is to soak two cotton pads in apple cider vinegar and apply them to the insides of your wrists while you sip the second dose. Breathing should be easier after this.

## Mullein Tea

Mullein is an expectorant, helping loosen phlegm, making coughing more productive. It also helps to soothe the mucous membranes. This simple tea is helpful for any kind of cough or respiratory problems.

### Ingredients:

1½ cups water
1–2 teaspoons fresh or dried mullein leaves and flowers
1 teaspoon honey

### Directions:

1. Place the dried mullein in a tea ball or make your own tea bag using cheesecloth and string.
2. Boil the water and pour over the tea. Allow to steep for 10–15 minutes.

---

### Herbs and Other Foods for Asthma Relief

The foods listed here have been found by many to help alleviate asthma symptoms, but are not suitable as use in place of an inhaler or other medical treatment, particularly in the case of an asthma attack or chronic asthma. Note that some herbs may interfere with other asthma medications, and some are not safe for children. Check with your doctor.

- Garlic
- Ginger
- Ginseng
- Honey
- Mullein
- Turmeric

*See Sage and Thyme sections, page 154 and 158*

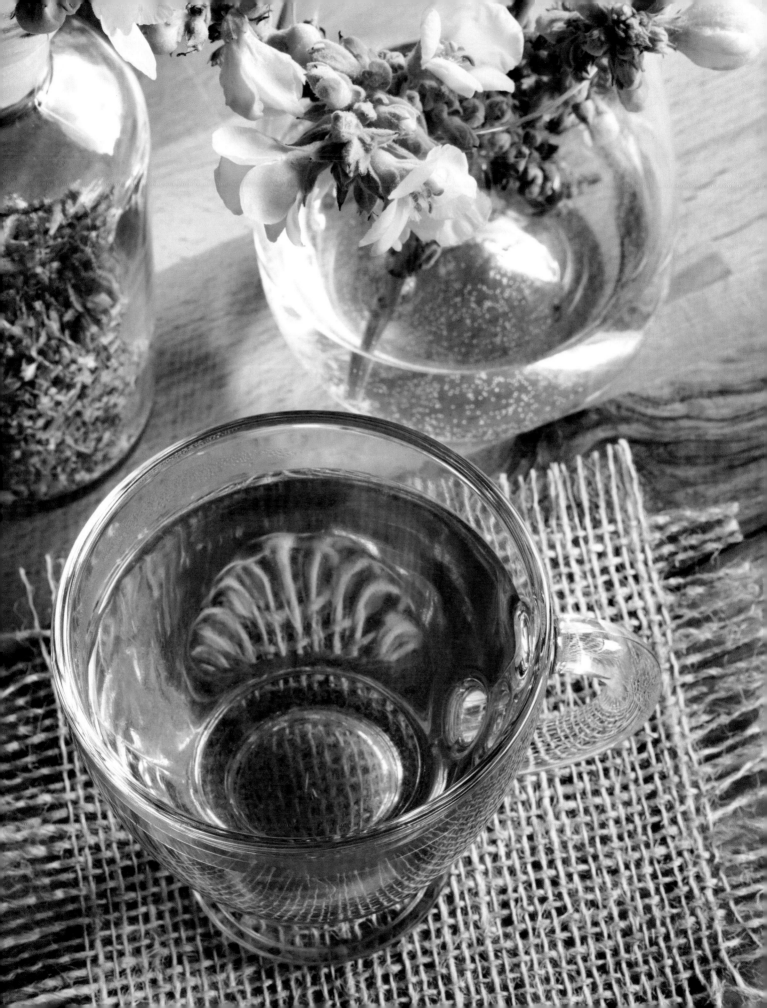

# Common Cold

## Yarrow Rose Hip Cold and Flu Relief

Ingredients:

3 tablespoons dried yarrow flowers
    (or 4 tablespoons fresh, chopped)
1 teaspoon dried spearmint leaves
1 teaspoon licorice root
2 teaspoons dried rose hips
3 teaspoons fresh ginger root
3 clove fruits
½ teaspoon cardamom seeds
2 cinnamon sticks, broken
Juice of 1 fresh lemon or orange
6 cups water
Cayenne powder—liberal shakes

Directions:

1. Combine ingredients in a large pot to consume throughout the day. Bring water up to a boil, then reduce to low heat and cover for 15 minutes. Strain.
2. Drink a cupful every 1–2 hours. Sweeten if desired. Use for children and adults alike at the onset of a cold or flu to minimize aches and pains and to encourage body sweating. Can assist with those under-the-weather symptoms such as head congestion, sore throat, coughing, headaches, fever, restlessness, watery eyes, stomachaches, and general aches and pains.

## Cold Care Syrup

The cinnamon, cloves, and ginger in this cold care syrup make a delicious addition to the herbal immune boosting power of elderberries and echinacea. Prepare for cold season by making a large batch of cold care syrup to store in the refrigerator. For immune boosting, most sources recommend that adults take up to one tablespoon of the syrup per day, while children should take one teaspoon. For acute illnesses such as colds or flu,

take the syrup several times per day. Note: Honey should not be given to children under one year.

Ingredients:

1 cup dried whole elderberries (You can also use ⅔ cup elderberry powder or 2 cups fresh elderberries)
2 tablespoons echinacea root
2 tablespoon fresh ginger root
1 cinnamon stick
½ teaspoon whole cloves
3½ cups water
¾–1½ cups raw honey (sweetened to your personal preference)

Directions:

1. Place all ingredients except honey into a heavy saucepan and simmer over low-medium heat for 30–45 minutes.
2. Strain the liquid using a mesh strainer or cheesecloth.
3. Allow the mixture to cool until it is just warm to the touch. Add honey and stir until well mixed. Refrigerate until use.

## Chest Congestion and Sinus Remedy

This very simple remedy will help soothe your throat, boost your immune system, and decrease your mucus buildup.

Ingredients:

1 mug of hot water
2 tablespoons lemon juice
2 teaspoons apple cider vinegar
1 teaspoon honey

Directions:

1. Heat the water to boiling and place in a mug.
2. Mix the lemon juice, apple cider vinegar, and honey into the hot water. This easy and refreshing drink will help with congestion, mucus, and phlegm and will boost your immune system and soothe your throat. Drink a few times a day when sick.

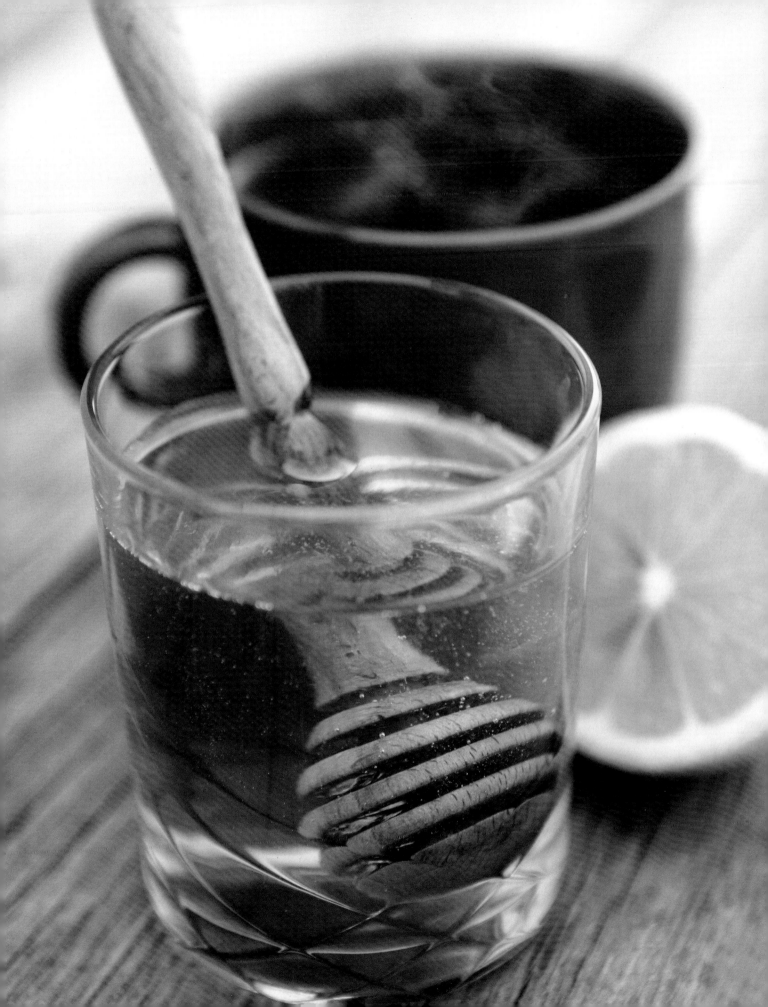

## Head Cold Tea

Sometimes when you get sick, it feels like your nasal cavities are fighting the virus all by themselves. The rest of your body feels fine, but your head feels ready to explode. This head cold tea will help clear your nasal cavities and support your immune system.

### Ingredients:
1½ cups water
2 green onions
1 drop ginger essential oil

### Preparation:
1. Heat water in a pan on high heat until it boils.
2. Reduce heat and add 2 green onions. Let onions simmer, covered, for five minutes.
3. Strain onion broth into a ceramic mug and let cool.
4. When the broth is close to a drinkable temperature, but still steaming, add one drop of ginger essential oil and stir with a metal spoon.

### Administration:
1. Inhale the steam from the mug for approximately one minute.
2. Drink the green onion and ginger essential oil mixture when it is cool enough to drink, but still warm.

### Benefits:
- Green onion and ginger root "tea" is a common folk remedy for colds. This recipe brings the concentrated benefits of ginger essential oil to the traditional recipe.
- Ginger essential oil has both antiviral properties and immune-supporting properties. This combination makes it ideal for supporting the body while it fights off the common cold.

## Cold and Flu Tincture

### Ingredients:
2 parts echinacea
2 parts elderberries
1 part goldenseal
1 part boneset
½ part ginger
½ part thyme
¼ part garlic
¼ part raw, local honey

See instructions for making a tincture on page 204. This formula is indicated when strong cold and/or flu symptoms are present, such as fever, body aches, lots of congestion, intense sore throat, and cough.

## Coconut Oil for Colds and Flu

The antiviral properties of coconut oil mean it is an excellent natural treatment for colds and related conditions. Consume between one and three tablespoons a day to boost your immunity. If you are feeling congested, try combining solid coconut oil with a few drops of essential oil and apply the mixture to your chest. When you have a headache or feel feverish, try massaging plain coconut oil into your temples. A dollop of coconut oil in a cup of hot tea will soothe and heal a sore throat. A daily dose of coconut oil is also soothing and beneficial for a cough, as the oil will destroy the bacteria causing the cough. Try stirring the coconut oil into a cup of hot tea for soothing and therapeutic refreshment.

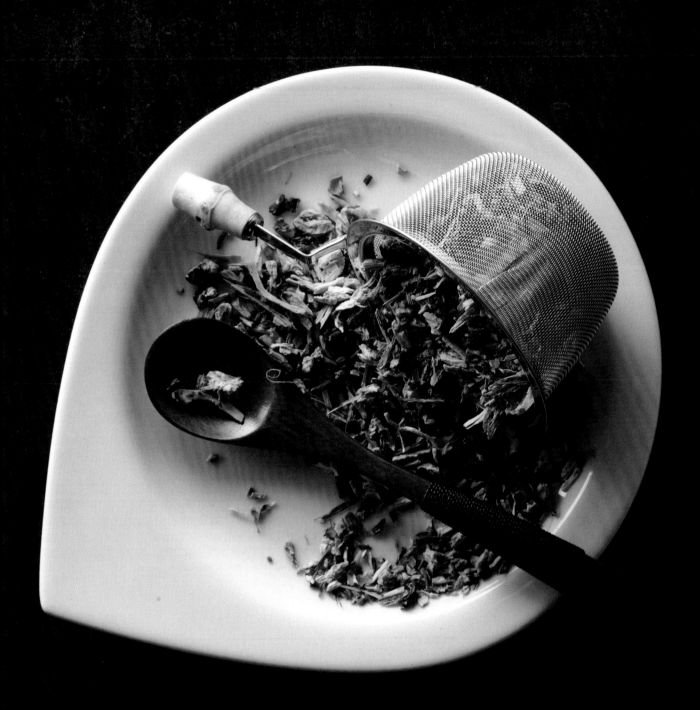

# Coughs

Daisy leaves are rich in chlorophyll and high in fiber with soothing mucilage properties. Both the leaves and flowers are welcome additions to soups, salads, mixed into stews, and added into sandwiches. Avoid during pregnancy and lactation.

## Daisy Restorative Lung Tea

### Ingredients:

2 teaspoons daisy flower and/or leaf
½ teaspoon thyme herb
1 teaspoon sweet violet herb and flower
½ teaspoon aniseed

### Directions:

1. Boil 1 cup of water and pour over herbs.
2. Infuse, covered, for 15 minutes, strain, and drink 3 cups per day as an adult dose.

## Decongestant Oregano Coconut Vapor Rub

### Ingredients:

1 drop oregano essential oil
1 drop lemon essential oil
1 tablespoon unrefined coconut oil

### Directions:

1. Mix with a spoon and store in a tightly covered container. The texture is best hardened for a topical rub.
2. Test on a small area of skin first before using this as a chest rub for seasonal allergies and congestion. It can also be rubbed onto the nostrils to hydrate dry skin; the volatile oils will assist with clearing the sinus passages for easier breathing.

When experiencing the initial symptoms of a cold, I suggest to clients to rub this mixture onto the soles of their feet prior to heading off to bed. The volatile oils will be absorbed through the thin skin on the arch of the foot and will disinfect the lungs, enhancing immune activity while sleeping; this simple application alone can go a long way in warding off a cold. Keep in mind that essential oils are highly concentrated and should be well diluted. If your skin is sensitive, increase the amount of coconut oil in the blend.

## DIY Vapor Rub

You can customize this rub to suit your own preferences by experimenting with different essential oils. Eucalyptus and peppermint will pack the most punch in terms of effectiveness, so use at least 40 drops (combined) of those. After that, choose from lavender, lemon, rosemary, camphor, cinnamon, and tea tree oils. If you intend to use the rub on a child, be sure the oil is safe for the child's age.

### Ingredients:

¼ cup coconut oil
¼ cup shea butter
60–75 drops essential oils (see above)

### Directions:

1. Scoop coconut oil and shea butter into the bowl of a stand mixer with a paddle attachment.
2. Mix until the oils turn into a whipped butter texture.
3. Add essential oils and mix to combine.
4. Store in an airtight glass jar. To use, rub a little on your chest.

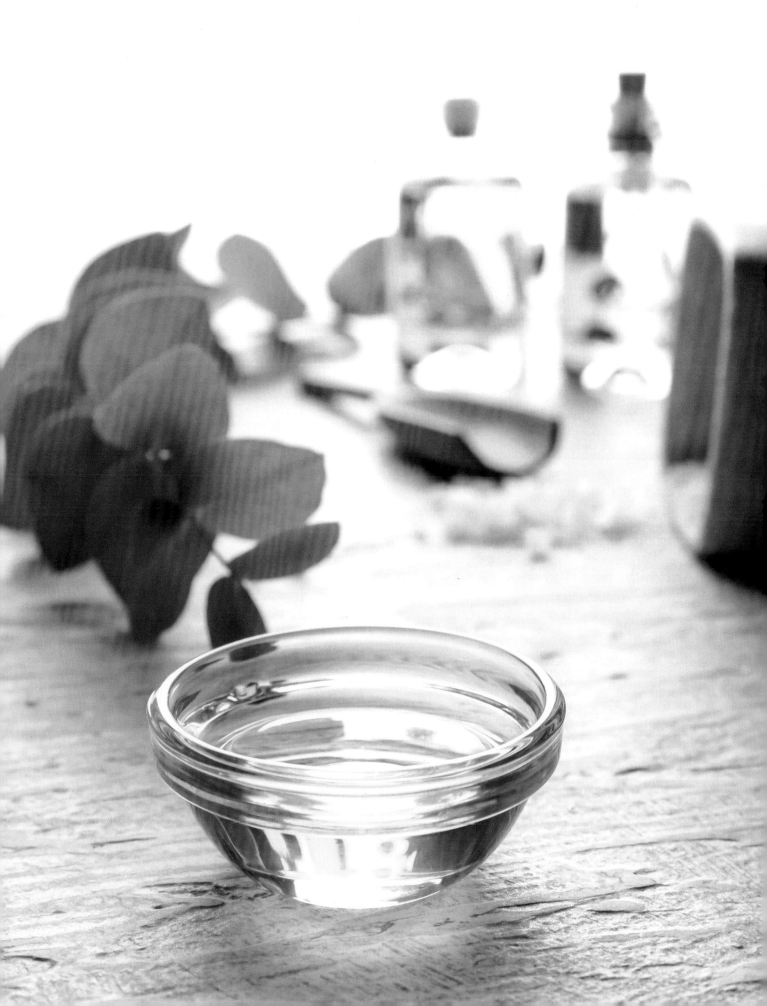

# Flu

## Flu Bomb Protocol

The flu, unlike the common cold, usually hits suddenly and seemingly out of the blue. You feel fine, and then within less than an hour, you're achy, feverish, and feel downright miserable. Luckily, this flu bomb protocol is there for you the moment you feel that tickle in your throat or ache in your neck that signals an upcoming bout of the flu. One of the other great benefits of this protocol is that it works on the common cold, too! Just make sure you start using it right away. The lower your viral load, the more effective this and any other supportive measure will be. And remember rest, rest, rest, rest, and more rest is the very best way for your body to focus on fighting the flu or any other infection.

There are four recipes within this protocol because your body needs multiple means of support when it is fighting off the flu. The recipes are listed with ingredients, preparation, and administration first, but use them all for the entire protocol.

## Antimicrobial Water

### Ingredients:
16 ounces of water
1 teaspoon honey
1 drop lemon essential oil
1 drop cinnamon essential oil
1 drop lemongrass essential oil

### Preparation:
1. In a pint glass, combine 1 teaspoon of honey and 1 drop each of lemon, cinnamon, and lemongrass essential oils.
2. Add 16 ounces of water.

### Administration:
1. Drink the entire contents of the pint glass.

## Flu-Fighting Gargle

### Ingredients:
1 ounce water
1 drop clove essential oil
1 drop rosemary essential oil
1 drop oregano essential oil
1 drop lemon essential oil
1 drop melaleuca essential oil
1 drop cinnamon essential oil

### Preparation:
1. In a 2-ounce glass, add one drop each of clove, rosemary, oregano, lemon, melaleuca, and cinnamon essential oils to 1 ounce of water.

### Administration:
1. Pour the Flu-Fighting Gargle into your mouth toward your throat.
2. Gargle for 1–2 minutes.
3. Spit.

## Flu-Fighting Neck and Chest Rub

### Ingredients:
2 teaspoons sweet almond oil (or other carrier oil)
3 drops cypress essential oil
2 drops black pepper essential oil
2 drops melaleuca essential oil
1 drop basil essential oil

### Preparation and Administration:
1. Take caps off essential oil bottles.
2. Pour 2 teaspoons sweet almond oil into the palm of your hand.
3. Add 3 drops cypress, 2 drops black pepper, 2 drops melaleuca, and 1 drop basil essential oils.
4. Rub your hands together, then rub your shoulders, neck, and chest with the Flu-Fighting Neck and Chest Rub.
5. Replace the caps on the essential oil bottles.
6. Inhale the aroma of the rub.

## Flu-Fighting Foot Rub

### Ingredients:
1 tablespoon extra-virgin olive oil
1 medium-large garlic clove, crushed
1 drop oregano essential oil

### Preparation:
1. Use a garlic press to crush 1 medium-large garlic clove.
2. Scrape crushed garlic into a small glass bowl.
3. Add 1 tablespoon extra-virgin olive oil.
4. Mix in 1 drop oregano essential oil.

### Administration:
1. Scoop a portion of the Flu-Fighting Foot Rub into your hand.
2. Rub onto the bottoms of your feet.
3. Rub between your toes to stimulate the reflexology points for your lymphatic system.
4. Focus on the outer balls of your feet to activate the reflexology points for your lungs.
5. Scoop the rest of the Flu-Fighting Foot Rub into your hand and massage your entire foot.
6. Put on clean socks.

## Soup Enhancer

### Ingredients:
2 cups chicken noodle soup
1 tablespoon extra-virgin olive oil
1 medium-large clove garlic, minced
2 drops food-grade lemon essential oil
2 drops food-grade black pepper essential oil

### Preparation:
1. Heat 2 cups of your favorite chicken noodle soup and 1 medium-large minced clove of garlic on the stove.
2. While the soup is heating, in a small glass bowl, combine 1 tablespoon extra-virgin olive oil and 2 drops each of lemon and black pepper essential oils.

3. Once soup is evenly heated, remove from the stove and pour into a bowl (not plastic)
4. Allow to cool to a consumable temperature, then add oil mixture. Stir.

### Administration:
1. Snuggle up and eat your soup as you inhale the steam it produces.

---

### Essential Oils for Fighting the Flu

- Cinnamon and lemongrass essential oils are highly antimicrobial against viruses, bacteria, fungi, and protozoans.
- Clove, oregano, rosemary, lemon, basil, and melaleuca essential oils have a wide range of antimicrobial effects, both killing and inhibiting a variety of bacteria, viruses, and fungi.
- Cypress and basil essential oils are stimulating to the respiratory and cardiovascular systems.
- Lemon essential oil stimulates the liver, which improves overall health.
- Black pepper is the most commonly used spice, not just due to its taste, but also because of its medicinal properties. Black pepper essential oil contains pet ether, a highly antioxidant substance, with health benefits ranging from anticancer to immunological support.

# Hay Fever

## Coconut Oil

Using a cotton swab, apply a light layer of coconut oil inside each nostril. This will prevent pollen from irritating the nasal cavity.

## Ingestible Hay Fever Relief*

### Ingredients:

1 tablespoon local wild raw honey
1 drop peppermint essential oil
1 drop lemon essential oil
1 drop lavender essential oil

### Preparation and Administration:

1. Pour 1 tablespoon local wild raw honey into a large metal spoon.
2. Add 1 drop each of peppermint, lemon, and lavender essential oils.
3. Swallow mixture.

*Be sure to use food-grade essential oils. Not all essential oils are safe to consume.

## Hay Fever Relief Diffuser Blend

### Ingredients:

water
4 drops lavender essential oil
4 drops lemon essential oil
4 drops peppermint essential oil

### Preparation and administration:

1. Fill your diffuser with water to the fill line.
2. Add 4 drops each of lavender, lemon, and peppermint essential oils.
3. Turn on diffuser.
4. Inhale vapors released by the diffuser.

### Benefits:

- Consuming local honey can reduce the allergic reactions to local pollen.
- Lemon cleanses the air and body.
- Peppermint opens your airways and reduces the effects of allergic rhinitis.
- Lavender is anti-inflammatory and soothes irritated nasal passageways.

### NOTES AND TIPS:

This protocol is intended for children and adults over the age of six years old. For children between six months and six years, simply omit the peppermint essential oil in the Hay Fever Relief Diffuser Blend and do not administer the Ingestible Hay Fever Relief. Instead, blend one drop each of lavender and lemon essential oils in a teaspoon of carrier oil and rub on the child's chest.

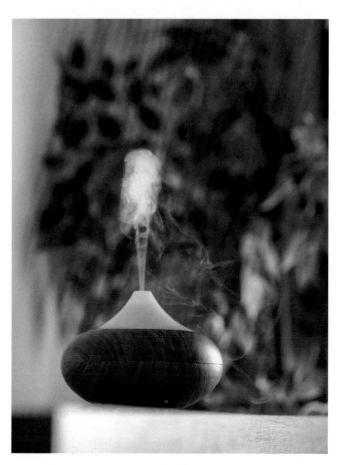

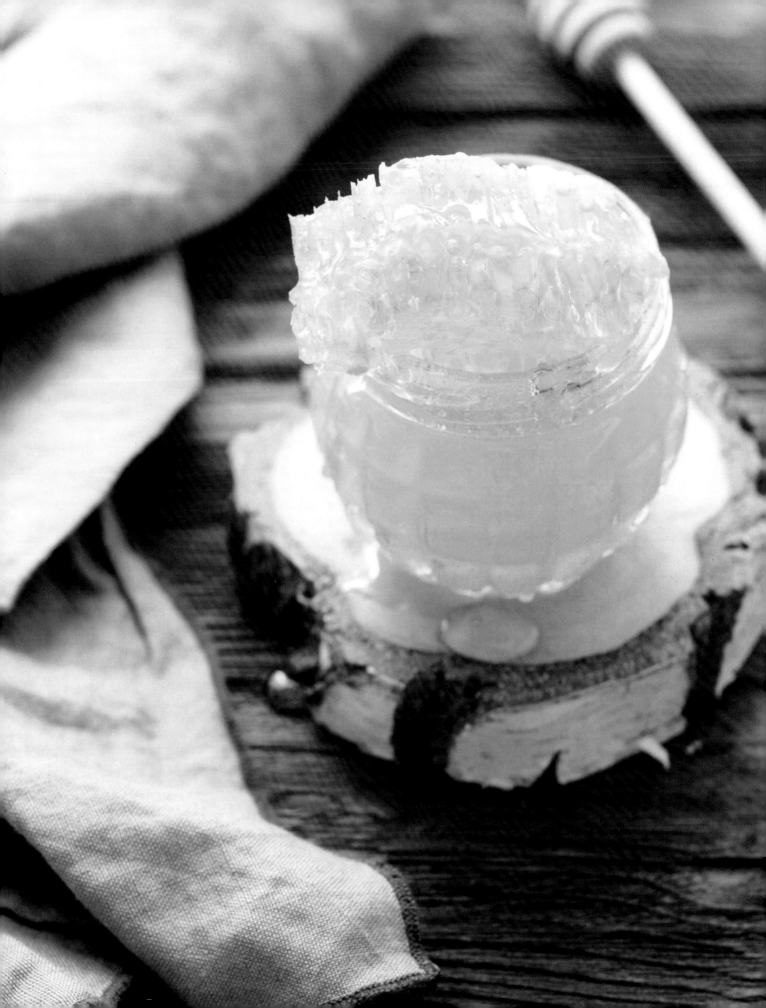

# Pneumonia and Bronchitis

## Bronchitis Elixir

This recipe is a variation of a Traditional Bronchitis Elixir referenced online from Mrs. Grieve's *A Modern Herbal*.

### Ingredients:

60 grams sunflower seeds, slightly browned/
  roasted
10 grams mullein leaf and flower
15 grams star anise or fennel seed
¾ cup brandy
½–¾ cup organic cane sugar

### Directions:

1. Boil slightly roasted seeds in 4 cups of water and simmer down to just over 1½ cups.
2. Ten minutes before removing from the heat, add the mullein and anise or fennel. Cover and simmer on low heat for an additional 10 minutes, then strain.
3. Add ¾ cup of brandy and ¾ cup of organic cane sugar. Bottle.
4. Adult dosages vary at 1–2 teaspoonfuls, three or four times a day as needed for a spastic cough.

## Sage Cherry Cough Syrup

A fantastic expectorant for spastic coughs, this formula can be taken for colds and flu, bronchitis, and pneumonia.

### Ingredients:

2 teaspoons sage leaf
2 teaspoons mullein leaf or flower
2 teaspoons plantain leaf
½ teaspoon fennel seed
1 teaspoon ginger root
4 cups water
Brandy
⅓ cup black cherry concentrate
Honey or sugar

### Directions:

1. Place the herbs in the boiling water, reduce heat, and simmer covered for 20–30 minutes until the mixture is reduced to about half the volume. Set aside the heat and infuse for an additional 10 minutes, covered.
2. Strain, measure, and add an equal volume (1:1 ratio) of honey to the tea.
3. Mix in black cherry concentrate. Brandy can be added in as a preservative and also for flavor.

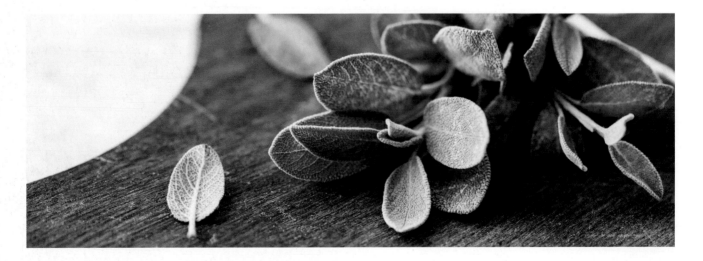

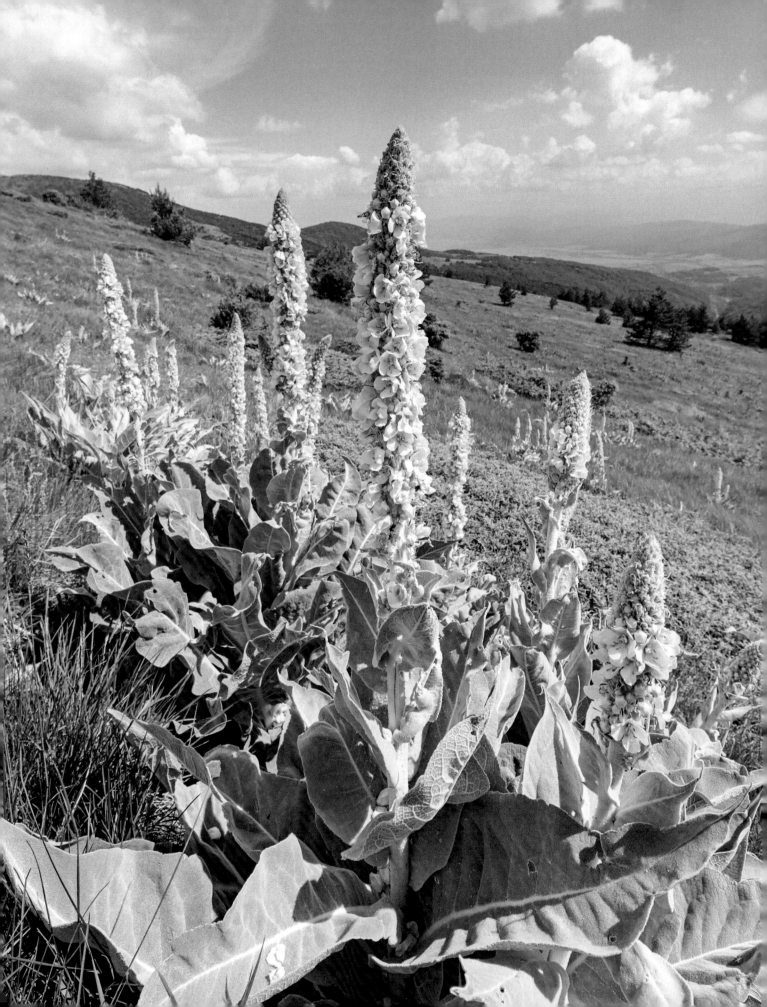

# Sinusitis

## Sinus Relief Herbal Steam

### Ingredients:

1 teaspoon dried chamomile flowers
1 teaspoon dried rosemary leaf
1 teaspoon dried spearmint leaf
4 drops eucalyptus essential oil

### Directions:

1. Boil water, pour into a basin, and add the herbs.
2. Steep, covered, at least 5 minutes. When ready to use, add the essential oil.
3. Be mindful not to burn yourself with the hot bowl or the hot steam. Put your head under a towel to trap the steam and inhale the vapors. You will feel immediate relief as the steam and disinfectant volatile oils open up the sinus passages. For children, place a towel around the bottom of the bowl to protect from burning. Always try out the heat from the steam first, by putting your wrist under the towel before putting a young child, with sensitive tissues, in direct contact with hot steam.

## Simple Ways to Alleviate Sinusitis

- Drink lots of water and other clear fluids
- Consume ginger, garlic, onions, raw honey, and spicy foods
- Take a hot shower and breathe in the steam
- Eat foods rich in vitamin C and/or take vitamin C supplements
- Use a humidifier in your bedroom at night
- Diffuse eucalyptus essential oil
- Use a neti pot
- Rest as much as possible

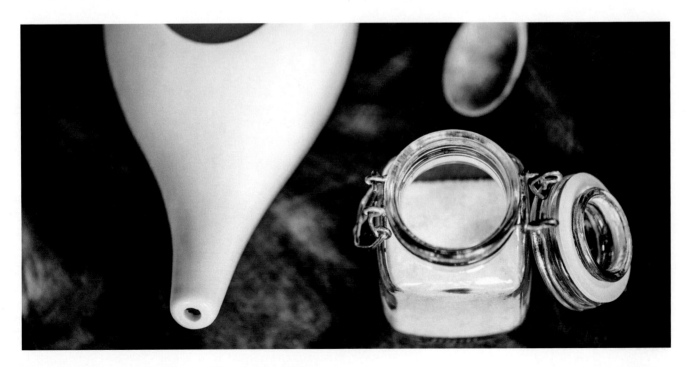

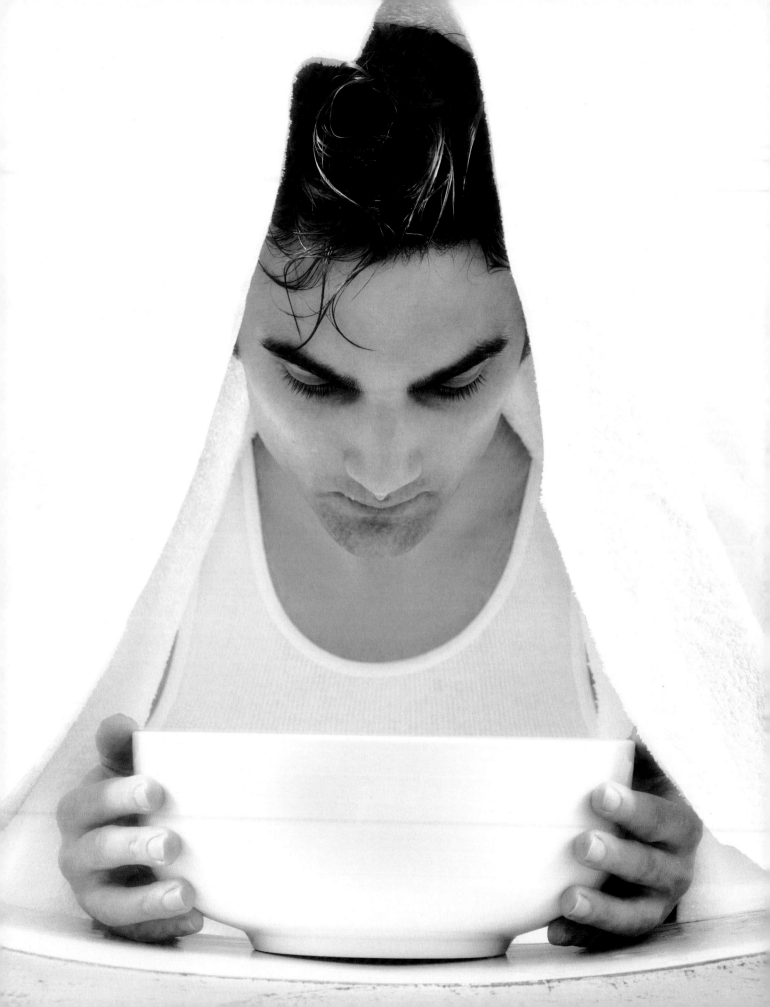

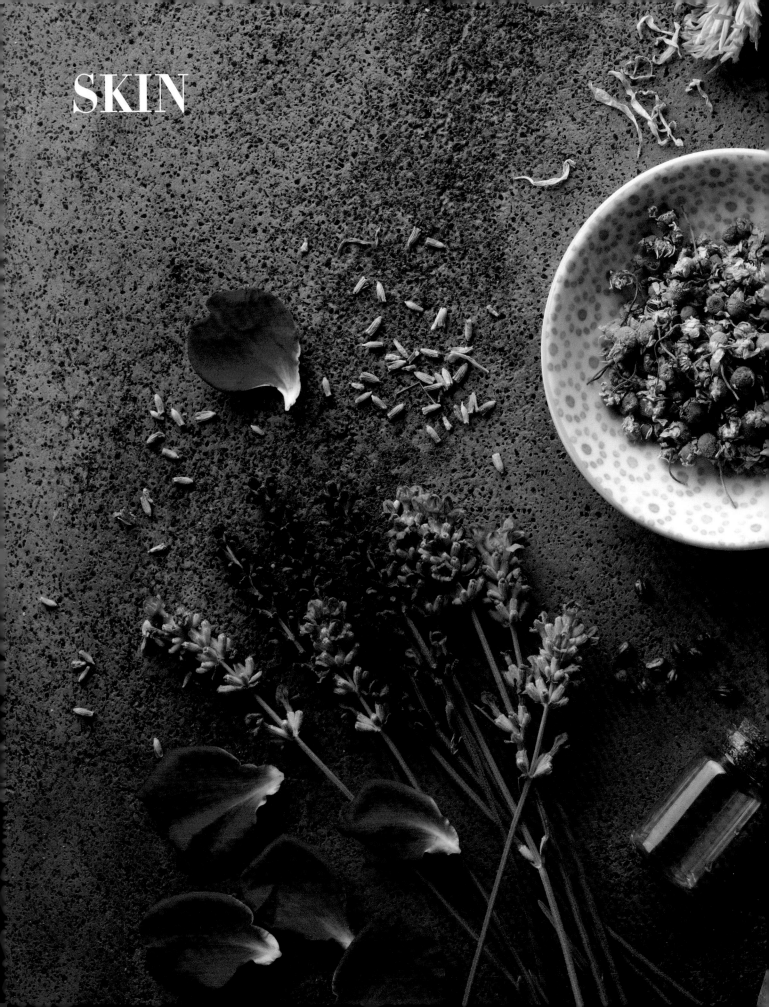

# SKIN

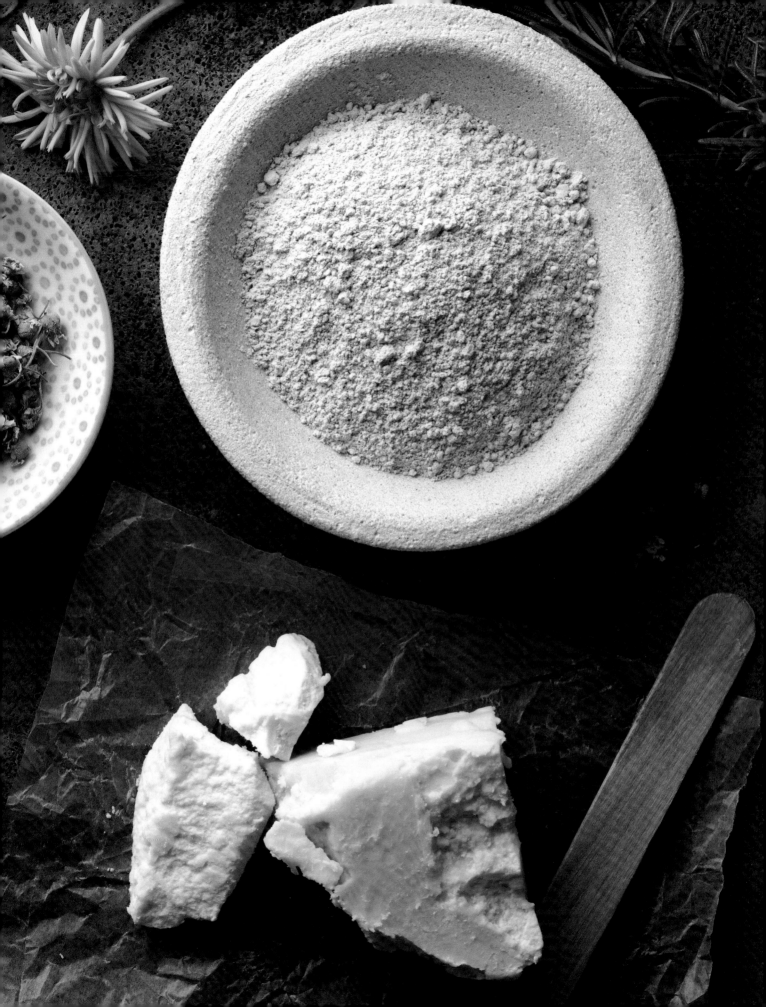

# Acne

## Aloe Vera Face Cream

We can't talk about aloe without creating an amazing face remedy with its amazing gel. By harvesting your own aloe gel, you are skipping out on all the additives, preservatives, and other unpronounceable additions to your store-bought aloe. With this recipe, you are getting pure, nature-made, skin-loving cream, plus the bragging rights to all your friends and family that you are "so DIY."

### Ingredients:

Aloe gel from a small leaf
½ cup extra-virgin coconut oil
A few drops essential oil of your choice (I prefer geranium, lavender, and ylang-ylang)

### Directions:

1. Take the gel from your small aloe leaf and place it in a blender. Blend the gel until it's light and frothy.
2. Place your blended aloe gel and ½ cup coconut oil into a bowl and whisk the two together using an electric hand blender for about five minutes until you get a consistency that's light, like a cake frosting.
3. Add a few drops of your choice of essential oil. I like using lavender, because it's great for the skin, can help heal irritations, and the scent is relaxing and calming. Geranium is a wonderful oil, which can balance oil production and condition the skin, and is a great addition to moisturizers. Ylang-ylang is a great oil to help treat acne and oily skin, and may help fight the effects of aging by stimulating cell growth! If

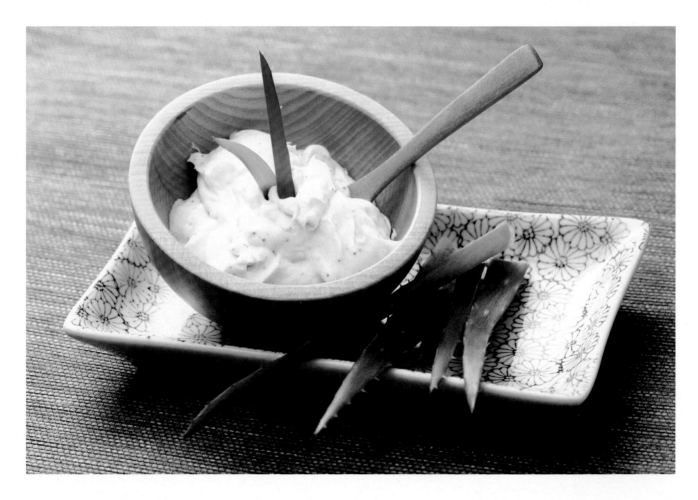

you're feeling extra saucy, why not add a drop of each to the cream?

4. Whisk the oil again with your potpourri of essential oils. After you're done, place your lotion into a glass container and store it in the refrigerator. You can use this anywhere on your body, in the morning, after a shower, before bed, when you're bored, literally whenever you want! The lotion should last for several weeks in your fridge, so make sure to use it before it expires.

## Don't Use Sparingly

This gooey mixture is wonderful for your skin, as it puts together two of the most skin-loving ingredients: coconut oil and aloe gel. Coconut oil is known for its antibacterial and antifungal properties, is an amazing and tropical-smelling moisturizer, and actually penetrates your skin on a deeper level than most other oils—this is due to its low molecular weight and how it bonds with proteins (science!). With that said, coconut oil can help reduce bacterial infections on the skin and help prevent acne breakouts; it's also a great protection from the sun, naturally providing you with a sun protection factor of four. This stuff is amazing; too bad it doesn't come from a houseplant. The mix of coconut oil with aloe gives you a moisturizing kick in the butt, helps you look younger, and makes you smell like the Garden of Eden. And remember, don't use sparingly. Slather this on your body like you're about to enter a mud-wrestling match. Your skin will thank you later.

## Acne Causes and Treatments

Adult acne can have a wide range of root causes included food allergies; sensitivity to ingredients in lotions, soaps, makeup, or laundry detergent; stress or hormone imbalances; lack of sleep; and more. You may need the help of more than one doctor and to do some experimenting to sort it out for yourself. Frustratingly, there's no one-size-fits-all solution for adult acne, and it may take several weeks to notice any difference after cutting out a food or making any other lifestyle change. You may wish to enlist a doctor in helping you sort out the contributing factors to the acne.

- Drink lots of water. Dry skin (as well as oily skin) can lead to acne, and water helps to flush toxins out of your body.
- Use coconut oil in place of face wash or lotion. Rub a little into your skin, rinse with lukewarm water, and dry your face.
- Make a mask of honey and cinnamon (2 parts honey, 1 part cinnamon). Rub into clean skin, leave for ten minutes, and rinse off.
- Mix one drop of tea tree oil with ten drops of water and dab on acne spots.
- Eat foods containing omega-3 fatty acids (salmon, chia seeds, walnuts, flaxseeds), or take a supplement.
- Mix together 1 part white sugar with 1 part coconut oil and use to exfoliate (rub into skin gently, rinse, and pat skin dry). Use once a day or less.
- Talk to your doctor about trying an elimination diet and keeping a food journal. Common acne triggers include gluten, dairy, sugar and other high glycemic foods, and chocolate.

# Athlete's Foot

## Coconut Oil

Coconut oil is an antifungal agent, so it is an excellent cure for athlete's foot. After showering at night, cover your foot with coconut oil and then place a plastic bag over your foot. Place a sock over the plastic bag to keep the bag in position. Keep the "coconut oil sock" on for at least three hours, preferably all night. In the morning, remove the sock and bag, and wipe your foot dry with a paper towel. Continue this nightly treatment until the fungal infection has disappeared. It should take around five applications to completely eradicate the condition.

## Apple Cider Vinegar

Soak your feet in a mixture of half apple cider vinegar and half water twice a day until symptoms subside or alternatively apply some apple cider vinegar directly to the affected areas a few times a day and at bedtime for relief.

## Tea Tree Oil

Combine one tea tree oil with one part jojoba, almond, or olive oil and rub on affected area two or three times a day. You can also add a few drops to a basin of water and soak your feet for 20 minutes.

## Baking Soda

Put about ½ cup baking soda in a basin containing about a gallon of water. Soak feet for 20 minutes. Do not rinse feet, but pat them dry with an absorbent towel. Repeat twice daily. Do not reuse the towel before washing, as athlete's foot can spread through contact.

### Foot Baths for Athlete's Foot

Soaking feet can be a very effective way of getting rid of athlete's foot. In addition to the apple cider vinegar and baking soda soaks described here, you can try adding these ingredients to a basin of water and soaking for 15–20 minutes.

- Fresh oregano leaves or a few drops oregano essential oil
- 2–3 tablespoons salt
- 1 teaspoon mustard powder
- Few drops camellia, cinnamon bark, tea tree, lavender, geranium, or coriander essential oil

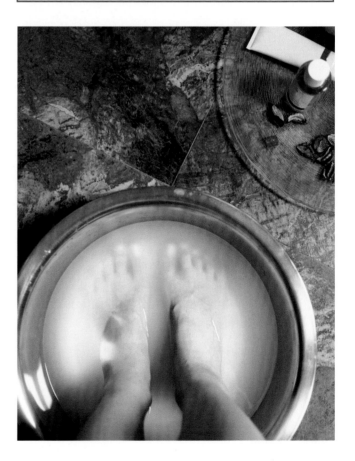

# Cold Sores

## Coconut Oil

The antiviral properties in coconut oil will help fight the herpesvirus that causes cold sores. Apply coconut oil up to three times a day, and take a daily oral dose of coconut oil to prevent or minimize further breakouts.

### Cold Sore Triggers

A cold sore outbreak may be triggered by a number of things, including a high fever, stress, hormonal shifts, lack of sleep, illness, or exposure to extreme weather.

### Simple Ways to Alleviate Cold Sore Symptoms

- Wrap ice in a light cloth and apply to sores.
- Dab aloe vera gel on sores.
- Several essential oils may be helpful in reducing the inflammation and promoting healing. Dilute one drop of food grade essential oil with several drops of an edible carrier oil such as almond, jojoba, or olive oil. Try lavender, lemon balm, peppermint, clove, chamomile, tea tree, or thyme essential oils.
- Apply vitamin E to sores.
- Make a paste of cornstarch and water and apply to sores.

*See Lemon Balm and Calendula sections, pages 143 and 132*

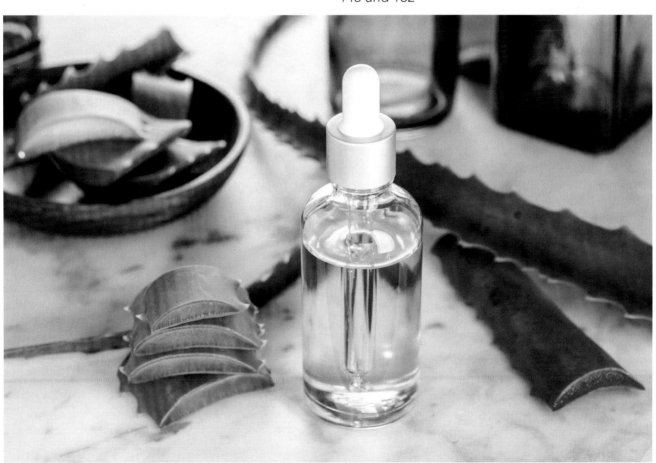

# Corns

## Coconut Oil

Corns are painful cone-shaped lumps of dead skin that accumulate on the feet, usually as a result of pressure from poorly fitting shoes. You can soften the corn with a nightly application of coconut oil.

The best way to remove corns permanently is to start by soaking the feet in a foot bath of warm water with ½ cup sea salt and ½ cup baking soda. After twenty minutes, rub the feet gently with a pumice stone and then apply coconut oil. For best results, cover the foot with a plastic bag and a sock and leave the "coconut sock" on overnight. Repeat nightly until the corn has dissolved.

## Foot Baths for Corns and Calluses

In addition to sea salt and baking soda, here are some other things you can add to your foot bath to soften corns and calluses:

- Epsom salt
- Few drops tea tree oil
- Few drops peppermint oil
- Few drops German chamomile

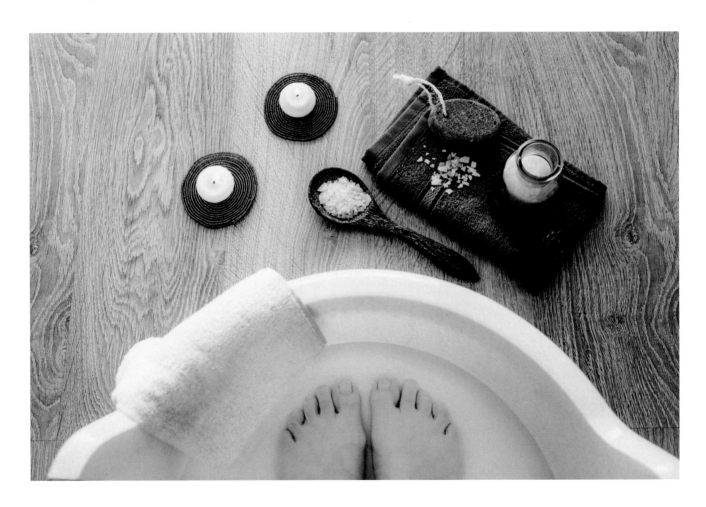

# Cuts and Sores

## Cayenne Pepper

Cayenne pepper is a hemostatic herb! What does it do? It stops bleeding! I keep this powder handy in the first aid cabinet for any open cut or wound. Sprinkle the powder over a bleeding wound and watch the blood clot in front of your eyes.

## Calendula Antiseptic Tincture

### Ingredients:

Calendula flowers, dried
Vodka

### Directions:

1. Pack the calendula flowers well into a glass container (if the flowers are whole, I suggest breaking them apart so there is more surface area to come in contact with the extraction liquid).
2. Follow the tincture-making instructions from the Tinctures section (page 204). Macerate for 3 weeks.
3. Strain and bottle. Use this tincture topically and internally for all antiseptic needs.

## Coconut Oil

Coconut oil is an effective natural antibacterial, so a thin layer of coconut oil applied to a wound will be soothing and will destroy any bacteria.

*See Thyme section, page 158*

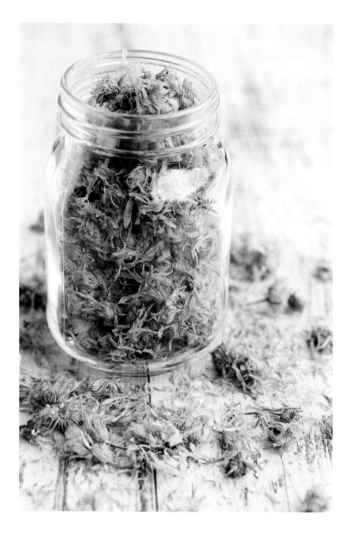

# Dandruff

## Apple Cider Vinegar

For dandruff, recycle an old shampoo bottle and fill it with apple cider vinegar. Apply full-strength apple cider vinegar to your hair and scalp and rub it in. Leave it to soak for half an hour before washing your hair. This will destroy the bacteria or fungus that could be causing your dandruff.

## Coconut Oil

Run a couple tablespoons of coconut oil into your scalp. Leave for about 15 minutes, then shampoo as usual.

## Lemon Juice and Aloe Vera

Rub a couple teaspoons of lemon juice into your scalp and wait about one minute before shampooing. Or combine lemon juice with a teaspoon of aloe vera and use the same way.

## Baking Soda

Sprinkle a tablespoon of baking soda on your scalp and massage in. Leave for one minute before shampooing.

## Green Tea

Soak scalp with green tea, or add green tea to the apple cider vinegar rinse above. Allow to sit about five minutes and then rinse or shampoo.

## Tea Tree Oil

Add a few drops of tea tree oil to any of the above treatments or to your shampoo.

> ### Cradle Cap
>
> Cradle cap is the baby form of dandruff and presents as thick scales or flakes on a baby's scalp. You can use a gentle brush or comb to loosen the flakes and sift them out of the hair. You can also massage some coconut oil into the scalp, leave it for about fifteen minutes, then wash out with baby shampoo. You may also want to try switching baby shampoos, as some brands may irritate your baby's scalp or cause it to become too dry.

*See Rosemary section (page 150) and Hair Treatments (page 274)*

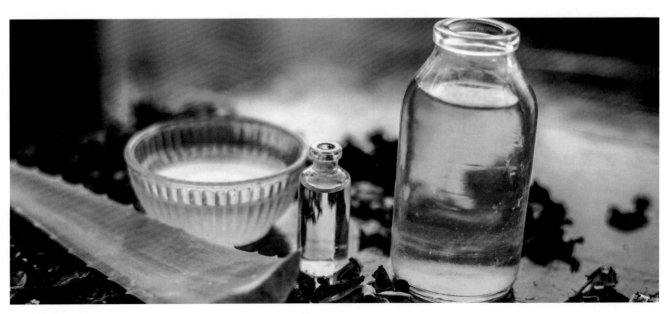

# Eczema

## Eczema Lotion Bar

Eczema is itchy and irritating to children and adults alike. Scratching at it only makes it worse, and it's hard to convince a six-month-old to stop scratching. Luckily, this eczema lotion bar is perfect for everyone over six months of age. So instead of staring at your or your child's dry, flaky, itching skin and trying to will it to stop hurting and itching, grab one of these eczema lotion bars and kiss the itch good-bye.

### Ingredients:

¼ cup beeswax
¼ cup shea butter
¼ cup evening primrose oil
1 tablespoon dried lavender (optional)
20 drops lavender essential oil
10 drops frankincense essential oil
10 drops Roman chamomile essential oil

### Preparation:

1. Create a mock double boiler by placing a heat-safe glass bowl in a pan of simmering water.
2. Melt ¼ cup beeswax in the bowl.
3. Add ¼ cup shea butter to the melted beeswax and allow it to melt as well.
4. Swirl to mix together beeswax and shea butter.
5. Remove from heat.
6. Add ¼ cup evening primrose oil and stir.
7. Allow to cool, but not so much that it hardens.
8. Add 1 tablespoon dried lavender (optional).
9. Add 20 drops lavender, 10 drops frankincense, and 10 drops Roman chamomile essential oils.
10. Stir together all ingredients.
11. Pour into silicone molds and allow to dry until hardened (about 1–2 hours).
12. Once hardened, remove from molds and store in an airtight glass container.

### Administration:

1. Remove lotion bar from airtight container.
2. Rub bar directly onto affected area.
3. Gently rub lotion into skin.
4. Return bar to airtight container.

### Benefits:

- Evening primrose oil, when used topically, has been found to reduce the severity of atopic eczema in children and adults.
- Shea butter is a traditional African moisturizer with anti-inflammatory and analgesic properties. The inflammation of the skin affected by eczema is subdued by the shea butter, as is the itching eczema causes.
- Lavender relieves the pain and itching caused by eczema.
- Lavender, frankincense, and Roman chamomile are all anti-inflammatory and antioxidant essential oils, which help to soothe, calm, and heal eczema.

## Coconut Oil

Eczema is characterized by dry, itchy, and inflamed skin. The antibacterial, antifungal, and antimicrobial properties of coconut oil can heal the skin and prevent secondary infection, while the texture of the coconut oil is soothing to the skin. Apply a thin layer to the affected skin daily until the eczema has cleared. A daily dose of coconut oil every day will boost the immune system, helping to heal and prevent further outbreaks of eczema.

*See Chickweed, Daisy, and Watercress sections, pages 136, 138, and 160*

# Hemorrhoids

## Coconut Oil

Coconut oil is soothing and clears infection. Dry the afflicted area carefully with a cotton ball and then gently apply a layer of coconut oil. Repeat after each bowel movement.

## Apple Cider Vinegar

Apple cider vinegar can be applied in its full-strength form to hemorrhoids to reduce stinging and promote shrinking. The daily use of apple cider vinegar tonic (See High Blood Pressure) can help to soften stools and reduce the strain during bowel movements. This will eliminate the main cause of hemorrhoids occurring.

## Simple Ways to Alleviate Hemorrhoid Discomfort

- Take a hot bath with Epsom salt.
- Apply witch hazel to the affected area.
- Apply aloe vera directly to the area.
- Apply a cold compress to the area.
- Wear loose clothing.

*See Watercress section, page 160*

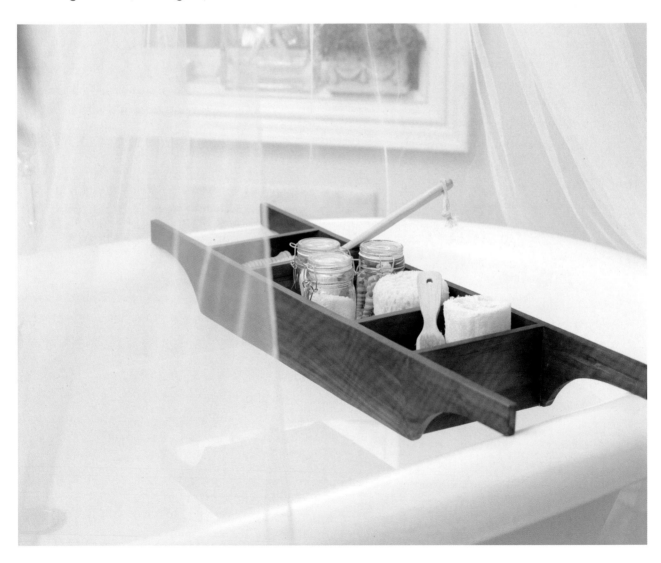

# Insect Bites

## Pineapple Weed Insect Repellent

### Ingredients:

25 grams dried pineapple weed
10 grams dried daisy flowers
200 ml grape-seed oil
4 drops citronella essential oil
4 drops lavender essential oil
4 drops cedar wood essential oil
10 drops of vitamin E oil

### Directions:

1. Prepare an infused oil using pineapple weed and daisy flowers.
2. Strain and add in essential oils and vitamin E. Bottle.
3. Rub into skin as needed, prior to needing insect-repellant properties.

## Bites Be Gone Anti-Itch Paste

Make up a new batch every time you need this so it doesn't lose its strength. But it's so simple to throw together you won't be itching for much longer than it would take you to find the tube of medicated commercial cream. The tea tree oil may sting at first (be warned if you plan to use this on children), but its antibacterial properties are important.

### Ingredients:

1 tablespoon baking soda
1 tablespoon bentonite clay
1–2 teaspoons shea butter, enough to make a paste
2 drops tea tree oil

Mix the ingredients well in a small bowl.

**To Use:** Smooth on itchy bug bites or rashes from being outdoors.

## Apple Cider Vinegar

Be sure to get appropriate treatment for spider bites and other bites and stings if you are allergic. Full-strength apple cider vinegar can be used to lessen the pain and swelling of bee stings, fire ant bites, mosquito bites, wasp stings, and spider bites. You can also use it on jellyfish stings if hot water is not available or the sting is not too severe. Apple cider vinegar would definitely be a prudent addition to your luggage when visiting the beach or nature parks.

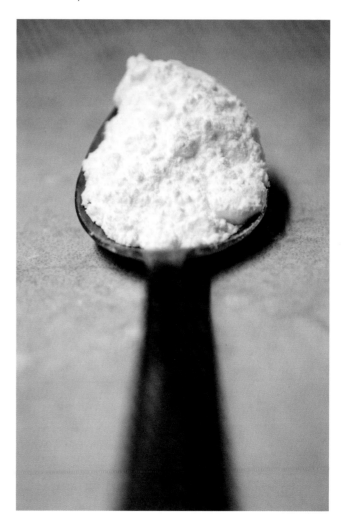

# Poison Ivy

## Poison Ivy Relief

### Ingredients:

2 cups Epsom salt
1 cup baking soda
Cool water in a bath
5 drops lavender essential oil
3 drops peppermint essential oil
Cotton washcloth

### Directions:

1. Add all ingredients to the tub. Dissolve the crystals in the bath, then ease your way in.
2. Add ice cubes to cool down the water. Soak the cotton washcloth and apply to the affected area as needed.

This application can also be prepared in a basin for more localized areas. Add in ice cubes for cooling relief. Apply a paste of baking soda powder (moistened with a little water to form a paste) to the rash after the bath. The baking soda and peppermint essential oil will be a welcome relief from the itchiness.

## Anti-Itch Oatmeal Paste

Just like preparing breakfast, cook a small amount of oatmeal on the stove. Cool slightly prior to applying to the skin, to ensure you do not burn (test by putting a small amount on your wrist), and apply it directly to the skin as a paste. Add just enough water so the oatmeal is thick and will cling or hold to the skin. Apply and wait until the oatmeal is completely cool. Rinse the skin. Baking soda and 1–2 drops of peppermint essential oil can be added for an extra itch-relieving effect. Soothing relief from poison ivy, itchy skin rashes, and dermatitis.

## Coconut Oil

Poison ivy contains a toxic resin called urushiol that causes an extremely irritating skin inflammation. Massage warm coconut oil into the area to soothe the itchiness and eradicate the toxins.

### Essential Oils for Poison Ivy

Dilute a few drops of any of these essential oils in a carrier oil (melted coconut, jojoba, olive, almond) and rub gently into affected area of skin. You can also add a few drops of essential oil to the Anti-Itch Oatmeal Paste.

- Cypress
- Eucalyptus
- Geranium
- Lavender
- Myrrh
- Peppermint
- Roman chamomile
- Rose
- Tea Tree

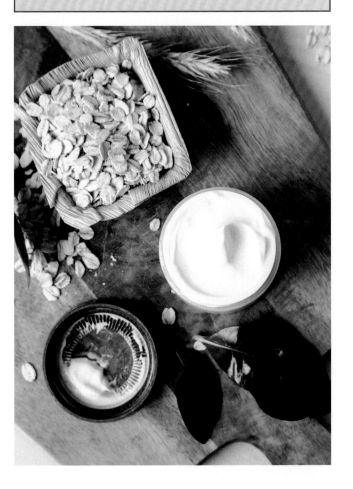

# Psoriasis

## Dandelion Abscess Poultice

Dandelions have been used for thousands of years to help treat abscesses, sores, eczema, psoriasis, rashes, and other joyless bodily manifestations we'd rather not talk about. Creating a dandelion-based poultice is a great way to heal and resolve these nasty issues. Poultices are topical applications typically made from herbs. Making poultices is simple, cost-effective, and fun, utilizing the amazing herbal remedies you have growing at your home.

This dandelion poultice is great to use on the skin for a variety of skin issues, such as itchy and dry skin, acne, eczema, rashes, and even bruises. Similar to making a mojito, you'll want to take out your mortar and pestle and get your muscles working, as you'll need to crush the herbs into a paste. Making a poultice doesn't have to be a chore; it's as simple as gathering your fresh leaves and chopping. The amount of herbs you use is up to you; it depends on how much of the skin needs to be covered.

### Ingredients:
Fresh dandelion leaves
Mortar and pestle or blender

### Directions:
1. Take the dandelion leaves and chop them into small pieces, then transfer to a mortar and pestle to further crush the herbs until they become a pulp. The end result doesn't have to be perfectly smooth and silky, just crushed with the juices flowing.
2. If you like, place the herbs in a blender or food processor to get the same results.
3. Spread the crushed herbs on the area of skin that needs treatment. Cover with gauze or muslin to hold the poultice in place. To relieve symptoms, you can leave the poultice on overnight or throughout the day.

## Coconut Oil

Psoriasis is a chronic skin condition, causing itchy, scaling skin. Consume two tablespoons of coconut oil a day to improve the condition of the skin and strengthen the immune system. You can also soothe the afflicted area by applying a thin layer of warm coconut oil.

*See Aloe Vera section, page 130*

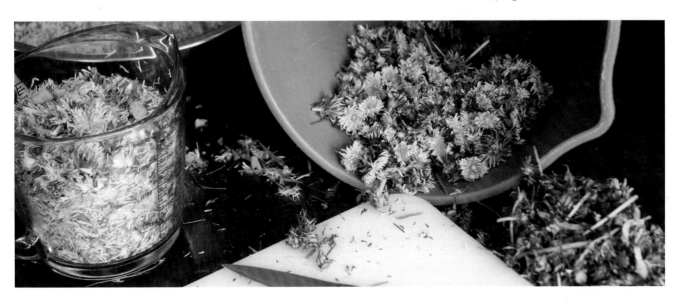

# Rashes

## Coconut Oil

Apply a thin layer of coconut oil to the affected area daily until symptoms subside. Additionally, take a daily dose of coconut oil to improve your immune system.

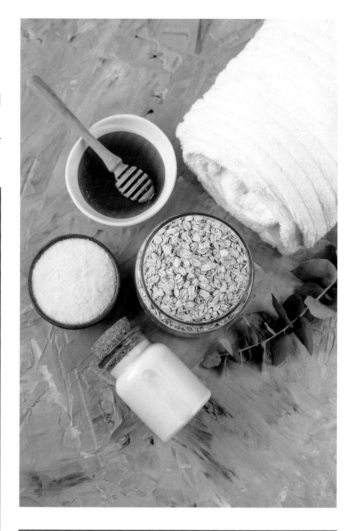

---

### Simple Ways to Soothe a Rash

Rashes can be caused by all manner of things, so it's a good idea to get them checked out by a doctor to try to determine what the root cause is. But here are several ways to soothe the inflammation and discomfort of most rashes.

- Add 1–2 cups finely ground oatmeal, Epsom salt, or baking soda (or any combination of the three) to a warm bath and soak for 20 minutes.
- Rub olive oil gently into the rash. You can also add a bit of honey if you don't mind being a little sticky.
- Make a paste of baking soda and water or baking soda and coconut oil. Apply to rash. Allow to sit for several minutes and then rinse off and pat dry.
- Apply alove vera to the affected area.
- Brew chamomile tea, allow to cool, and use a clean cloth to dab the tea onto the skin.
- Apply calendula oil to the rash.

---

*See Aloe Vera, Daisy, and Calendula sections, pages 130, 138, and 132*

### Hives from Stress

If you've ruled out illness or an allergic reaction as causes of your rash, stress might be the culprit, particularly if you're experiencing the red welts or patches that we call "hives." Hives may be your body's way of telling you that you need more rest or exercise or to find another way to cope with life's stresses.

# Sunburn

## Soothe Away the Ouch Sunburn Blend

### Ingredients:

50 ml aloe vera juice or gel
20 ml witch hazel, distilled
10 drops of lavender essential oil
3 drops peppermint essential oil
20 ml spearmint herb infusion
10 ml distilled water

### Directions:

1. Mix together all ingredients in a spray bottle. Shake well.
2. Apply liberally and frequently to cool a burn.

## Coconut Oil

Coconut oil can stimulate the renewal of cell growth, and this is particularly necessary when the skin cells have been damaged by the elements. Apply a thin layer of coconut oil to the areas on the body that are affected by sunburn or windburn. Reapply when needed until symptoms disappear.

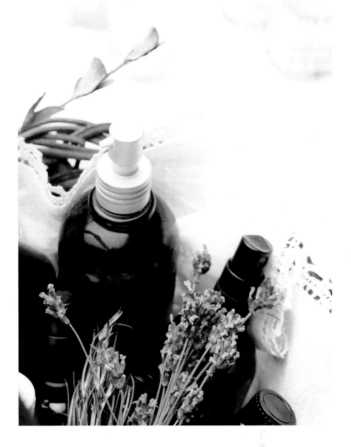

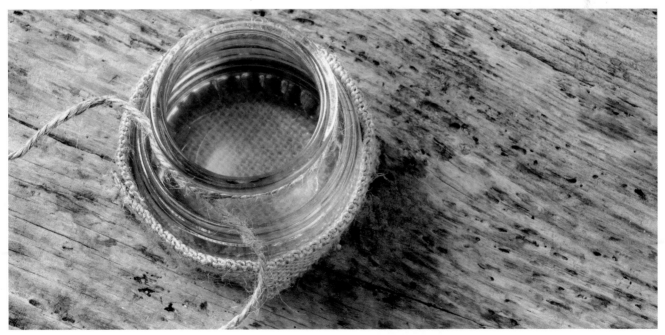

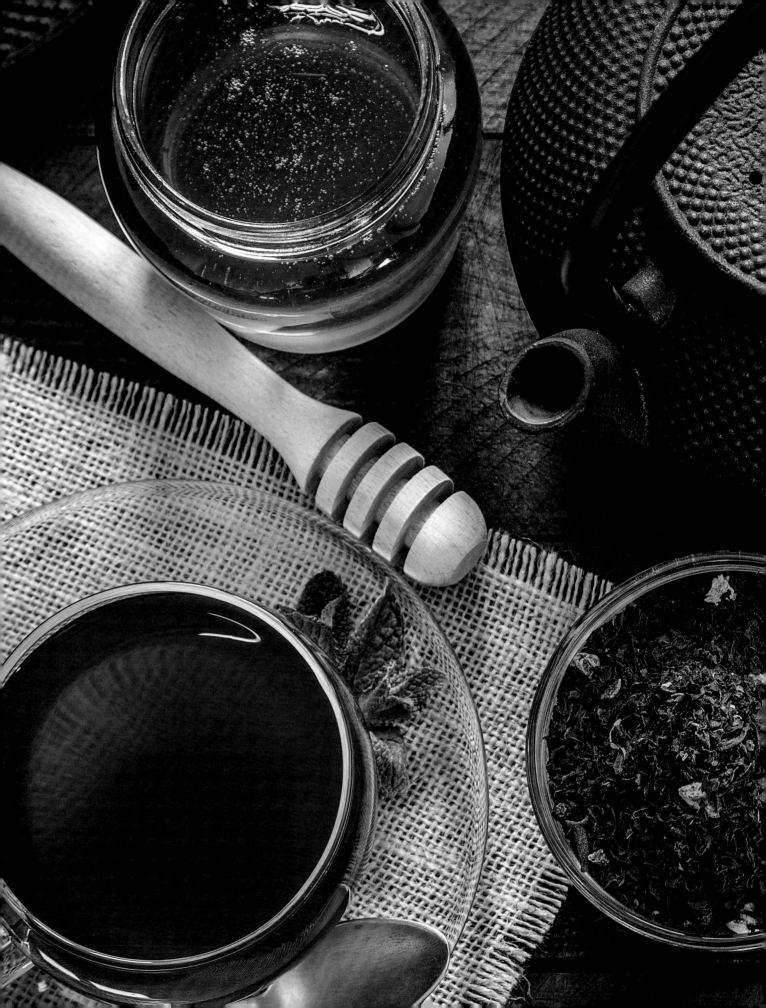

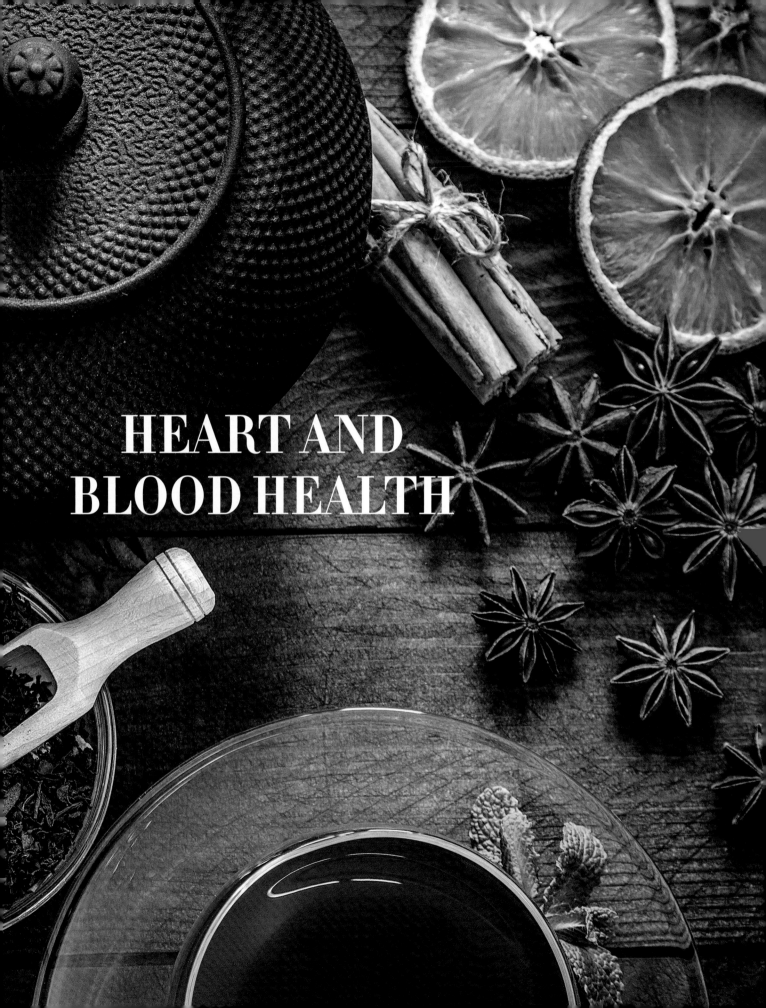

# HEART AND
# BLOOD HEALTH

# Anemia

## Iron and Energy Syrup

### Ingredients:

2 parts yellow dock
1 part nettle
1 part dandelion root
¼ part kelp
¼ part blackstrap molasses

This is a great syrup to take daily, especially when experiencing low iron levels that lead to fatigue. It's great during pregnancy, when levels are likely to dip down.

## Anti-Anemia Cocktail

### Ingredients:

2 cups water
1 tablespoon blackstrap molasses
½ lime

### Directions:

1. In a tall glass or jar, mix the water and molasses.
2. Squeeze the ½ lime into the beverage and stir.

Blackstrap molasses is high in iron and the lime juice is high in vitamin C, which will help you absorb the iron.

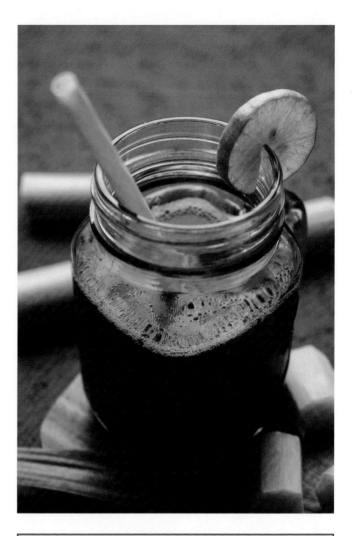

### Symptoms of Anemia

Below are some of the common symptoms of anemia.

- Cold hands or feet
- Difficulty concentrating
- Difficulty sleeping
- Dizziness
- Fatigue or weakness
- Headache
- Irritability
- Leg cramps
- Pain in your bones, joints, or belly
- Pale skin
- Shortness of breath

### Foods that Help the Body Absorb Iron

Eating more iron-rich foods won't help if your body isn't absorbing the iron properly. Try consuming foods full of vitamin C and A in addition to eating iron-rich meats, beans, and vegetables.

- Apricots
- Bell peppers
- Broccoli
- Carrots
- Citrus fruits and juices
- Dark leafy vegetables
- Melons
- Peaches
- Strawberries
- Sweet Potatoes

# Cholesterol

## Cholesterol-Lowering Tea

### Ingredients:

1 part ginger root
2 parts green tea leaf
8 oz. hot water

### Directions:

1. Combine dried herbs and steep in water, covered, for 10–15 minutes.
2. Remove herbs from water, and sip tea slowly.

Many of the cholesterol-lowering commercial drugs on the market today (statins) come with considerable side effects. The herbs listed below can help lower cholesterol naturally and are generally deemed a safer alternative in the world of holistic medicine. As with blood pressure, ginger, ginseng, and green tea are go-to herbs for this job. Population-based clinical studies have found that when comparing men who drink green tea on a regular basis to those who don't, the green tea drinkers had significantly lower cholesterol levels. Ginger has also been deemed helpful, as has ginseng.

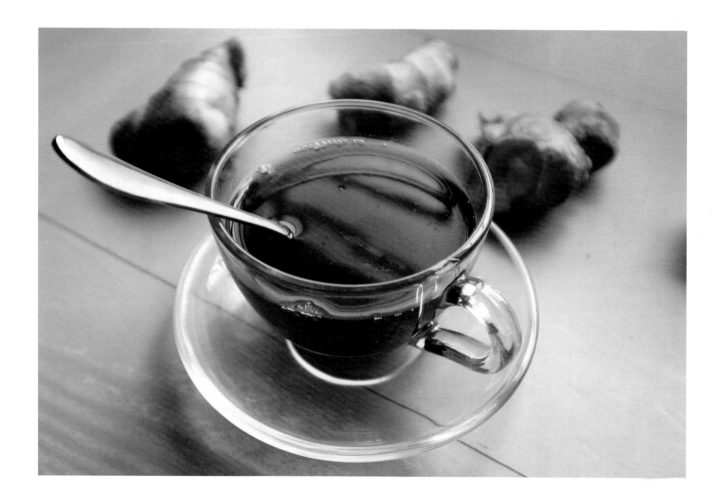

# High Blood Pressure

## Apple Cider Vinegar Tonic

Apple cider vinegar contains potassium. Potassium helps to balance out the body's sodium levels and thus helps to lower blood pressure. Take the general tonic on a regular basis for long-term effective relief from the unpleasantness of high blood pressure. Apple cider vinegar also contains magnesium which helps to relax the walls of the blood vessels, effectively lowering blood pressure.

*Yields: 1 Serving*

### Ingredients:
250 ml water
1–2 tablespoons apple cider vinegar
Raw organic honey to taste (optional)

### Directions:
1. Mix the ingredients together in a large glass.
2. Sip it at your leisure.
3. Feel the difference!

- Eat foods rich in magnesium such as whole grains, legumes, and organic meats
- Eat moderate amounts of dark chocolate or cocoa
- Reduce intake of refined sugar and carbs
- Exercise regularly
- Sleep eight or more hours a night
- Find ways to reduce stress
- Don't smoke

### Simple Ways to Lower Blood Pressure

- Reduce alcohol intake
- Instead of coffee, drink a cup or two of green tea each day. In general, caffeine can raise blood pressure, but green tea has been shown to be effective in lowering blood pressure.
- Eat foods rich in potassium such as avocadoes, bananas, leafy greens, sweet potatoes, nuts, seeds, and beans
- Eat foods rich in calcium such as organic dairy products, leafy greens, beans, and tofu

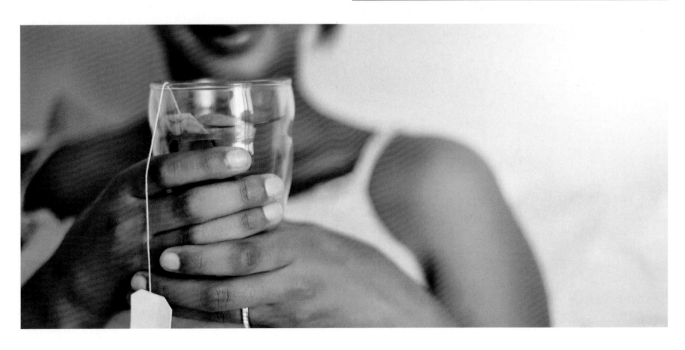

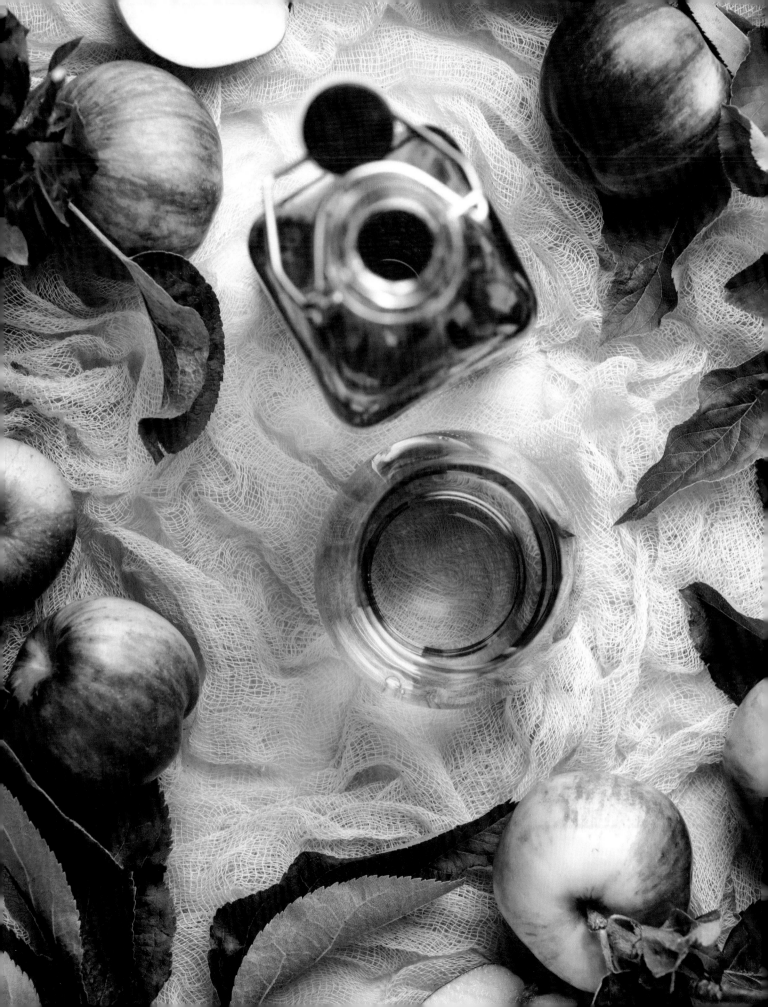

# Varicose Veins

## Calendula Vein Liniment

### Ingredients:
2 tablespoons dried calendula flowers
2 tablespoons yarrow flowers
1 tablespoon self-heal herb
Approx. 100 ml distilled witch hazel water
(available from a health food store or
drugstore)

### Directions:
1. This liniment is prepared exactly like a tincture, except it is intended for external use only. Mention this on the label. Pour enough witch hazel over to cover the dried herbs and macerate for 2 weeks.
2. Strain and bottle. Keep in the fridge.
3. Apply topically to areas of inflammation and varicose veins. The easiest application is to moisten muslin with water, cutting large enough to cover the inflamed area. Pour on the liniment and wrap the area. Provides immediate cooling relief and anti-inflammatory support to the inflamed tissues.

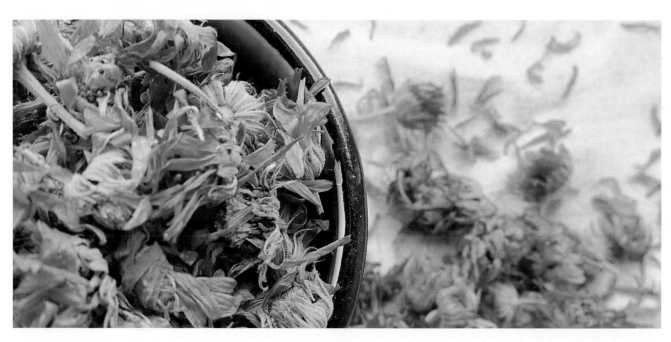

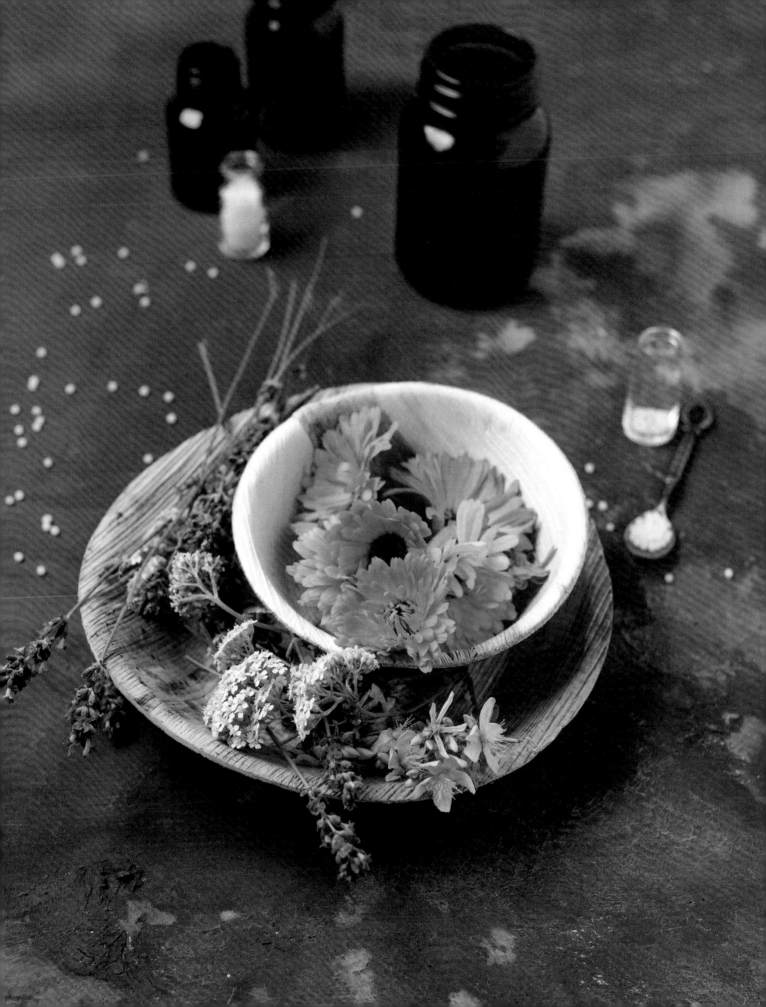

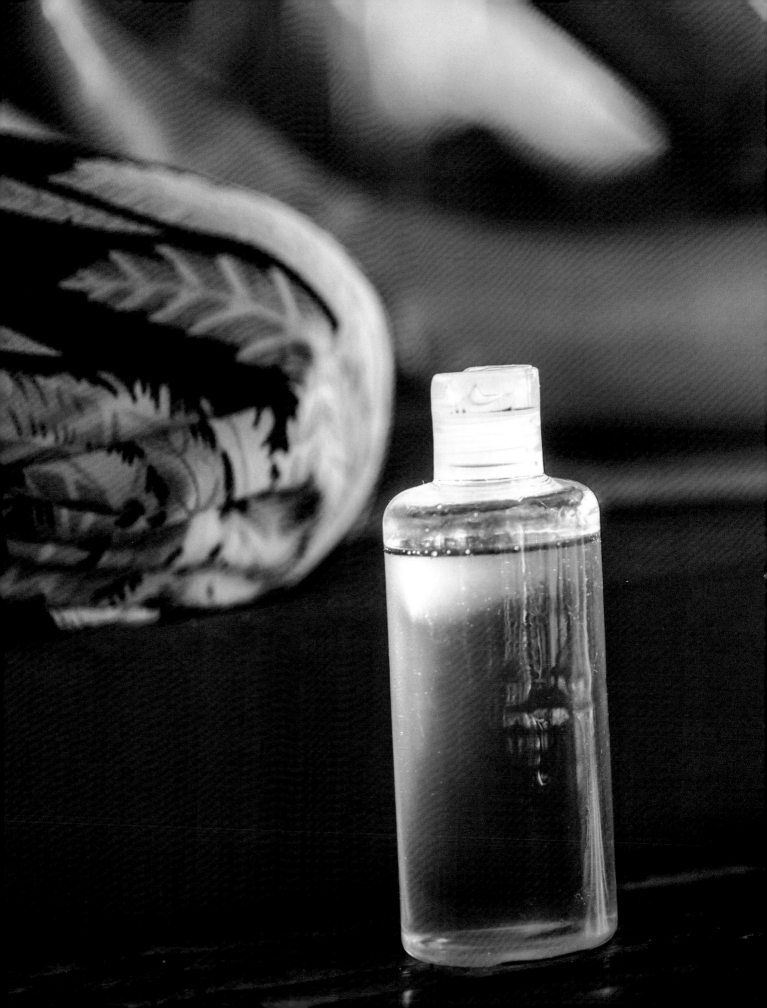

# BONES, MUSCLES, AND JOINTS

# Arthritis

## Arthritis Joint Rub

Arthritis is a painful condition that comes in multiple forms, most prevalently osteoarthritis and rheumatoid arthritis. These two forms of arthritis have different causes: wear and tear causes osteoarthritis, while rheumatoid arthritis is an autoimmune disease. However, both forms of arthritis cause joint pain and inflammation. Massage can reduce the severity of both types of arthritis. Adding essential oils to massage improves the anti-inflammatory and pain-management aspects of massage.

### Ingredients:
1 teaspoon sesame oil
1 drop frankincense essential oil
1 drop ginger essential oil
1 drop juniper berry essential oil
1 drop myrrh essential oil
1 drop Roman chamomile essential oil

### Preparation and Administration:
1. Remove the caps from the oil bottles.
2. In the palm of your hand, pour 1 teaspoon sesame oil.
3. Add one drop each of frankincense, ginger, juniper berry, myrrh, and Roman chamomile essential oils.
4. Massage the Arthritis Joint Rub into any joints affected by arthritis.
5. Recap the oil bottles.

### Benefits:
- Sesame oil works as an analgesic and has been found to relieve the inflammation associated with arthritis.
- Roman chamomile is anti-inflammatory and relieves rheumatic pain.
- Frankincense supports the maintenance of cartilage, therefore slowing down the progression of osteoarthritis.
- Myrrh is traditionally used in India, East Africa, and Saudi Arabia to treat rheumatoid arthritis due to its anti-inflammatory properties.
- Juniper and ginger essential oils are antinociceptive, inhibiting the sensation of pain. Like the other essential oils in this recipe, they also have anti-inflammatory properties.

## Coconut Oil

Coconut oil is a powerful anti-inflammatory and it helps increase the absorption of magnesium, an excellent mineral for muscles, joints, and the neurological system. Take a daily oral dose of coconut oil to relieve symptoms both in the short term and the long term.

## Apple Cider Vinegar

While apple cider vinegar cannot cure arthritis, it can certainly help to relieve the pain and many people have attested to its effectiveness. The potassium in apple cider vinegar is thought to help prevent the buildup of calcium in the joints, which causes the stiffness and pain. Furthermore, it has been suggested that the painful joints characteristic of arthritis may actually be caused by an accumulation of toxins in the joints. Specifically the pectin in apple cider vinegar helps to absorb the toxins and remove them from the body. Apple cider vinegar is a natural detoxifier and will help to purify your whole body. It is recommended to take a dessert spoonful of apple cider mixed in water at mealtimes for relief from pain.

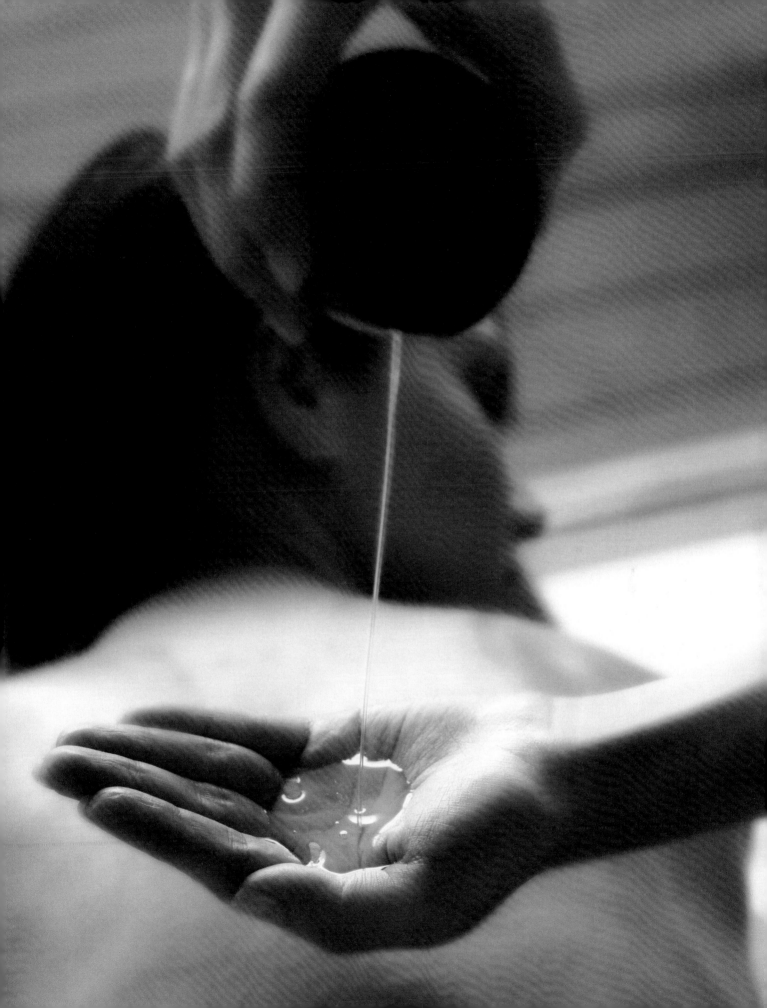

# General Pain

## Lavender Bath Salt

Bath salts are a wonderful way to relax and unwind after a long day, not to mention they're incredible for your muscles. In fact, Epsom salt is known to be high in magnesium and to be a natural anti-inflammatory. Many athletes soak in Epsom salt after a hard workout, and the benefits don't stop there. By some estimates, up to 80 percent of people are deficient in magnesium, a mineral necessary for regulating over three hundred enzymes in the body, aiding in the detoxification process, and repairing your DNA! This is no small task.

The mix of Epsom salt and lavender will give you a relaxing combo, allowing your mind to rest, your muscles to relax, and your body to detox.

### Ingredients:
¾ cup Epsom salt
½ cup Dead Sea salt
2 tablespoons dried lavender buds
1 tablespoon safflower oil
⅛ teaspoon vitamin E oil
8 to 10 drops lavender essential oil

### Directions:
1. Combine all your ingredients in a bowl and mix well.
2. Place your mixture in an airtight container, preferably glass.
3. Let the mixture sit for several days so the essential oils and fresh herbs can infuse into the salts. That's it! Pour the salts into a hot tub for a restorative soak.

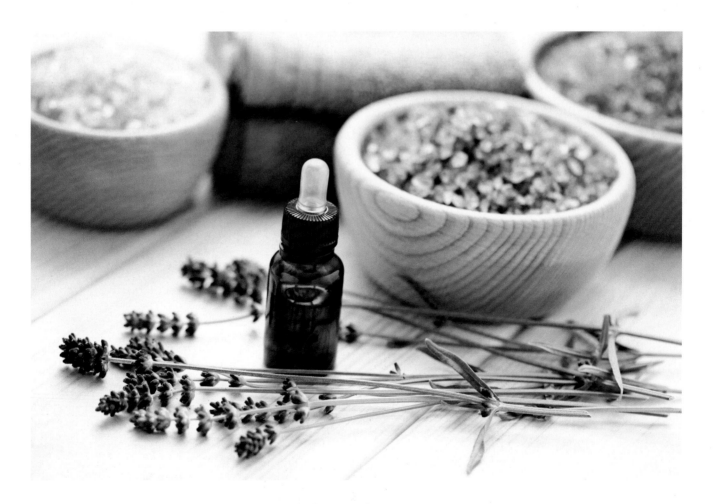

# Osteoporosis

## Apple Cider Vinegar

Apple cider vinegar contains such minerals as magnesium, manganese, phosphorus, calcium, and silicon, which are important for strong and healthy bones. It also contains the trace mineral boron. Boron works to support the metabolism of calcium and magnesium and elevates the levels of estrogen and testosterone in the body, both of which lead to strong bones. Taking the apple cider tonic (see High Blood Pressure) regularly will be a good dietary source of these minerals, which will sustain bone mass density and will help ward off degenerative bone diseases like osteoporosis.

## Bone Up Tea

### Ingredients:
1 part horsetail leaf
1 part red clover
8 oz. hot water

### Directions:
1. Combine dried herbs and steep in water, covered, for 10–15 minutes.
2. Remove herbs from water, and sip tea slowly.

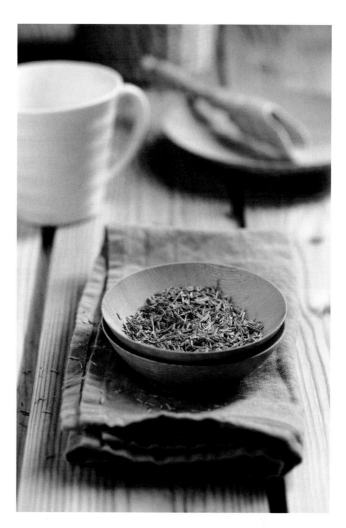

### Horsetail

Horsetail is an amazing herb for bone building and repair as it directly stimulates the production of bone cells, which helps increase formation of bone tissue. Horsetail also supplies large amounts of readily absorbable calcium to the body and is rich in other minerals that the body uses to repair and rebuild injured tissue. Red clover is also hypothesized to support good bone health. Milk may not do a body good, but these herbs most definitely do.

# Sprains and Pulled Muscles

## Super Pain Balm

This solid balm is portable and great to have for aches and pains from physical activity such as sports, hikes, or farming. It provides fast relief for joint and muscle pain of any kind.

*Makes: 8oz (240ml) solid balm*

### Ingredients:

1 handful (about 50g) of whole dried spice blends: cloves, black peppercorn, ginger OR turmeric, *Boswellia serrata*, black peppercorn (This will lend a slight golden color to the skin when applied.) Blend the spices as you desire with the fragrance profile that you prefer.

⅓ cup (80ml) coconut oil

3 tbsp (45ml) beeswax

½ cup (120ml) CBD-infused murumuru butter

2g or 2ml liquid sunflower lecithin

### For the spiced aromatic coconut oil:

1. Fill a canning bath or stockpot with water. Prepare a clean glass canning jar and new lid. Add the whole dried spices of your choice to the canning jar along with the coconut oil. Affix the lid tightly and place in the canning bath or stockpot.

2. Bring the canning bath or stockpot to a simmer and process the jar for 45 minutes.

3. Turn off the heat and carefully remove the jar from the water. Allow it to cool until warm to the touch on a towel on the counter, but do not allow the oil to harden. Once the jar has cooled sufficiently, carefully open it; it may have sealed during the processing of the oil.

4. Strain the oil from the herbs through cheesecloth and gently squeeze to release as much of the oil from the spices as possible into the small pan that you will use to make the balm.

### Make the balm:

1. In the pan with the spiced coconut oil, apply low heat and melt the beeswax, CBD-infused murumuru butter, and the sunflower lecithin together with the spiced coconut oil, combining thoroughly.

2. Pour the mixture immediately into balm containers. Rest on the counter for 5 minutes, affix the lid, and then place in the freezer for 20 minutes to fully harden. The freezer step is necessary to prevent the balm from having a grainy texture.

3. Remove from the freezer and the balm is ready to use and is shelf-stable. Use within 6 months for best results.

## Coconut Oil

Coconut oil lubricates muscles and joints by increasing blood circulation. You can take a daily dose of coconut oil to improve your muscle strength and tone, and you can treat painful areas by using warm coconut oil as a massage lotion, to soothe and heal the afflicted area.

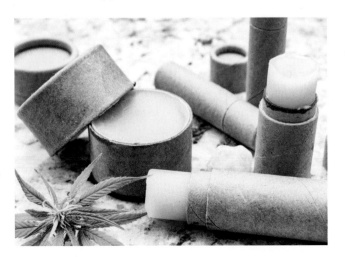

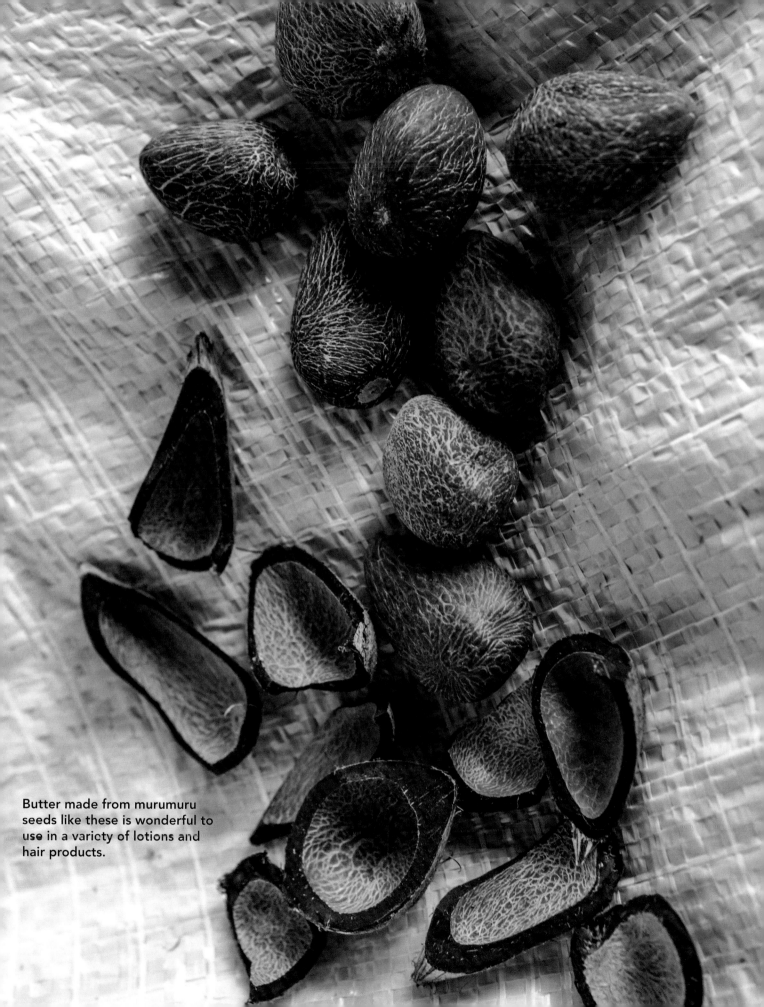

Butter made from murumuru
seeds like these is wonderful to
use in a variety of lotions and
hair products.

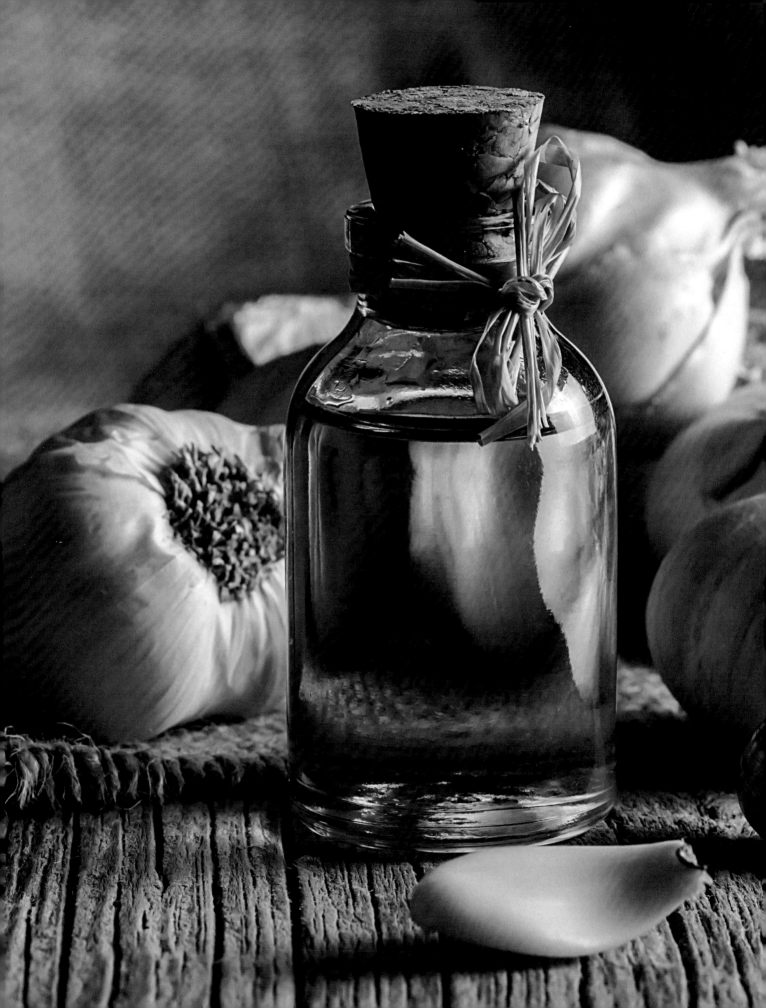

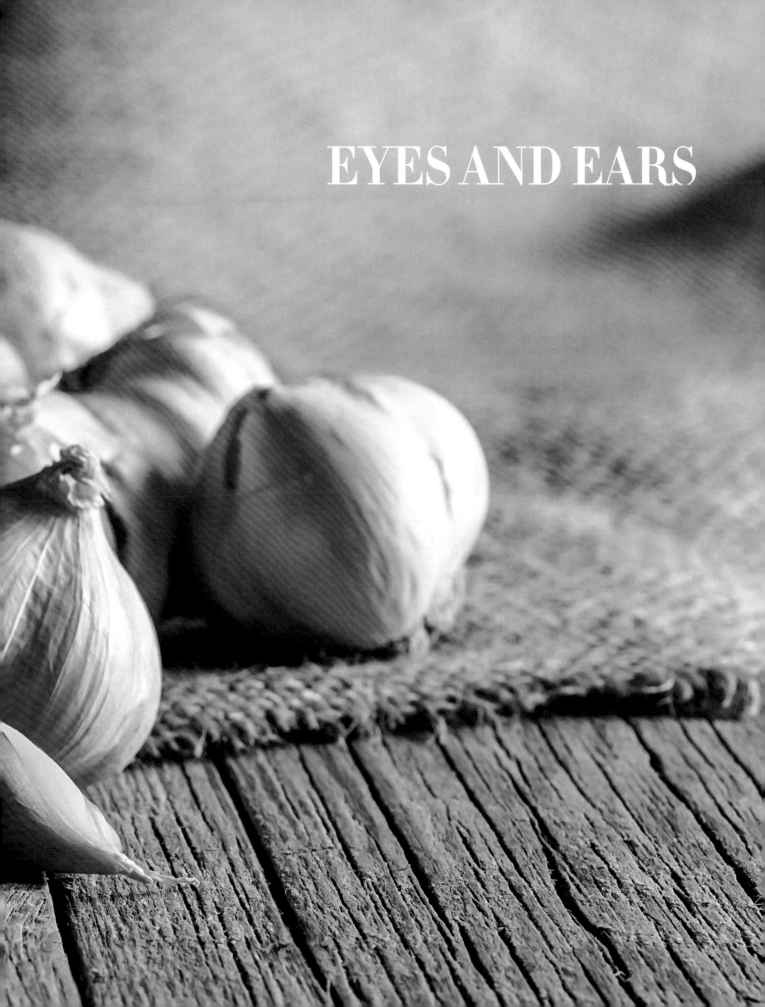

EYES AND EARS

# Earwax Buildup

## Mullein and Garlic Ear Oil

### Ingredients:

5 grams dried mullein flowers
5 grams dried self-heal flowers or herb
2 cloves of garlic, peeled and finely minced
50 ml olive oil
4 drops tea tree essential oil

### Directions:

1. Cover mullein, self-heal, and garlic with olive oil and let sit for 3 days.
2. Strain and add in tea tree essential oil.

## Administration:

Use drop dosages into the ear for middle-ear infections, glue ear, or cold and flu symptoms.

## Ear Oil

Ear oils are applied by drop dosages to the ear canal and are effective for middle ear afflictions, symptoms related to a cold or flu, respiratory infections, mumps, glue ear, or infections. The blend offers antimicrobial and anti-inflammatory herbs to reduce swelling and pain, clear up infections, and moisten impacted earwax in the ear canal.

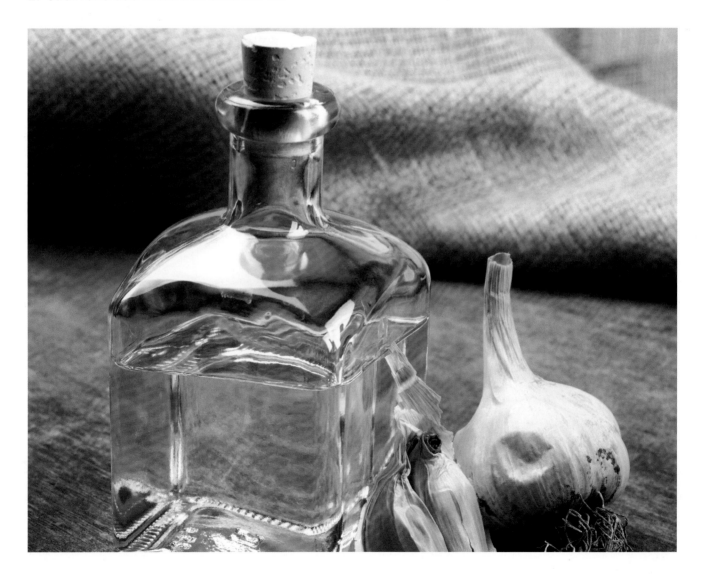

# Eyestrain

## Soothing Chamomile Astringent Eyewash

**Ingredients:**

1 teaspoon chamomile dried flowers

1 teaspoon calendula dried flowers

1 teaspoon red raspberry dried leaf

**Directions:**

1. Prepare as an infusion (see page 194) using distilled water.
2. Strain very well before pouring, lukewarm, into an eyecup and bathing the eyes.

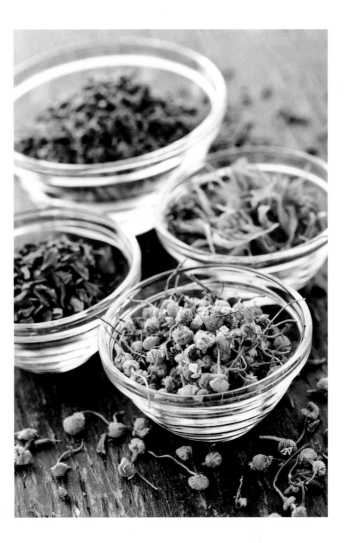

### Carrots for Eyesight

Can carrots really help you see better in the dark? Yes, to some degree. The beta-carotene found in carrots is necessary for your body to make vitamin A, and vitamin A helps the brain process light through the eyes. Vitamin A is also essential for the health of the cornea, the protective outer layer of your eye.

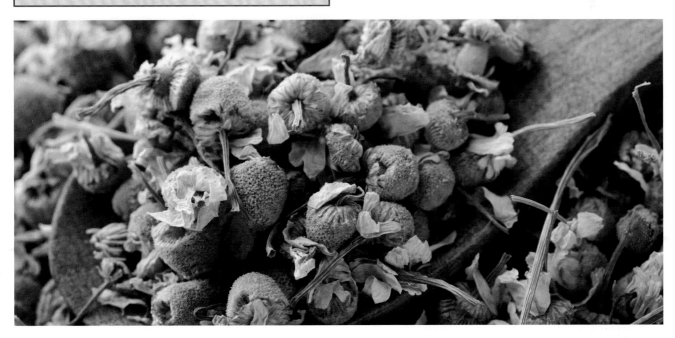

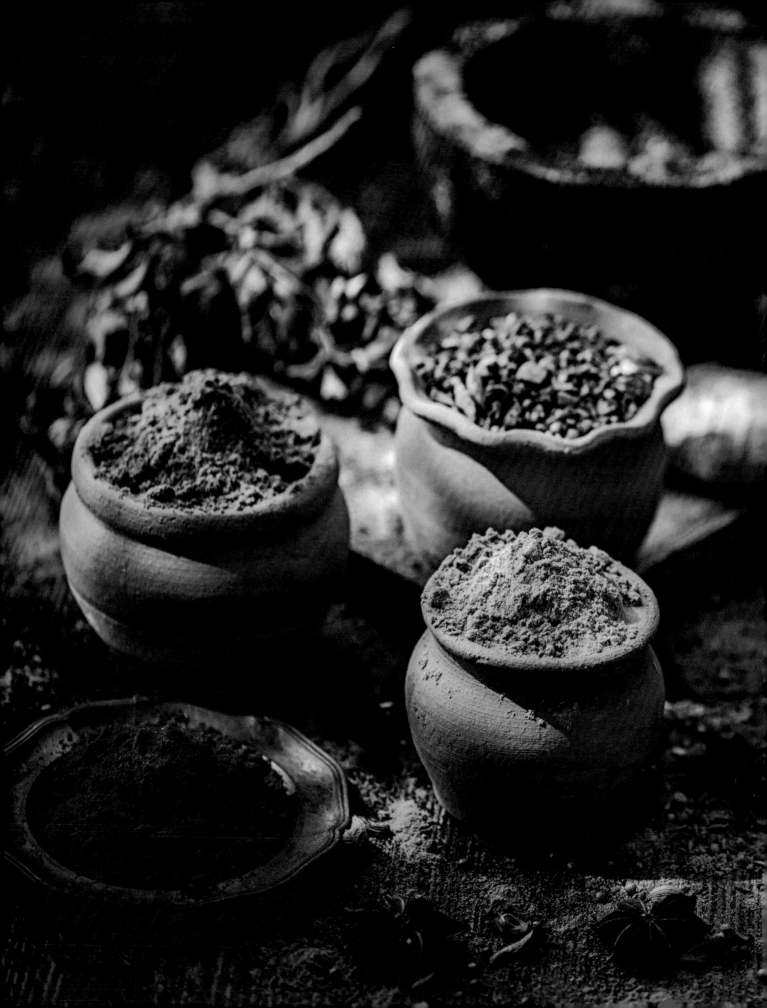

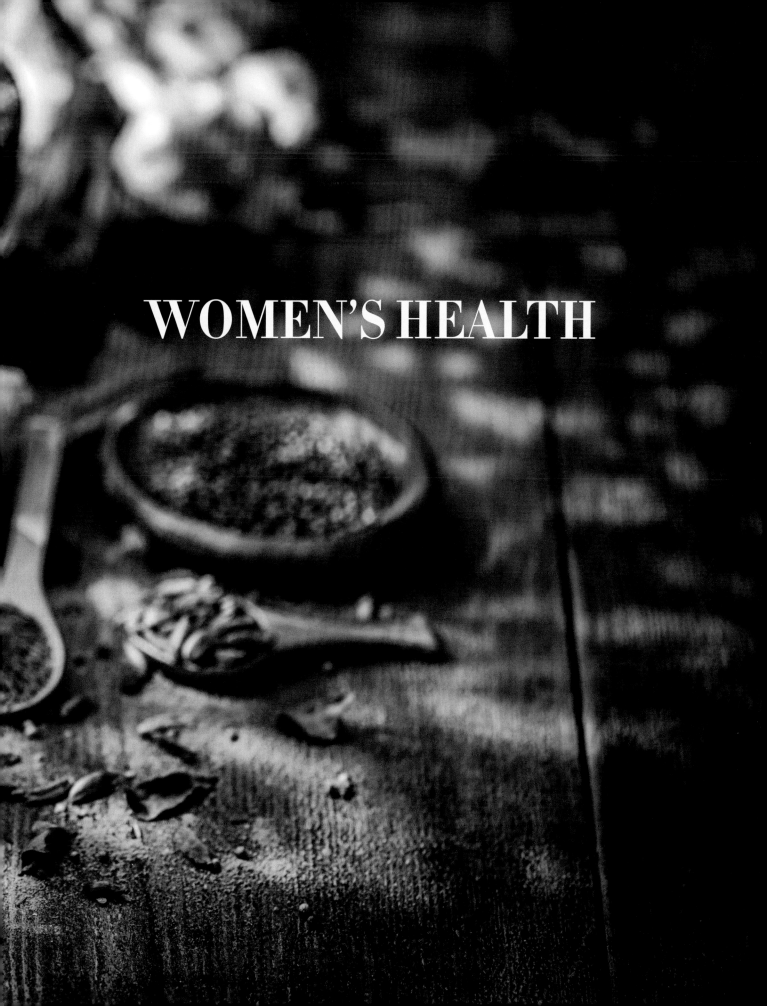

# WOMEN'S HEALTH

# Breastfeeding

## Sore, Cracked Nipples

### Peppermint

For women trying to breastfeed, peppermint water may be effective in preventing nipple cracks and nipple pain for first-time mothers. While breastfeeding is an optimal method to feed your child, it's not necessarily kind to a new mother's breasts. Soaking nipples in mint-infused water can be the difference between painful and sore nipples and smooth sailing.

### Calendula

As a cream, poultice, herbal wash, or infused oil, calendula reduces inflammation and ensures immediate healing for nipples that are raw from breastfeeding. For the inflammation of mastitis or for mumps or gland inflammation, prepare a poultice.

## Lactation Stimulation

There are many herbs that have been proven safe and effective when used to stimulate and increase milk production by new mothers. These are called galactogogues.

As with all herbal use while pregnant and/or breastfeeding, one should consult with an herbalist prior to self-administering.

### Helpful Herbs

- Anise
- Fennel
- Fenugreek
- Nettle

## Lactation Tea

### Ingredients:

1 part anise seed
1 part nettle leaf
2 parts fenugreek seed
8 oz. hot water

### Directions:

1. Combine dried herbs and steep in water, covered, for 10–15 minutes.
2. Remove herbs from water, and sip tea slowly.

---

### Breastfeeding and Calories

Breastfeeding burns around 200 to 500 calories a day. If you find that your milk supply is dropping, you're frequently very hungry, or you're losing too much weight, you may need to increase your caloric intake. Focus on healthy fats and grains, and include a range of fruits and vegetables in your diet. Avocados, nuts, and seeds are easy to eat without a lot of preparation and are full of good nutrients to support your breastfeeding journey.

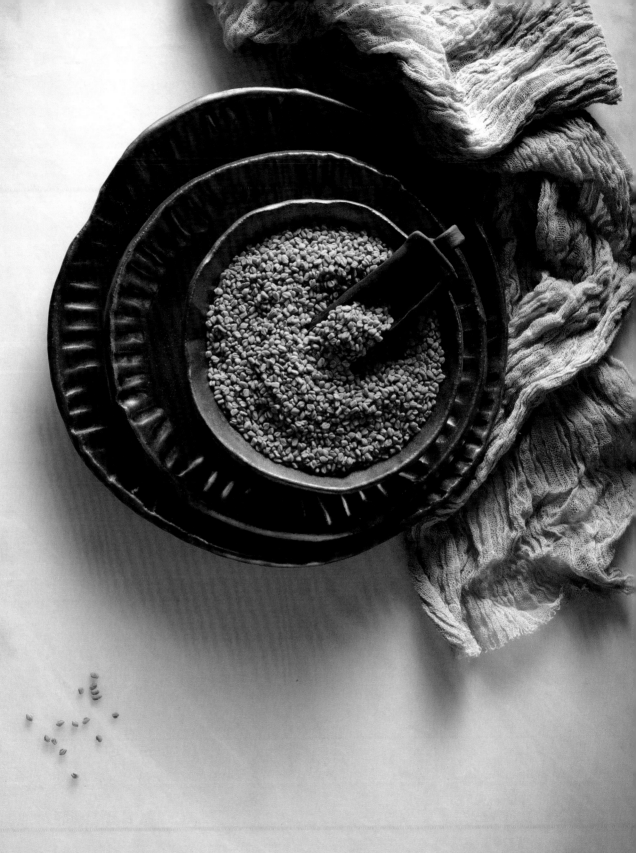

Fenugreek seed is one of the better known galactogogues that is often found in lactation supplements and teas.

# Infertility

## Folic Acid

If you are trying to conceive, a crucial element of your diet is your intake of folic acid. This should be taken as a vitamin supplement from the time you stop using contraception. Otherwise known as vitamin B9, folic acid is also found in fortified foods such as breakfast cereals. You should also try to eat foods that are naturally rich in folic acid.

### Dosage:
- Take folic acid at least two months before you start trying to conceive
- Take for at least 12 weeks into pregnancy
- Dosage: 0.4 mg every day

### A higher does of 5 mg is recommended if:
- You are taking other medication, e.g. for epilepsy, which may inhibit absorption of folic acid
- You have already had a child with a neural tube defect
- You have a BMI of over 30
- You have a history of diabetes

### Which foods contain naturally occurring folic acid?
- Green, leafy vegetables
- Avocado
- Raspberries
- Citrus fruits
- Asparagus
- Beans, peas, and lentils
- Brown rice

## Calcium and Fatty Acids

As well as increasing your intake of folate-rich foods and folic acid supplements, and eating a diet rich in vegetables and protein, you can enhance your chance of conceiving by eating plenty of foods high in fatty acids and calcium.

Recent studies have shown that calcium is vital for triggering the growth of the embryo. This mineral helps alkalize the cervix, creating a less hostile environment for both the sperm and the egg. You should consume around 1,000 mg a day through eating dairy products and leafy greens, or with supplements

Fatty acids, otherwise known as the "good" fats—omega-3, omega-6, and omega-9—are an essential part of a healthy diet, particularly when you are trying to conceive. The most important of these three fatty acids is omega-3 in terms of fertility health.

### Omega-3:
- Regulates hormones, increases cervical mucus, and increases blood flow to the uterus
- Found in oily fish, such as mackerel, and in green, leafy vegetables

### Omega-6:
- Strengthens cell structure and reduces inflammation in the body
- Found in seeds, nuts, and most vegetable cooking oils

### Omega-9:
- Helps strengthen the immune system and balance cholesterol levels
- Found in seeds, nuts, and avocados, with highest levels in olive oil

## Lifestyle Changes

Women and men who want to conceive can improve their chances by improving their lifestyles. Unhealthy lifestyle choices include smoking, drinking alcohol to excess, and using illegal drugs—these behaviors have been shown to reduce fertility, negatively affect fetal health, and increase the risk of miscarriage. Though lifestyle changes may be hard, it is worth it for your own health as much as your baby's.

### Smoking:

- Women who smoke are 1.5 times more likely than nonsmokers to take more than a year to conceive.
- The 7,000 chemicals in cigarette smoke (including nicotine) damage a woman's eggs and reproductive organs, creating problems with ovulation.
- Smoking while pregnant increases the risk of premature birth, low birth weight, and SIDS.
- Male smokers often have problems with erectile dysfunction, and their sperm is known to be damaged by smoking.

### Alcohol:

- Studies have shown that women who consume more than six units of alcohol per week are 18 percent less likely to conceive.
- Even when a woman does conceive, excessive alcohol consumption can lead to fetal alcohol syndrome, an umbrella term for a range of abnormalities such as impaired growth, intelligence, and sensory perception.
- There is no known safe amount or safe time to drink alcohol during pregnancy.

### Drugs:

- For some legal and illegal drugs, the evidence on their harmfulness to fertility and pregnancy is clear; for others, less so.
- Some studies indicate that cannabis use hinders ovulation in women.
- The use of amphetamines, methamphetamine, cocaine, and heroin has been linked to placental abruption (separation from the uterus) and miscarriage.

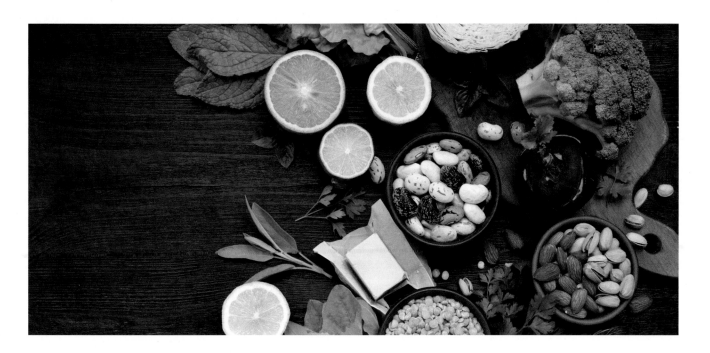

# Menstrual Cycle and PMS

## Pain Relief Tonic

### Ingredients:

2 tablespoon yarrow herb
1 tablespoon red raspberry leaf
2 tablespoon feverfew leaf
1 tablespoon ginger rhizome
2 tablespoons hops rhizome
Vodka to cover (approximately 150–200 ml)

### Directions:

1. Use as a menstrual regulator and astringent herb for painful and irregular menstruation. Prepare as a tincture (page 204) and after 2 weeks, strain and use as a pain tonic. Beginning 2 days prior to menses, take a teaspoon 3 times daily as prevention and hourly as needed for pain.

## Menstrual Relief Massage Blend

Menstrual cramping and pain can range from mild to crippling. Painful menstruation is referred to as dysmenorrhea, which can negatively affect the daily lives of women around the world. Essential oils and massage have long been used to combat the pain and cramping associated with dysmenorrhea. The Menstrual Relief Massage Blend soothes menstrual pain, reduces menstrual cramping, and even helps with potential mood effects of the menstrual cycle.

### Ingredients:

1 tablespoon virgin coconut oil
3 drops geranium essential oil
3 drops ginger essential oil
3 drops lavender essential oil
2 drops clary sage essential oil
2 drops fennel essential oil
2 drops marjoram essential oil
1 drop cinnamon essential oil
1 drop clove essential oil

### Preparation:

1. Put 1 tablespoon virgin coconut oil into a small glass, ceramic, or metal container.
2. Add 3 drops each of geranium, ginger, and lavender essential oils.
3. Add 2 drops each of clary sage, fennel, and marjoram essential oils.
4. Add 1 drop each cinnamon and clove essential oils.
5. Mix well with a metal spoon or fork.

### Administration:

1. Pour ⅓–½ the Menstrual Relief Massage Blend into your hand.
2. Massage into your pelvic region.
3. Pour another ⅓–½ the Menstrual Relief Massage Blend into your hand.
4. Massage into your lower back.
5. Use the rest of the Menstrual Relief Massage Blend to focus on any areas with particular cramping or pain.

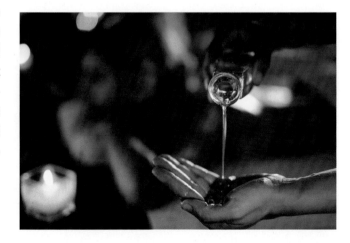

**Benefits:**

- Clove, marjoram, and lavender essential oils are analgesics and reduce the sensation of pain. Lavender also plays a psychological role in the perception of pain by reducing anxiety about pain and by affecting the way the brain acknowledges feelings of pain.
- Clary sage and geranium are hormone-balancing essential oils. They reduce pain and mood imbalances that result from menstruation.
- Ginger and cinnamon are warming, anti-inflammatory essential oils.
- Fennel essential oil reduces overconstriction of the uterus, which reduces the cramping and pain associated with menstruation.
- Virgin coconut oil has analgesic and anti-inflammatory properties.

## Healthy Moon Cycle Blend

### Ingredients:

2 parts raspberry leaf
1 part nettle
½ part cinnamon
¼ part vitex
¼ part dong quai
¼ part fennel seed
¼ part parsley

### Directions:

1. Combine dried herbs and steep in water, covered, for 10–15 minutes.
2. Remove herbs from water, and sip tea slowly.

A blend for an easeful female cycle, this tea promotes a regular rhythmic cycle, in addition to helping with cramps, and PMS. It's packed with vitamins and minerals for toning the reproductive system and healthy blood.

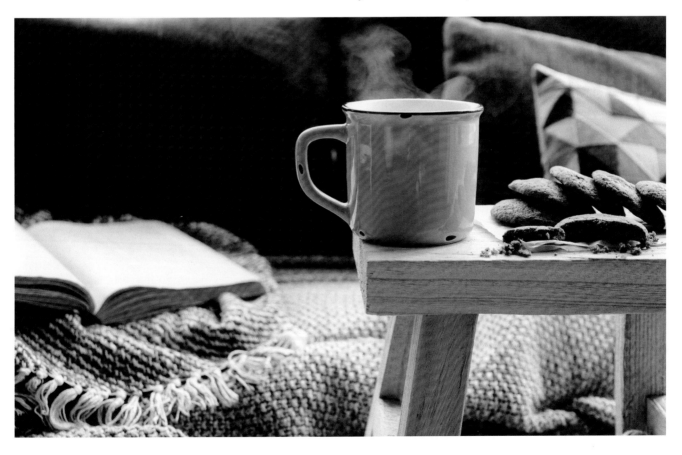

# Morning Sickness

## Prevention and Treatment

There are several things you can do to both help prevent and alleviate morning sickness:

1. Get plenty of rest, as tiredness can trigger nausea
2. Try wearing acupressure bands on the wrists
3. Have some crackers by your bed to eat as soon as you wake in the morning
4. Avoid strong-smelling foods and chemicals
5. Eat up to five small meals a day in order to keep the stomach full—hunger quickly turns to nausea
6. Herbal teas, such as fennel, peppermint, or chamomile, may help*
7. Consuming anything containing ginger, such as tea, biscuits, or flat ginger ale can help settle the stomach
8. Stay well hydrated—always keep a bottle of water with you

*Not all herbal teas are considered safe to consume while pregnant. Check with your doctor if you are unsure.

## Apple Cider Vinegar

Like indigestion is at times a problem of too little stomach acid, morning sickness is sometimes the result of too little stomach acid. This is caused by there being no stimulus to produce digestive acids after a night of inactivity. Sipping a glass of apple cider vinegar tonic (See High Blood Pressure, page 72) in the morning can help bring about a comfortable balance of stomach acids.

### Essential Oils and Pregnancy

Some oils are not safe for pregnant women. Avoid using any in your first trimester. For second and third trimester, research any herbs or oils you wish to use prior to use. Among those considered safe for the second and third trimesters are:

- Bergamot
- Chamomile
- Eucalyptus
- Frankinscence
- Geranium
- Ginger
- Grapefruit
- Lavender
- Lemon
- Lemongrass
- Lime
- Mandarin
- Neroli
- Patchouli
- Petitgrain
- Peppermint
- Roman chamomile
- Rose otto
- Rosewood
- Sandalwood
- Sweet orange
- Tea tree
- Ylang-ylang

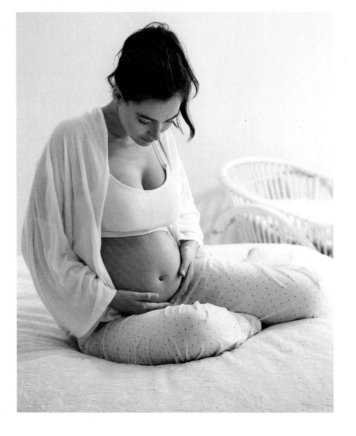

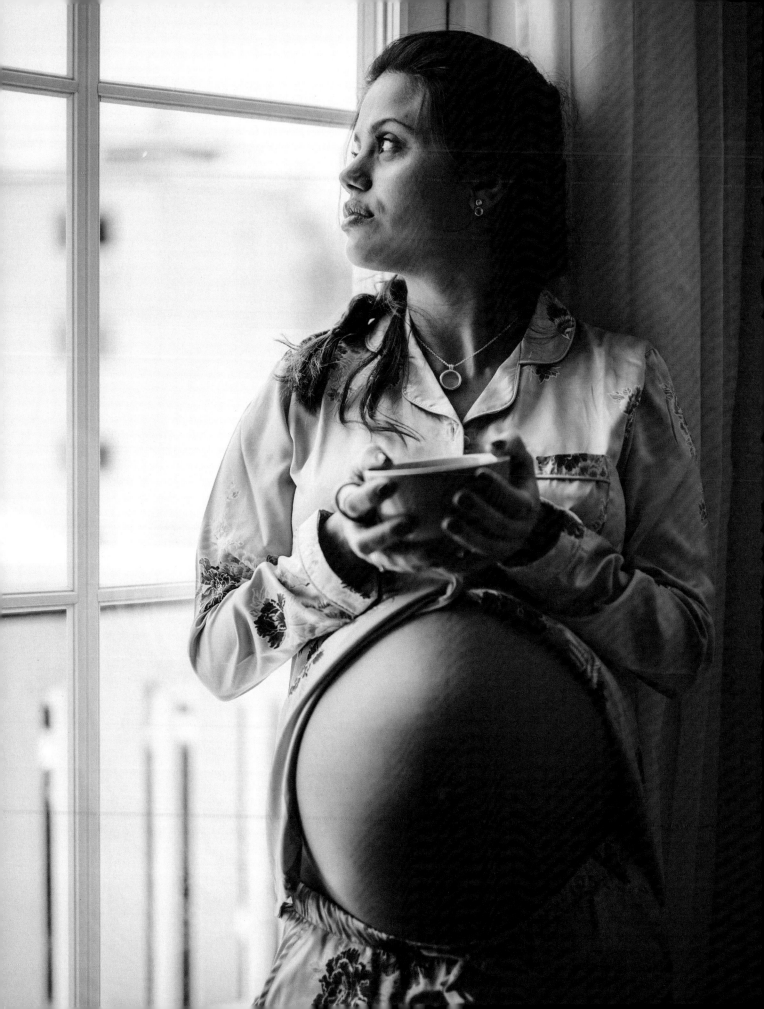

# Urinary Tract Infection

## Coconut Oil

A UTI is characterized by frequent, painful urination and can be associated with fever, nausea, or bleeding. It is important to treat a UTI promptly to prevent the infection from traveling into the kidneys. Coconut oil is an excellent natural remedy, particularly when combined with coconut water. The coconut oil will kill the bacteria and soothe the urinary tract. The coconut water assists in soothing and healing the urinary tract, while ensuring you retain the right level of electrolytes. Take three doses of coconut oil daily, and drink three generous glasses of warm water with coconut oil throughout the day.

## Calendula Tea

Tea made from calendula is a great option for the treatment of urinary tract infections, those amazing reminders of womanhood which make you want to urinate every five minutes for days on end. If you are someone prone to these infections, drinking this tea on a regular basis can help prevent future occurrences.

The tea is also beneficial for those with sore throats, providing a soothing feeling to a sore and itchy throat, as well as aiding digestion, helping with canker sores or mouth ulcers, and more.

Making tea from your own flowers is an extremely easy way to attain major health benefits from your indoor plants. Just dry your flowers and steep them in hot water. Done!

### Ingredients:
Small handful of dried calendula blossoms
Hot water

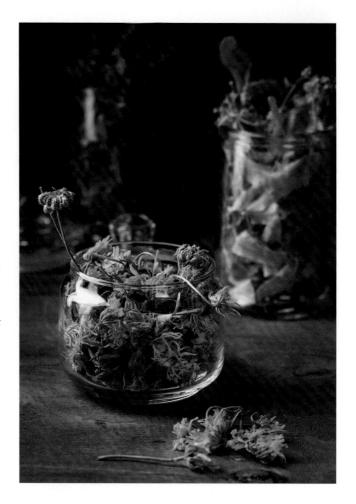

### Directions:
1. Simply pour boiling water over your dried calendula blossoms and steep for fifteen minutes.
2. After fifteen minutes, strain off the flowers and drink your tea!

### Cranberry Juice for UTIs

Cranberry juice may help protect or heal from UTIs by making it harder for bacteria to stick to your uterine walls. Look for cranberry juice that is sweetened with other fruit juices and doesn't contain high-fructose corn syrup. Note that if you suffer from kidney stones, cranberry juice isn't the best option, as it's high in oxalates.

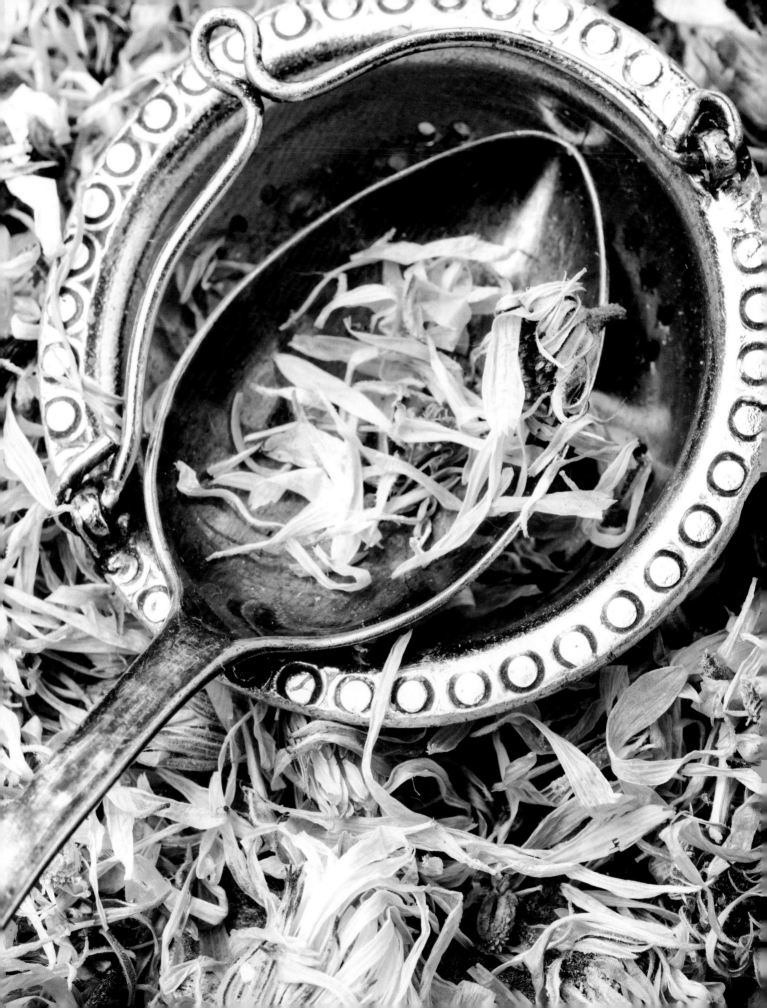

# Yeast Infection

## Topical Wash

For candida yeast infection and leukorrhea: prepare an infusion (see page 194) of calendula, thyme, and chamomile—using equal parts—as a topical wash.

## Apple Cider Vinegar

Use a douche of 2 tablespoons apple cider vinegar to 1 quart warm water, twice daily until the symptoms have stopped. Adding a cup of apple cider vinegar to your bath will provide external relief.

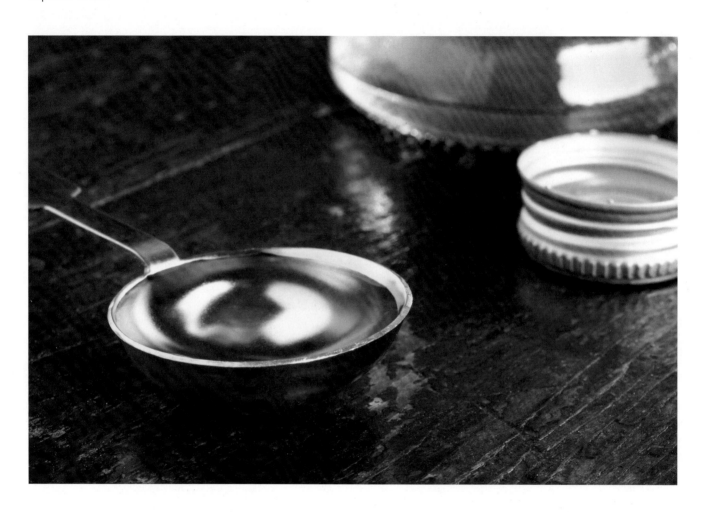

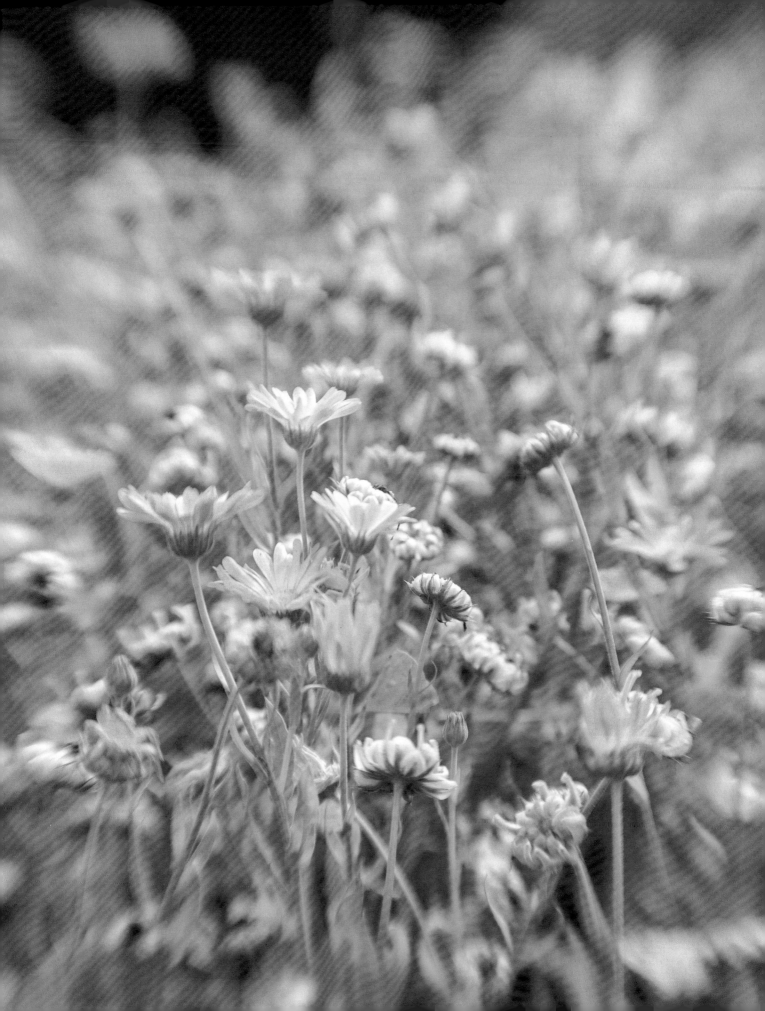

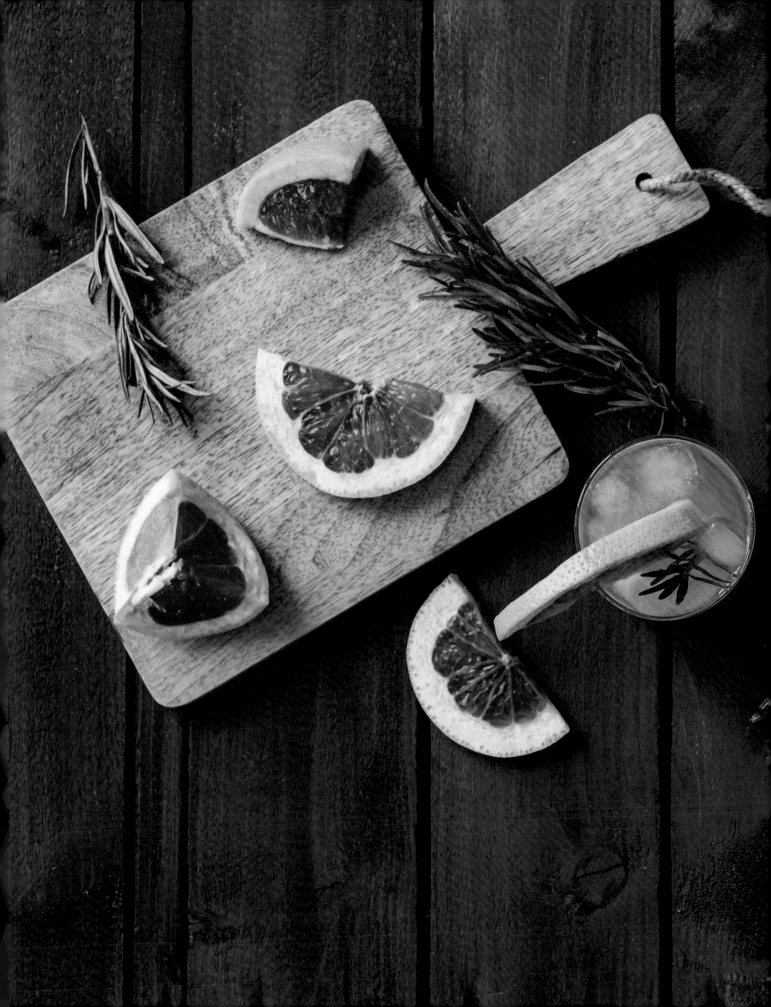

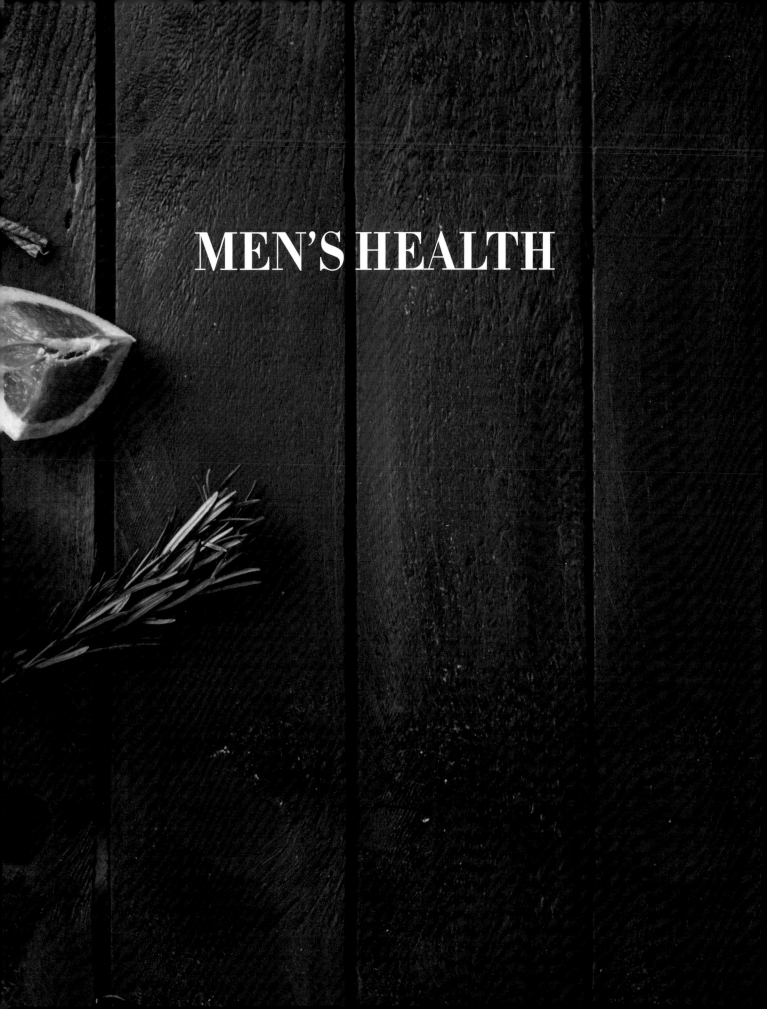

# MEN'S HEALTH

# Baldness

## Rosemary Shampoo

You can quickly make your own hair-stimulating shampoo that not only smells great, but helps rejuvenate your follicularly challenged scalp.

### Ingredients:
¼ cup distilled water
2 tablespoons dried rosemary
shampoo bottles
¼ cup liquid castile soap
1 teaspoon vegetable glycerin
½ teaspoon jojoba oil
7 drops rosemary essential oil
5 drops peppermint essential oil

### Directions:
1. Boil the distilled water in a pot and remove from heat. Steep 2 tablespoons of dried rosemary for twenty minutes.
2. After twenty minutes, strain the rosemary tea, let it cool down completely, and pour it into a shampoo bottle.
3. Using a funnel, pour the liquid castile soap into the bottle, followed by the vegetable glycerin, jojoba oil, and rosemary and peppermint oils.
4. Close the bottle and shake well to combine.
5. Your homemade rosemary shampoo is done, simple as that. Store your shampoo in a cool, dry place, preferably the refrigerator, and use within a month. Shake well before each use.

## Hair Rinse

### Ingredients:
2 teaspoons yarrow leaf and flowers
2 teaspoons rosemary herb
3 cups boiling water

### Directions:
1. Prepare as an infusion (see page 194) using herbs intended to encourage circulation to the scalp. The astringent properties may assist with preventing hair loss.

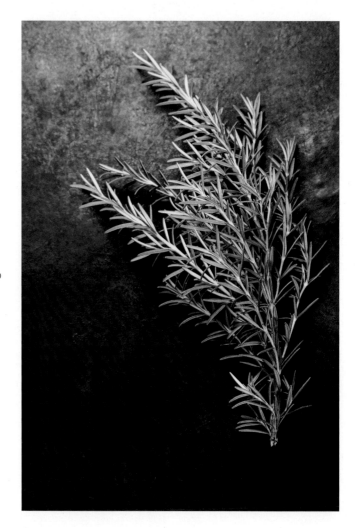

# Infertility

## What Can Men Do?

Men can make a number of changes in their everyday lives to aid their fertility by boosting their sperm count and sperm motility, giving themselves the best chance of successfully fathering healthy children.

1. Consider your job—try to make adjustments if your work involves exposure to harsh chemicals such as fertilizers. Some studies have found that regular contact with chemicals can affect motility and increase the risk of sperm abnormalities.
2. Eat a healthy, balanced diet, rich in whole and unprocessed foods—this will provide your body with vitamins and minerals, notably zinc, which are essential for the production of healthy sperm.
3. Get regular exercise—as well as the proven benefits of exercise for overall health and reducing stress, this will increase your body's levels of the hormone testosterone, which will give your libido a helpful boost.
4. Aim to ejaculate every other day—every day would mean testicles would struggle to keep up with production.
5. Make changes as early as possible—sperm production takes a while (typically sixty-four days until maturation) so sooner is better to allow the changes to take effect.

## What Should Men Avoid?

Avoid too much exposure to heat, including laptops and hot baths, to regulate the temperature of your testicles.

Stop smoking, as it has an adverse effect on your sperm count and it has been shown to damage the membrane around the sperm.

Avoid too-tight underwear to allow air to circulate around your testicles.

Reduce your consumption of alcohol—drinking to excess can reduce sperm production and lower your body's testosterone levels.

Avoid drugs and junk food—these can affect your libido and ability to get an erection.

Avoid stressful situations—stress can lead to erectile dysfunction and may affect the quality of your sperm's work.

## Fertility Foods

### Zinc
- Keeps testosterone levels high and improves sperm health
- Found in red meat, pumpkin seeds, and vegetables such as peas

### Folic Acid
- Studies have shown men with higher levels of folic acid have fewer abnormal sperm
- Highest levels found in asparagus and lentils

### CoQ10
- An antioxidant enzyme found in nuts and seeds, particularly sesame seeds
- Taking a CoQ10 supplement can boost fertility by 13 percent, as it helps the motility of the sperm

### Selenium
- This antioxidant helps form healthy sperm and increases sperm motility
- Found in Brazil nuts and fish such as salmon and tuna

### Vitamin E
- Sperm quality is improved by having plenty of vitamin E in your diet
- It is commonly found in almonds and other nuts

## Vitamin C

- As well as helping with general health, vitamin C increases both sperm count and the health of the sperm
- The best source is citrus fruits

## Fatty Acids

- Omega-3 fatty acids are needed to produce plenty of prostaglandins in the semen. These suppress the female immune system's attack on the sperm when they enter the cervix
- Found in walnuts and oily fish such as sardines and salmon

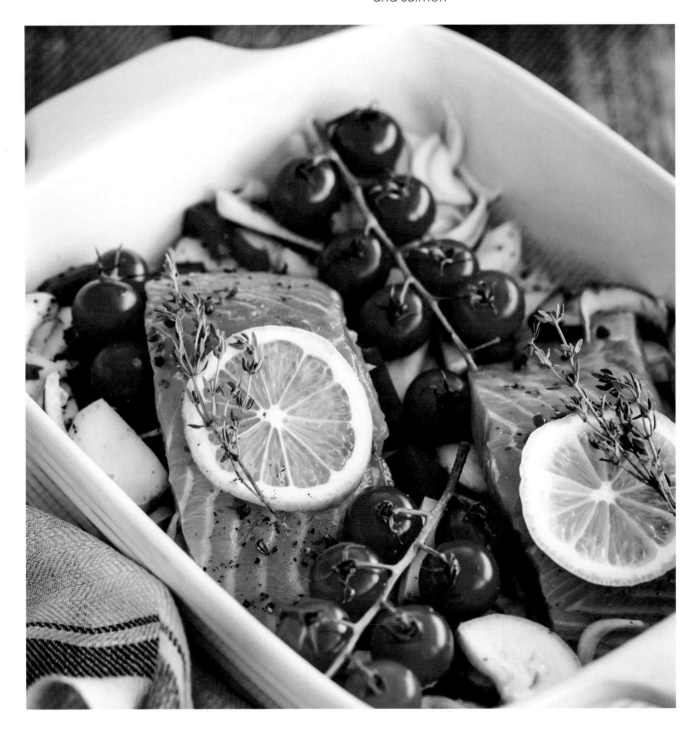

# Shaving Care

## Warm and Woody Shaving Cream

Shaving your face is a bit of an art form, requiring a steady, agile hand and the right tools. Those tools not only include the right razor, but also the right shaving cream. The Warm and Woody Shaving Cream is the shaving cream you need to achieve a close, smooth shave. It's moisturizing, healing, and will leave you feeling like a million bucks.

### Ingredients:
### Shaving cream base:

⅓ cup shea butter
1 tablespoon raw or Manuka honey
⅓ cup sweet almond oil
2 tablespoons unscented liquid castile soap (optional)

### Essential oils:

15 drops sandalwood essential oil

### Preparation:

1. Create a double boiler using a sauté pan and a medium glass bowl or large glass measuring cup. Fill the pan with ½–1 inch of water and bring to a soft boil on low-medium heat. Place the glass bowl/measuring cup into the water.
2. Melt ⅓ cup shea butter in the glass bowl/measuring cup.
3. Add 1 tablespoon honey and let it melt into the shea butter.
4. Remove from heat and mix in ⅓ cup sweet almond oil.
5. Place bowl in refrigerator and let contents solidify. This takes about 30 minutes to an hour.
6. Remove from refrigerator and use a hand mixer to whip the mixture until soft peaks form. Use a spatula to scrape the sides of the bowl to ensure that none of the mixture sticks to the sides.
7. (Optional) Add 2 tablespoons unscented liquid castile soap and whip until fully incorporated into the mixture.
8. Add 15 drops of sandalwood essential oil to the shaving cream base and whip for 20–30 seconds.
9. Use a metal spoon or spatula to transfer the shaving cream into one 8-ounce mason jar or two 4-ounce mason jars.
10. Apply the lid(s) and label.
11. Store away from heat and moisture.

### Benefits:

- Shea butter is incredibly moisturizing and protects skin from free radicals. It heals oxidative damage that has already occurred.
- Honey is a powerful antibiotic and will protect your skin from bacterial colonization. If you do receive any nicks while shaving, the honey will protect them from infection.
- Almond oil is easily absorbed into the skin.
- Sandalwood essential oil acts as an astringent for your skin, while at the same time soothing your face with its cooling, antioxidant, and antispasmodic properties.
- Sandalwood essential oil also increases attentiveness and mood, which brings a feeling of zen to your shaving routine.
- The santalol and santyl acetate in the sandalwood essential oil are both antimicrobial, protecting your skin in case of abrasion.

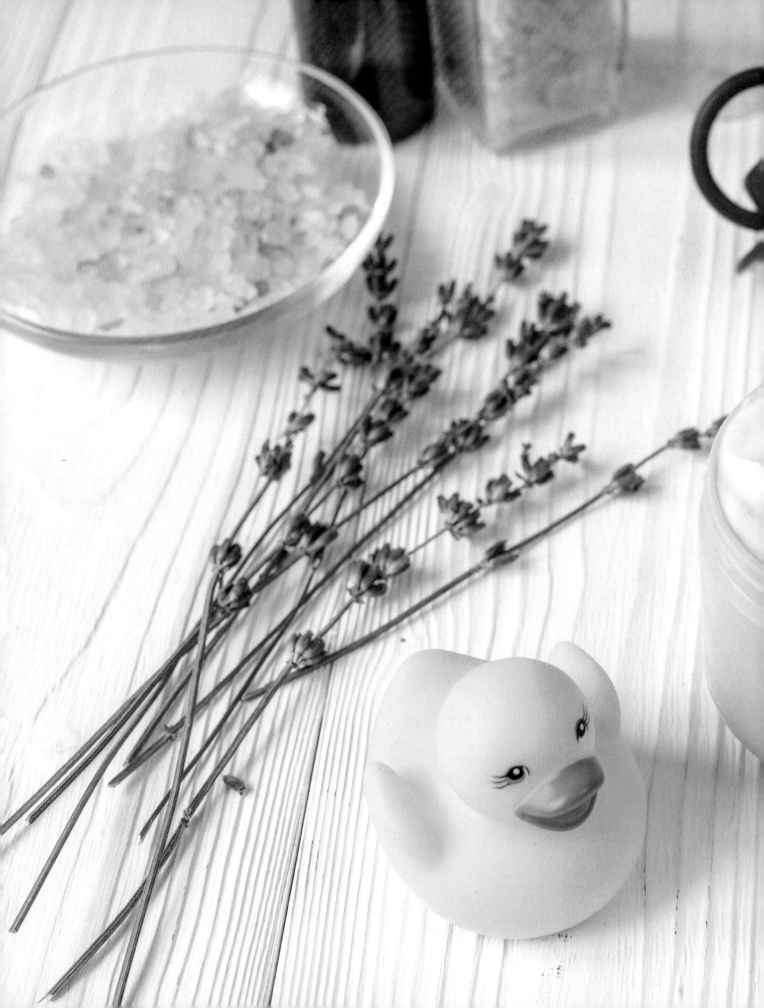

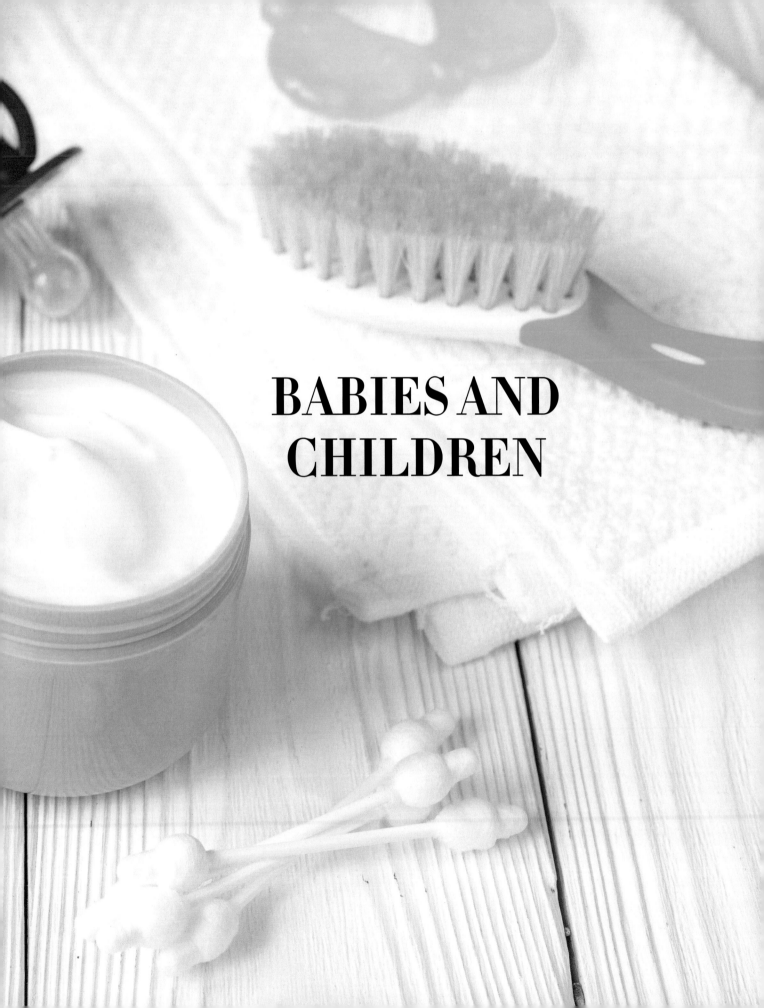

# BABIES AND CHILDREN

# Diaper Rash

## Comforting Diaper Cream

Changing babies diapers regularly and keeping a baby's bottom dry are the best ways to prevent diaper rash, but sometimes that's not enough. Diaper rash can be painful for babies and toddlers, making diaper changes difficult and the whole family unhappy. The Comforting Diaper Cream soothes sore bottoms and prevents diaper rashes from occurring in the first place.

### Ingredients:

½ cup virgin coconut oil

½ cup cornstarch

8 drops lavender essential oil

6 drops Roman chamomile essential oil

4 drops melaleuca essential oil (six months and older)

### Preparation:

1. In a glass bowl, use an electric hand mixer to whip ½ cup solid virgin coconut oil until it makes peaks. This takes about 10 minutes depending on the weather.
2. Add 8 drops lavender and 6 drops Roman chamomile essential oils.
3. If your child is six months or older, add 4 drops melaleuca essential oil.
4. Mix until oils are evenly distributed.
5. Stir in ½ cup cornstarch. Mix until an even consistency is obtained.
6. Divide between 2–3 four-ounce mason jars.

### Administration:

1. Using dry hands, scoop a small amount of Comforting Diaper Cream into your hand.
2. Gently rub onto your baby's clean, dry bottom.
3. Allow your baby to spend some time diaperless or put on a new diaper.

### Benefits:

- Coconut oil is soothing to the skin and protects against fungal infections, including candida infections.
- Melaleuca essential oil is also effective against candida and other fungal infections.
- Lavender and Roman chamomile essential oils are calming to the skin and relaxing for babies.
- Lavender essential oil acts as a mild analgesic, reducing the pain babies feel when they have a diaper rash.
- Cornstarch whisks moisture away from your baby's skin.

## Apple Cider Vinegar

Apple cider vinegar is an effective cure for many forms of rashes due to its fungicidal and antibacterial properties. It can be used in a half-water, half-apple-cider-vinegar mixture which you dab on with a soaked cotton ball at each diaper change. Another remedy is to mix it half-and-half with freshly brewed and cooled rooibos/red bush tea, which in itself is an effective diaper rash remedy. This mixture is also applied with a soaked cotton ball at each diaper change.

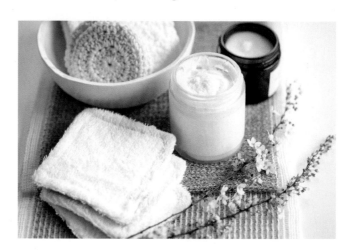

# Earache

## Coconut Oil

The medium-chain fatty acids in coconut oil will fight both viral infections and bacterial infections, while the warmth of gently heated oil will also be soothing to the painful site. Melt the oil and apply carefully with an eyedropper.* However, seek medical advice before any application if the ear drum is damaged.

*Test the temperature of the oil on your wrist to ensure it's not too hot before using it in a child's ear.

## Apple Cider Vinegar

Earaches are normally the result of ear infections and always require the attention of a physician as soon as possible. Often there is a wait before you can get the patient to see the physician or for the effects of the medicine to take hold. Relief from discomfort and healing benefits can be obtained by holding the affected ear over a steam bath with 1 part apple cider to two parts water. Be careful not to hold the ear too close to the steam. This is effective for young children, but not babies, who may not be able to communicate if the steam is too hot.

> If an infant of three months or younger has a temperature of 100.4°F, call your doctor or go to the ER. If you're unable to get a good temperature reading but suspect a fever, go to the doctor. It's better to be safe than sorry, as fevers in newborns can be very serious. For older babies and toddlers, a temp of over 102°F is worth a call to your doctor.

## Simple Ways to Ease Earaches

- Fill a sock with beans, rice, or coarse salt, and tie the open part of the sock into a knot. Heat in the microwave until warm (but not too hot). Use as a warm compress on the painful ear. You can also add a little lavender essential oil to the sock.
- Garlic and mullein oil can be purchased in a small glass bottle with a dropper. Run the bottle under hot water to warm the oil. Test the warmth on your wrist. If the temperature is a pleasant warmth, have the child lie on their side with the aching ear facing up. Place two or three drops in the aching ear. It's best if the child can stay in that position for about 15 minutes as the oil sinks in. You can also make garlic oil by chopping a fresh garlic clove and heating it together with a few tablespoons of olive oil on the stove top using low heat. You don't want the oil to smoke. When the oil becomes fragrant, remove from heat and allow to cool until just barely warm. Carefully strain out every bit of the garlic clove before using. Store extra in the refrigerator.
- Gently massage behind the ears and down the neck to help drain excess fluid.
- Allow nursing babies to nurse as much as possible. They may experience some relief from the sucking motion, and the milk may strengthen their immune system to fight whatever is causing the pain.

See also Garlic and Mullein Ear Oil, page 86

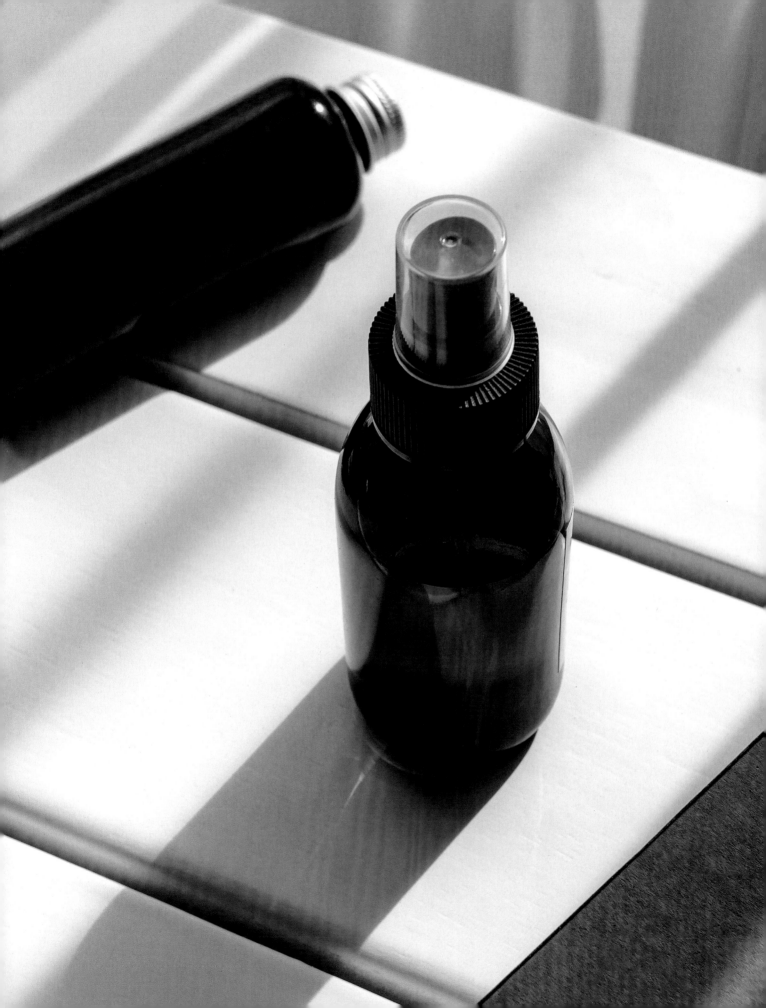

# Head Lice

## Apple Cider Vinegar

If over-the-counter lice preparations are not available or are too toxic for your skin, try rinsing your hair with full-strength apple cider, then allow it to dry naturally. This will kill the adult lice and dissolve the glue that binds the eggs to the hair shaft. Now wash your hair with shampoo and then apply olive oil to your hair. The olive oil will allow you to see any remaining lice or eggs; you must then pick them out with a comb and rewash your hair. Repeat this daily until all the lice are gone.

## Lice Repellant

Fill a 16-ounce glass spray bottle with distilled water. Add 30 drops tea tree oil, 5 drops eucalyptus essential oil, 5 drops peppermint essential oil, and then 10 drops your choice of geranium, lavender, cinnamon leaf, or thyme essential oil. Fill the rest of the bottle with witch hazel. Shake gently and then spray on scalp and back of neck. You can also spray hats, scarves, hairbrushes, and anything else likely to carry lice home. The recipe can easily be halved if you have a smaller spray bottle or don't need as much.

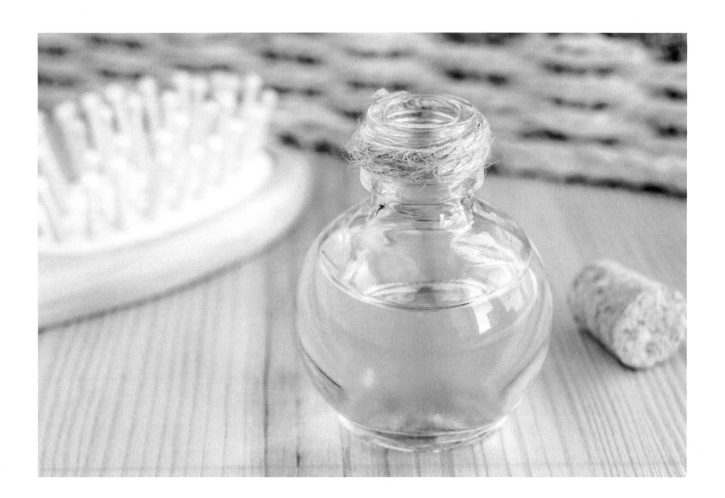

# Sore Throat

## Soothe My Throat Gargle

This is a great remedy for children who are old enough to safely gargle. Do not use for babies or very young children.

### Ingredients:
1 part thyme herb or rosemary
1 part calendula flower
1 part cleavers herb
½ part salt
2 cups boiling water

### Directions:
1. Prepare an infusion (see page 194) of equal parts of the herbs or any one of the herbs above.
2. Pour boiling water over the herbs and steep, covered, for 15 minutes.
3. Strain, and stir in the salt.
4. Gargle with warm tea until liquid is used completely. Repeat 2–3 times per day or hourly for acute conditions.

Too often a sore throat can be the beginning of a deeper immune assault. This potent blend containing volatile oils offers potent antiviral and antibacterial properties.

## Honey Lemon Ginger Drops

These little candies double as throat lozenges. Made with honey rather than processed sugar and spiked with vinegar and lemon juice, they are healthier than most store-bought lozenges, and as tasty as any candy you'll try. Don't give these to babies or young children who could choke on them.

Makes a little less than 1 pound of drops.

### Ingredients:
½ cup water
3-inch piece of ginger root, peeled and finely diced
1 cup honey
2 tablespoons apple cider vinegar
2 teaspoons fresh-squeezed lemon juice
½ teaspoon slippery elm powder (optional)

### Directions:
1. Line a cookie sheet with parchment paper and spray lightly with cooking spray.
2. In a small saucepan, simmer the water and ginger for about half an hour. Strain, reserving the liquid. (You can toss the ginger bits in sugar, let them dry on a cookie sheet, and enjoy them as chewy ginger candies.)
3. In a medium saucepan, combine the ginger water, honey, and vinegar. Stir with a metal spoon until honey liquefies.
4. Stop stirring and insert the candy thermometer. Don't stir the syrup again until it's removed from the heat. Allow mixture to come to a boil. If sugar crystals form on the sides of the pan, wipe them away with a damp pastry brush.
5. When the syrup reaches 300°F, remove from heat. If you're not using a candy thermometer, this is hard crack stage. Allow mixture to cool slightly until boiling has ceased. Add the lemon juice and stir.
6. Working quickly, use a ½ teaspoon measure to drop the syrup onto the lined cookie sheet, leaving a little space between each one. If desired, sprinkle with slippery elm powder. Let cool for at least ½ hour. Store for about a week at room temperature or refrigerate for longer storage.

### Simple Ways to Soothe a Sore Throat
- Gargle with salt water
- Eat a small spoonful of raw honey. (Babies under one year should not be given honey.)
- Take a hot shower and breathe in the steam
- Drink warm fluids
- Sip ginger, licorice root, turmeric, or chamomile tea

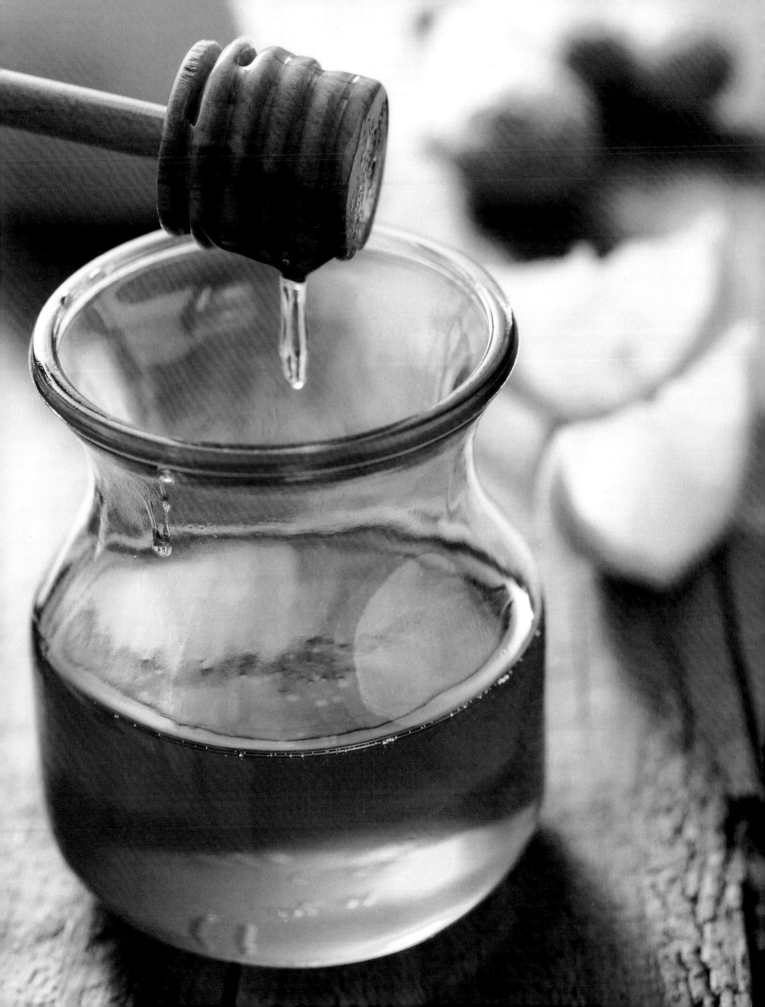

# Teething

## Tummy and Teething Calm Popsicle

### Ingredients:
1 part spearmint leaf
1 part fennel seed
1 part feverfew herb

### Directions:
1. Brew equal portions as an infusion (see page 194) and sweeten with a little honey,* or add in sliced fruit such as chopped mango or peaches.
2. Pour into popsicle molds and freeze. These make ideal support for the pain of teething (omit the fruit and use fruit puree unless a child is eating solid food) and for a sore throat.

*Omit honey if child is under a year old.

## Simple Teething Soothers
- Rub a peeled slice of ginger root on your baby's gums to reduce inflammation.
- Mix cloves with coconut oil and chill in the refrigerator. Then rub on baby's gums. Cloves have a numbing effect.
- Dampen a washcloth and then refrigerate it until it's chilled. Allow your baby to chew on it to soothe his or her gums.
- A large, refrigerated carrot can be great for gnawing on. Don't use baby carrots as they're harder for a baby to grasp in her little hands and easier for a baby to choke on.

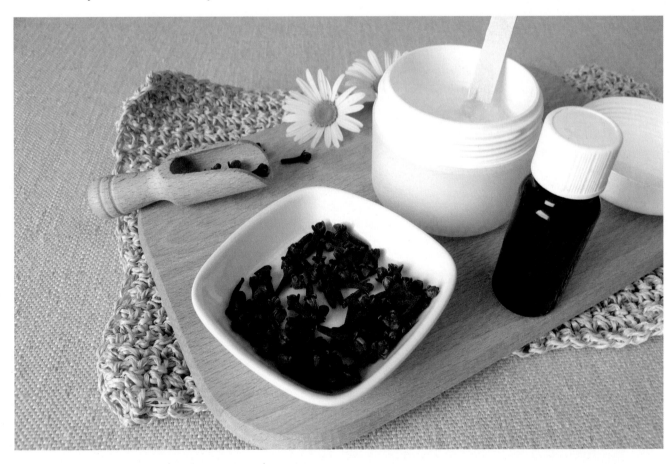

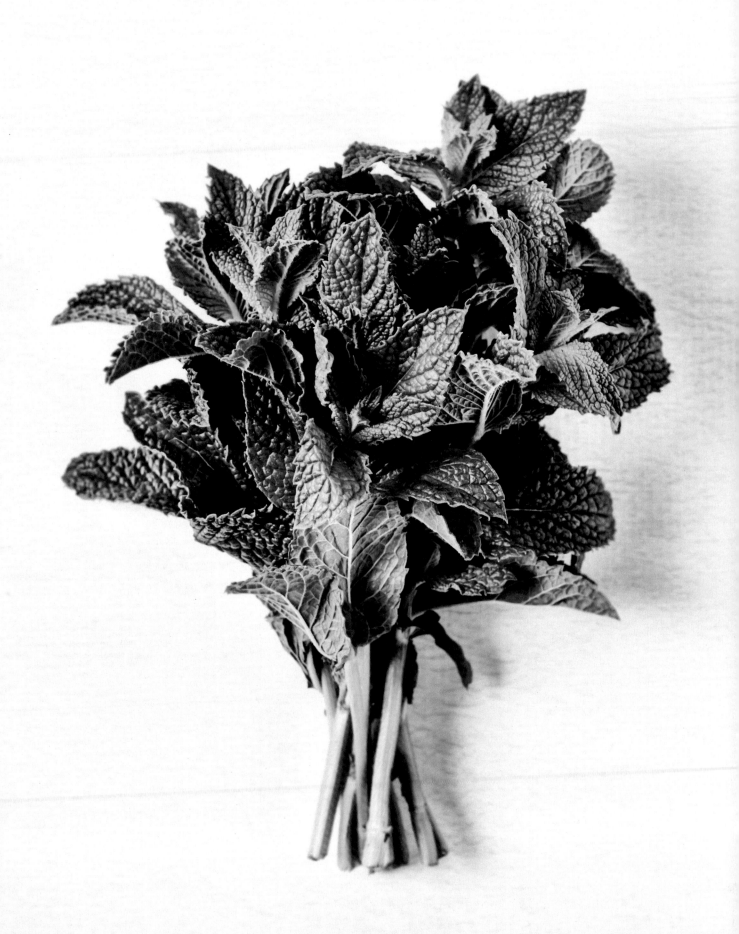

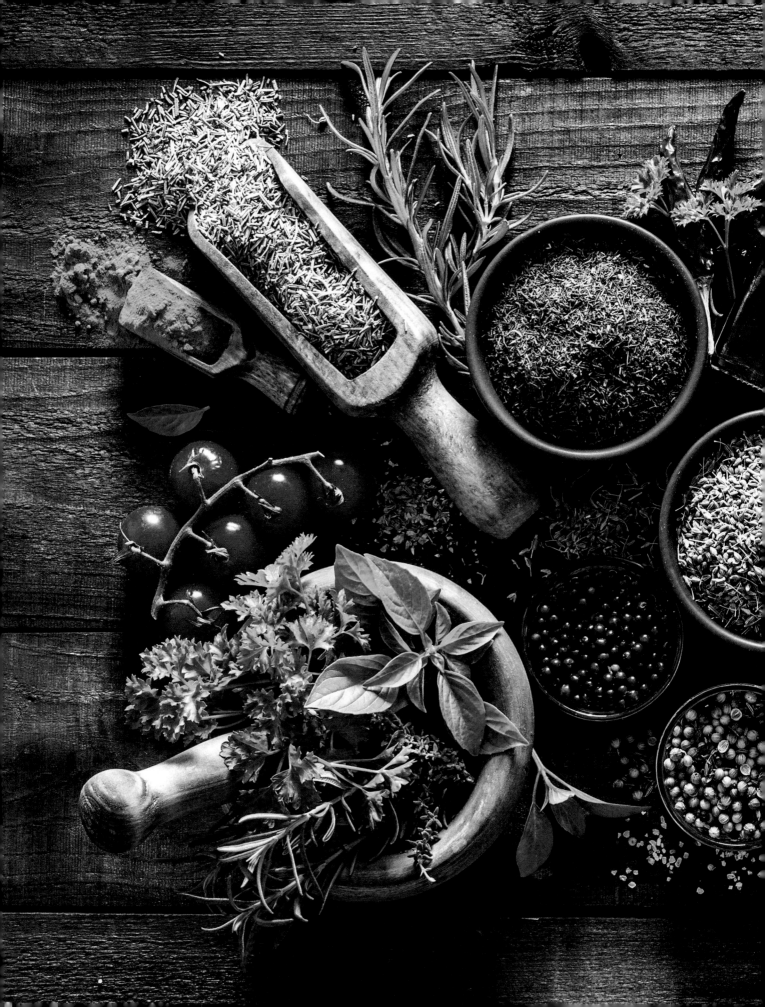

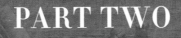

# PART TWO

# HEALING HERBS, SPICES, AND SUPERFOODS

| | | | |
|---|---|---|---|
| Herbs | 121 | Tonics and Shots | 207 |
| Juices and Cleanses | 167 | Broths | 219 |
| Smoothies | 185 | Medicinal Cooking | 233 |
| Teas and Elixirs | 193 | Natural Baby and | |
| Tinctures | 203 | Toddler Treats | 253 |

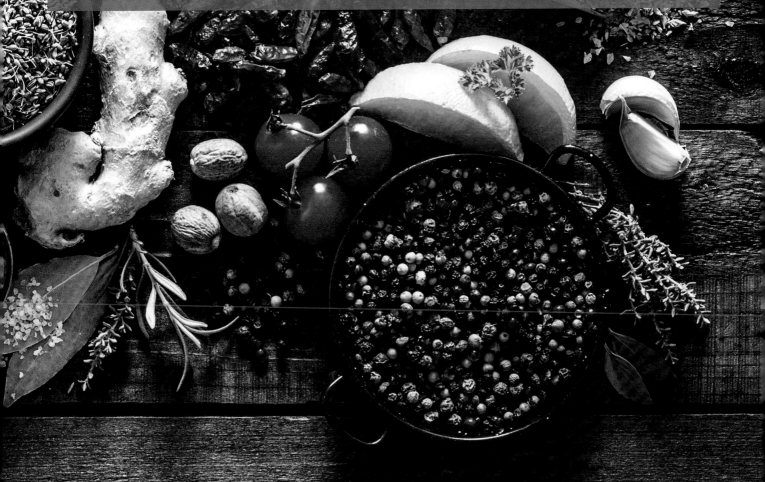

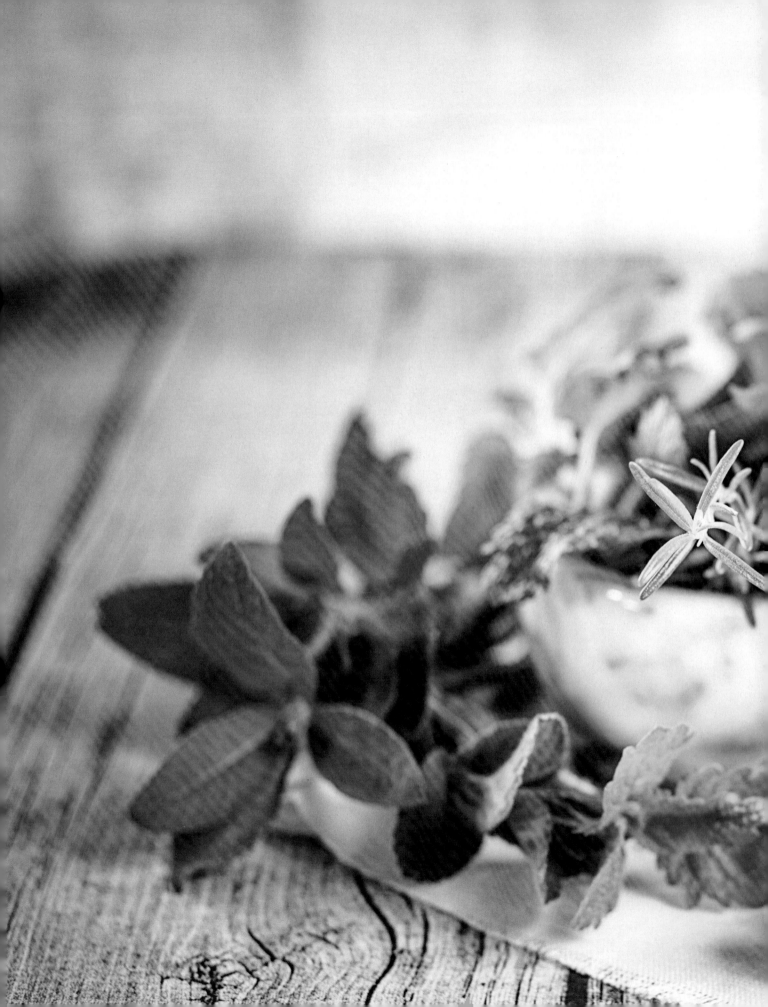

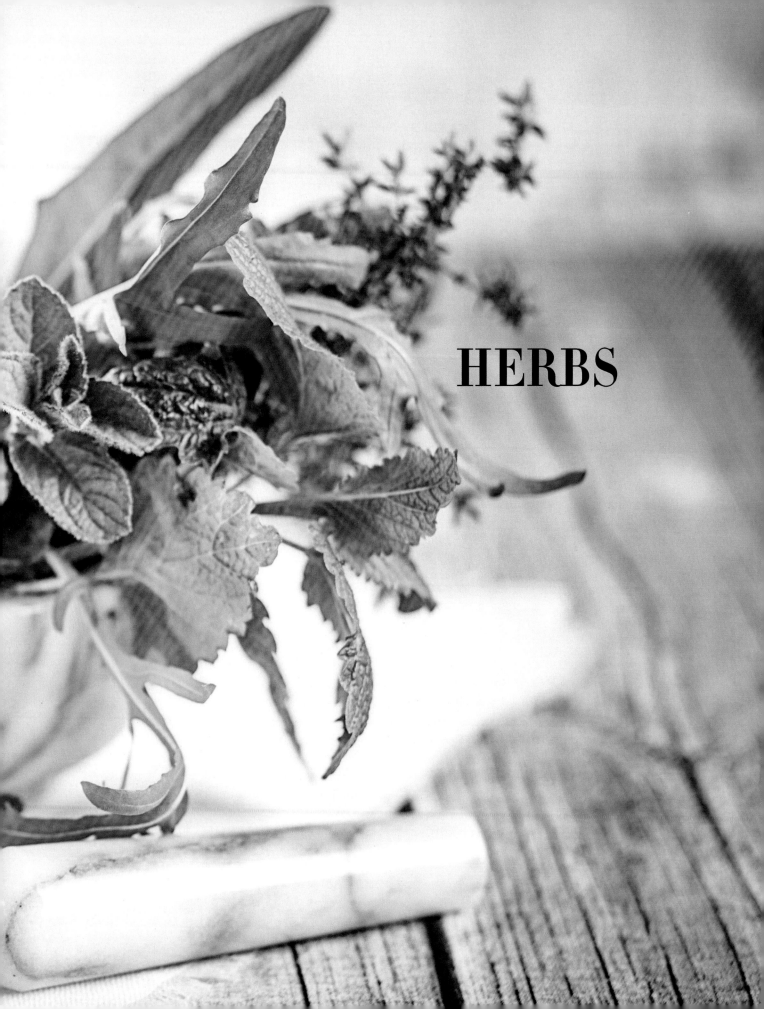

HERBS

# Planning an Herb Garden

## Herb Garden Designs

Once you have a good idea what plants you will be growing and have chosen a site for your garden, designing the garden is in order. Before turning ground, making beds, and adding compost and other amendments, designing on paper is a good idea. Think about what shape you want, what size, whether to do raised beds or not, etc.

Herb gardens can be very simply designed or very intricate. Think of your garden as an empty palette where you can mix and match colors and moods and reflections to your own individual needs and desires. Another way to consider the layout of your garden is to imagine yourself sculpting the earth. You are an earth sculptor! Here are a couple of unique possibilities to get the creative juices flowing.

## Moon Garden

A moon garden is a garden bed shaped like a crescent moon, with a couple of walkways for access. The moon garden could include plants that are used for women's moon cycles and/or plants that display whitish leaves and white flowers. Enjoying a moon garden is easy: one can walk through the garden at night and take in the view, especially if the moon is out. According to the Farmer's Almanac, the age-old practice of performing farm chores by the moon stems from the simple belief that the moon governs moisture. Pliny the Elder, the first-century Roman naturalist, stated in his Natural History that the moon "replenishes the earth; when she approaches it, she fills all bodies, while, when she recedes, she empties them."

## Mandala Garden

A mandala garden is a series of garden beds set up in a circular fashion. In one example, the beds are arranged splaying out from the middle of a circle. Plants of specific colors are in certain places, with specific plants blooming at certain times. Traditionally in the small backyard herb garden, the perennials form the structure or "skeleton" of the garden, and the annuals fill in around them. Annuals are planted each year, and so there are times where areas are bare, either before planting or after harvesting. This general design keeps the garden feeling full, even when there are no annuals growing. Perennials grow bigger each year, so leaving plenty of room around them for spreading is important.

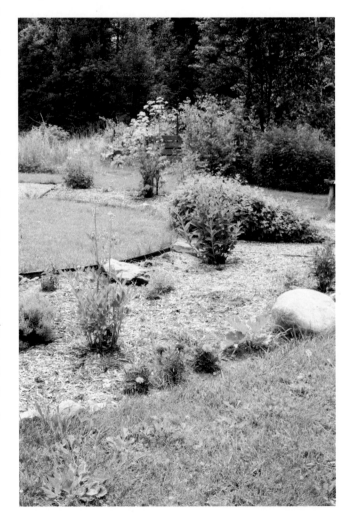

## Medicine Wheel Garden

A medicine wheel garden is a circular garden, usually divided into four quadrants, one for each of the four compass directions. The four directions have many representations and symbols that correspond with them in many cultures around the world.

As a simple example, east represents new life, birth, beginnings, and morning. South represents fire, heat, the middle of life, and passion. North represents the elder years, coldness, and winter. West represents the end of the day, sleep, rejuvenation, and death. These are just some representations that I have taken from various traditions (mostly earth-based spirituality) and incorporated into my intention when designing and planting my medicine wheel garden.

After you have done your own research on medicine wheels around the world, looked into the symbolism of the four directions, and thought about what is meaningful to you—maybe from your heritage or rituals and symbols that resonate with you—then you can start connecting the plants to them. Consider all of these things, as well as the size of your gardening space, and then choose your plants. This type of garden is meant to be a sacred space, an art project really. It is enjoyable to create something that is so customized to you and to really make it your own.

Herbs (especially perennials) spread, so make sure to leave plenty of space around each one, and cover the ground between them with either wood chip mulch or straw or whatever else you like.

Here are some ideas for coordinating plants and compass directions:

**For the East**: motherwort, calendula, sage, lavender, catnip, St. John's wort.
**For the South**: echinacea, thyme, boneset, astragalus.
**For the North**: parsley, lemongrass, oregano, basil, rhubarb.

**For the West**: valerian, lemon balm, chamomile, feverfew, holy basil.

These herbs, for me personally, correspond with the directions as I mentioned earlier. They are used in different stages of life, as well as different times of day. Along with planting herbs in the medicine wheel garden, it's fun to also collect many stones to place around, perhaps making a border with them, as well as stumps to sit on, a grassy area in the middle, an altar of some sort in the middle, prayer flags, etc. The options are endless—have fun with it!

If you want to dive deep into the world of medicine wheels and learn how to incorporate them into your life, I recommend *The Medicine Wheel Garden: Creating Sacred Space for Healing, Celebration, and Tranquility* by E. Barrie Kavasch.

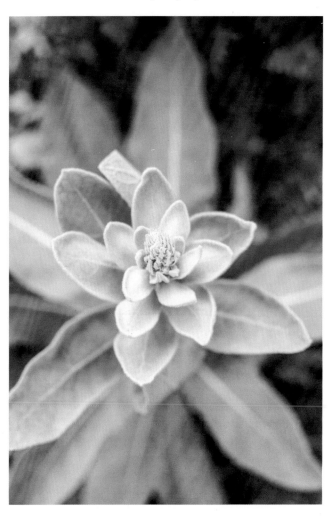

# Herbs to Avoid During Pregnancy

There are very few accounts of any herbs leading to adverse side effects during pregnancy. However it is responsible to consider a few general guidelines when pregnant. Avoid ingestion of any herbs that encourage menstruation (emmenagogues). Avoid ingestion of strong bitter herbs used to activate digestion, as they will also increase muscular contractions in the digestive tract, and avoid antiparasitic and laxative herbs. These herbs are too stimulating to use. The very best advice is to consult an herbal practitioner for specific guidance when using any herbs during pregnancy. This is a list of some commonly used Western herbs that should not be ingested during pregnancy. Some herbs are dose- or circumstance-dependent and are not included in this list.

- Arnica (*Arnica montana*)
- Barberry (*Berberis vulgaris*)
- Bayberry (*Myrica cerifera*)
- Belladonna (*Atropa belladonna*)
- Black cohosh (*Cimicifuga racemosa*)
- Bloodroot (*Sanguinaria canadensis*)
- Blue cohosh (*Caulophyllum thalictroides*)

- Buchu (*Agathosma betulina*)
- California poppy (*Eschscholzia california*)
- Chaparral (*Larrea divaricata*)
- Coltsfoot (*Tussilago farfara*)
- Comfrey (*Symphytum officinalis*)
- Dong quai (*Angelica sinensis*)
- Feverfew (*Tanacetum parthenium*)
- Ginseng (*Panax, Eleutherococcus*)
- Goldenseal (*Hydrastis canadensis*)
- Greater celandine (*Chelidonium majus*)
- Juniper (*Juniperus communis*)
- Licorice (*Glycirrhiza glabra*)
- Ma huang (*Ephedra sinica*)
- Mistletoe (*Viscum album*)
- Myrrh (*Commiphora molmol*)
- Nutmeg (*Myristica fragrans*)
- Parsley (*Petroselinum crispum*)
- Pennyroyal (*Mentha pulegium*)
- Pokeweed (*Phytolacca decandra*)
- Rue (*Ruta graveolens*)
- Sage (*Salvia officinalis*)
- Sassafras (*Sassafras albidum*)
- Scotch broom (*Sarothamnus scoparius*)
- Senna (*Cassia senna*)
- Tansy (*Tanacetum vulgare*)
- Tree of life (*Thuja occidentalis*)
- Wild carrot (*Daucus carota*)
- Wormwood (*Artemisia absinthium*)

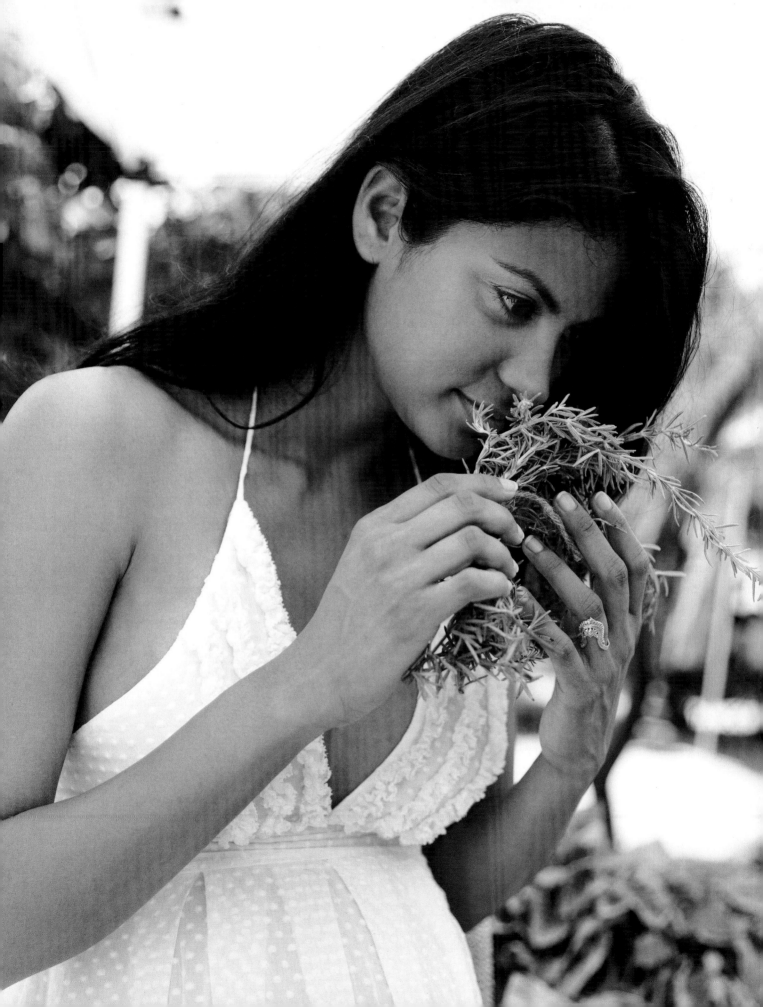

# Properties and Actions of Herbs

Included here are descriptions of some of the many properties and actions of herbs, with examples of specific herbs to follow.

**Abortifacient**: Can cause expulsion of the fetus, and if not, can cause other damage to fetus.
Blue cohosh, mugwort, pennyroyal.

**Adaptogen**: Helps our body adapt to and deal with stress in all areas—body, mind, spirit. Helps keep balance and conserve energy.
Astragalus, ashwaganda, ginseng, eleuthero.

**Alterative**: Blood purifiers, cleansers, builders, tonics. Helps the body deal with toxic substances and assimilate nutrients.
Burdock, comfrey, nettle, plantain.

**Analgesic**: Relieves pain.
Chamomile, skullcap, valerian.

**Anodyne**: Relieves pain (see Analgesic).

**Antiarthritic**: Relieves inflammation and joint pain. Protects joints from degeneration.
Turmeric, juniper, black cohosh.

**Antibacterial**: Inhibits the growth of or destroys bacteria and viruses.
Echinacea, elecampane, garlic, goldenseal.

**Anticatarrhal**: Decreases mucous production.
Elder, mullein, sage.

**Antipyretic**: Cooling to reduce or prevent fever.
Boneset, basil, chickweed.

**Antidepressant**: Relieves depression, supports the nervous system.
Lemon balm, oat tops, St. John's wort.

**Antiemetic**: Prevents vomiting.
Chamomile, ginger, peppermint.

**Antifungal**: Inhibits or destroys growth of fungi.
Garlic, tea tree, yarrow.

**Anti-inflammatory**: Reduces inflammation.
Cayenne, chamomile, turmeric, yarrow.

**Antilithic**: Prevents kidney stones.
Corn silk, gravel root, hydrangea.

**Antimicrobial**: Reduces microbial growth, same as antibacterial.

**Antioxidant**: Prevents damage from free radicals.
Astragalus, ginger, sage, turmeric.

**Antiparasitic**: kills parasites. Not to be used in excess.
Clove, elecampane, wormwood, garlic.

**Antiseptic**: Cleansing to the skin topically to prevent microbes and infection.
Calendula, sage, plantain, yarrow.

**Antispasmodic**: reduces muscle spasm, relaxes muscles.
Chamomile, cramp bark, kava, valerian.

**Antitussive**: Relieves coughing.
Elecampane, coltsfoot, poppy, thyme.

**Antitumor**: Suppresses growth of tumors.
Astragalus, burdock, echinacea, garlic, red clover.

**Antiviral**: Supports the immune system and suppresses the growth of viruses.
Elder, lemon balm, garlic, echinacea, osha.

**Aphrodisiac**: Tones reproductive organs and/or stimulates sexual desire.
Astragalus, ginseng, damiana, burdock.

**Astringent**: Constricting of tissues, used to bind swellings, bleeding, and mucous membranes.
Mullein, red raspberry, sage, yarrow.

**Bitter**: Stimulates digestion, by increasing production of bile.
Burdock, dandelion, motherwort, yarrow.

**Bronchodilator**: Relaxes bronchial muscles, to create easier breathing.
Chamomile, elecampane, peppermint, thyme.

**Calmative**: Calming to the nervous system.
Chamomile, hops, lavender, valerian.

**Carminative**: Relieves gas and griping.
Fennel, ginger, peppermint.

**Cholagogue**: Promotes bile flow from the gall bladder. These herbs also have laxative properties.
Burdock, dandelion, goldenseal.

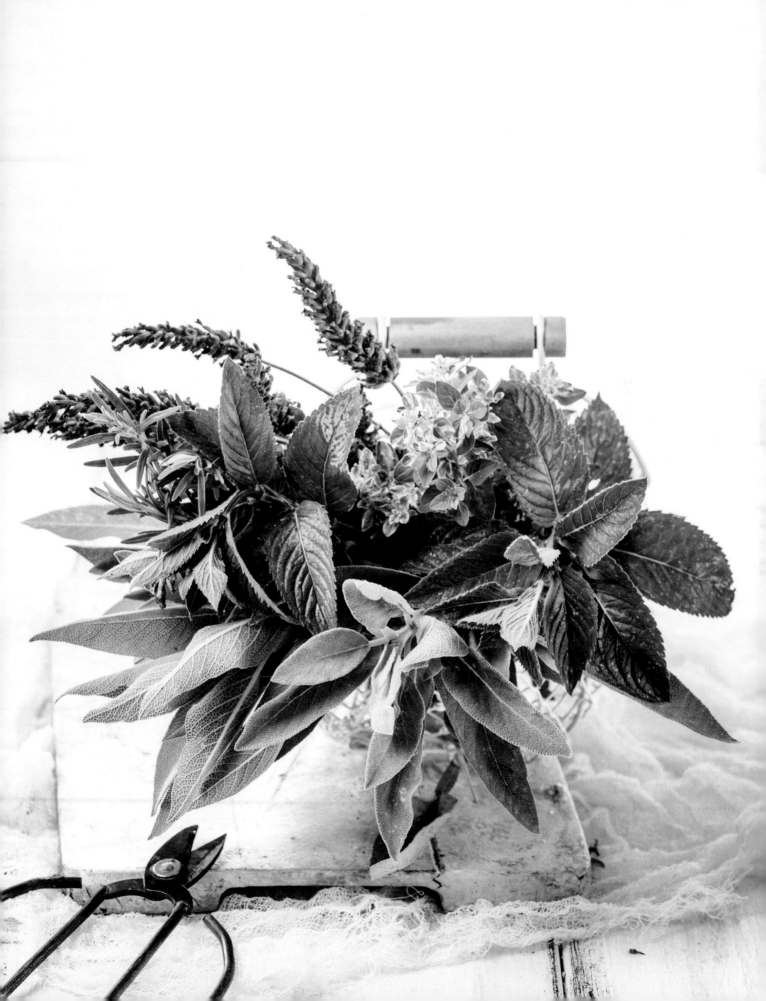

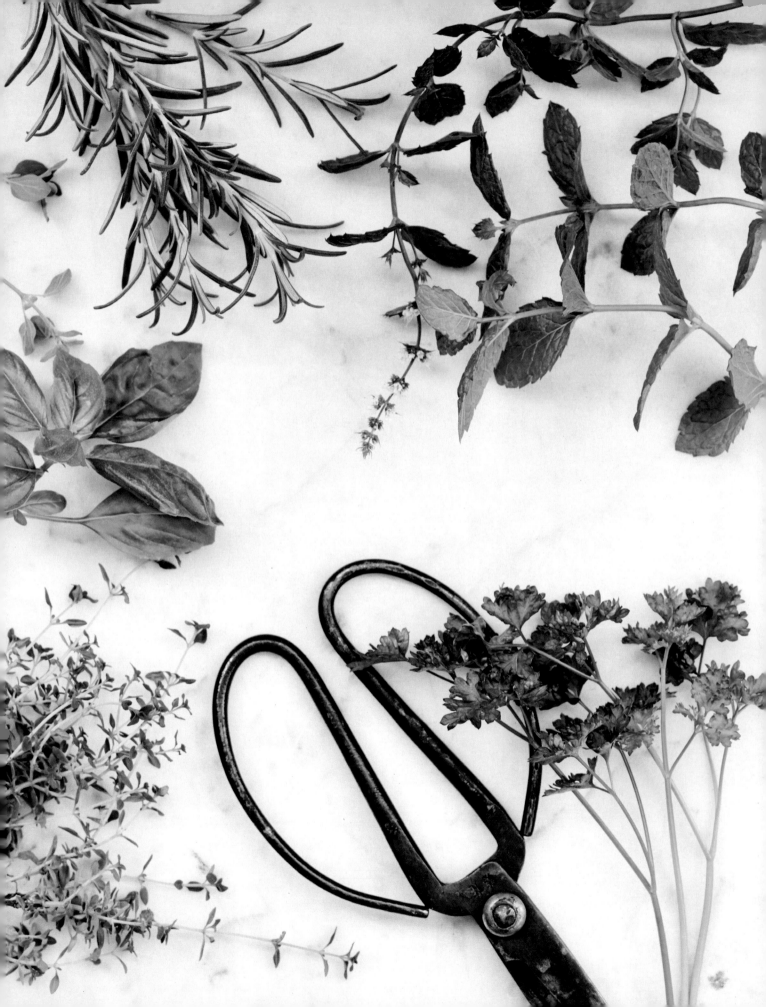

**Choleretic**: Stimulates bile production in the liver. (See Bitter and Cholagogue herbs).

**Demulcent**: Soothes and heals mucous membranes.
Marshmallow, comfrey, slippery elm, burdock, fenugreek.

**Diaphoretic**: Induces sweating.
Elder, peppermint, yarrow.

**Diuretic**: increases and stimulates urination.
Burdock, dandelion, elder, nettle, parsley.

**Emmenagogue**: Stimulates suppressed menstruation.
Blue cohosh, pennyroyal, yarrow.

**Emetic**: Induces vomiting.
Bloodroot, ipecac, lobelia.

**Emollient**: Protects, soothes, and softens the skin.
Oils of almond, apricot, sesame, and olive. Comfrey root, slippery elm, chickweed.

**Expectorant**: Expels mucus.
Comfrey, elecampane, coltsfoot, mullein, horehound.

**Galactagogue**: Increases milk flow.
Blessed thistle, fennel, dandelion, alfalfa, oat tops.

**Heart tonic**: Supports and strengthens natural functions of the heart.
Hawthorn, motherwort.

**Hemostatic**: Stops bleeding.
Cayenne, mullein, goldenseal, yellow dock.

**Hepatoprotective**: Supports normal liver function.
Burdock, dandelion, turmeric.

**Hypotensive**: Lowers blood pressure.
Garlic, ginger, hawthorn, motherwort.

**Immunomodulator**: Strengthens the immune system.
Astragalus, echinacea, garlic, St. John's wort.

**Laxative**: Promotes bowel movements.
Dandelion, yellow dock.

**Lymphagogue**: Helps lymph system to cleanse and strengthen.
Burdock, calendula, mullein, red clover.

**Nervine**: Calms the nerves.
Chamomile, motherwort, valerian.

**Nutritive**: Nourishes and strengthens the entire system.
Burdock, dandelion, nettle, plantain.

**Sedative**: Strong relaxing support to the nervous system.
Valerian, chamomile, catnip, skullcap.

**Stimulant**: Increases energy.
Echinacea, ginseng, dandelion, elecampane, sage.

**Stomachic**: See Bitter and Tonic.

**Tonic**: General promotion of functions of the entire body, or specific systems. Boosts energy on a deep level.
Nettle, dandelion, burdock, ginseng, skullcap.

**Vulnerary**: Encourages the healing of wounds and irritated tissues.
Aloe, comfrey, calendula.

# Aloe Vera

## Health Benefits

As with most plants, aloe contains a whole host of vitamins that the body needs, including A, C, E, B1, B2, B6, and B12. It also contains many minerals, such as calcium, sodium, iron, magnesium, potassium, and copper, but that's just to name a few. There are over seventy-five active components in aloe, including vitamins, minerals, amino acids, and organic compounds. It's pretty incredible what one spiky houseplant can do for your health.

Also found in aloe is a polysaccharide called acemannan, which is known to have antiviral properties as well as ease gastrointestinal problems and boost the immune system. Aloe vera also has twenty amino acids, of which seven are essential fatty acids. There's a lot packed into the aloe vera plant, but how do these components translate to your health? What do they actually do for you?

## The Ultimate Skin Remedy

We already know aloe's claim to fame of rehabilitating our chapped, burned, flaking, bodies after hours of basking in the sun—hello lobsters!—and for its ability to help heal irritations—hello rashes! When used topically, aloe gel is very effective as a treatment for a variety of skin conditions, not just the ones caused by our spring break in Cancún. The gel is able to help with a number of conditions, including cold sores, burns, abrasions, and psoriasis.

As a topical, it's been suggested as an effective treatment for first- and second-degree burns. The use of aloe is well established; the FDA approved aloe vera ointment for skin burns in 1959, and

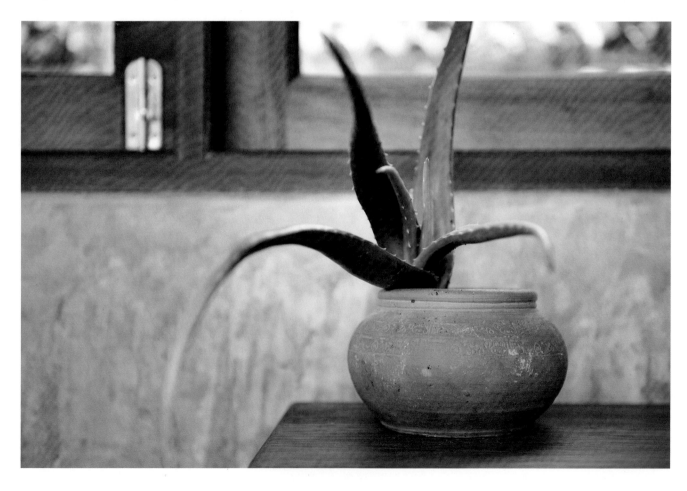

we've all been slathering it on our bodies ever since. In fact, four studies found that aloe may reduce the healing time of burns by nine days compared to conventional treatments; however, when it comes to wound healing, studies are pretty inconclusive.

## Reduces Dental Plaque

You read that right, your teeth might benefit from the delightful oozing gel of aloe. A study found that those who used aloe vera juice as a mouthwash compared to those who use standard mouthwash found that after four days, aloe was just as effective at reducing plaque as the standard products containing chlorhexidine.The results were repeated in another study during a longer time period. Apparently, aloe is able to kill the plaque-friendly bacterium *Streptococcus mutans* in the mouth as well as the yeast *Candida albicans*. Give me some aloe!

And if you are wondering why you would ever switch from your minty, delicious-tasting, last-minute toothpaste-replacement mouthwash to gross aloe juice, here are some side effects of your standard mouthwash: brown staining of teeth, increased formation of tartar, oral dryness, that awful burning sensation you get while rinsing, and the inability to drink orange juice after rinsing away.

## Antiaging

If you want yet another product for your beauty regimen, why not try aloe? One very small study found that women over the age of forty-five who topically applied the gel to their face showed an increase in collagen production and improved skin elasticity over a ninety-day period.

Collagen is found in our muscles, bones, tendons, skin, digestive system, and even our blood vessels. In fact, it's the most abundant protein in our body, and it helps our skin have elasticity and strength. Collagen helps build us, hold us together, and keeps us youthful. However, as we age, our collagen production decreases and leads to wrinkles, sagging skin, chicken legs, and other qualities no one is waiting in line for. Supplementing with products that contain collagen, such as aloe, can help us reduce the number of wrinkles and age better. Who doesn't want that?

## Ulcers and Canker Sores No More

Are you a canker sore person? What about mouth ulcers? These annoying reminders of pain are never welcome inside one's mouth and can last for over a week. A week of pain. However, some studies have shown that aloe may be a viable treatment for mouth ulcers and even speed up the healing process. It was found that an aloe vera patch applied to the area was effective at reducing the size of these unwelcome guests. And a different study found that not only did the aloe speed up the healing process, but it also reduced pain levels.

# Calendula

Newcomers to herbal medicine are often confused by the three interchangeable names, English marigold, pot marigold, and calendula, which all refer to the same plant. Although both are in the daisy family, it is important to note that the edible medicinal calendula is not the same plant as French marigold, which has a different Latin name, *Tagetes patula*, and limited medicinal use. Reputed to be the most hardy and easy-to-grow flower, it is known to ward off aphids in the garden. Collect the vibrant yellow orange petals when blooming throughout the summer and use as edibles in salads or dried for numerous applications in herbal medicine.

**Constituents**: volatile oils, flavonoids (quercetin, rutin), triterpenes (saponins), carotenoids, bitter principles, polysaccharides

**Medicinal Actions**: Calendula is an antiseptic, disinfectant, and wound healer. I always pack calendula tincture for travel as well as for a home first aid antiseptic and vulnerary for healing open cuts and wounds. It is anti-inflammatory, astringent, antimicrobial, antiseptic, cholinergic, emmenagogue, diaphoretic, digestive, hemostatic, bitter, anticatarrhal, antifungal, antispasmodic, antibacterial, anthelmintic, and immune stimulant.

**Applications**: infusion, tincture, poultice, infused oil, herb bath, poultice, cream, salve, throat gargle, syrup, fomentation, salve, spray

Think of calendula as the go-to wound healer for reducing inflammation and irritation and for preventing infection. The tincture or a cream is all you really need for open wounds. As a wound healer and antiseptic herb, the actions of calendula are unprecedented. Calendula helps speed up rapid epithelization of tissues, stimulating skin healing and preventing infection from any open wound, scratches, and ulcers. I use this herb topically for any and all nicks in the skin instead of over-the-counter

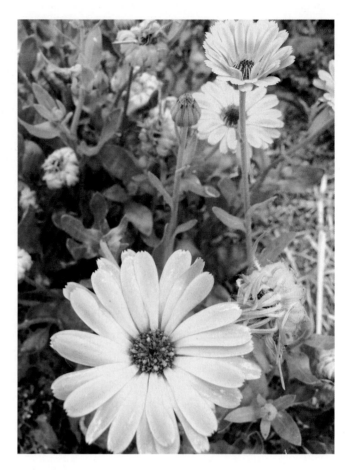

medicated creams, such as Polysporin. As an antiseptic and for speeding up the healing of wounds, it is an excellent base cream to which additional tinctures or essential oils may be added to create a custom cream.

Think of calendula as an internal and external antiseptic. Its antimicrobial properties offer value for both internal immunity as well as skin infections such as athlete's foot, abscesses, cold sores, and the virus that causes shingles.

Prepare an infused oil of calendula for cradle cap in an infant, and ever so gently massage the infused oil into the crusty, scaly areas of excess sebum. After a day or so, the crusts will dry out and separate from the scalp and can then be gently lifted off the scalp.

As a cream, poultice, herbal wash, or infused oil, calendula can be used to treat the skin of dry, cracked heels. It even reduces inflammation and ensures immediate healing for nipples that are raw from breastfeeding. For the inflammation of mastitis or for mumps or gland inflammation, prepare a poultice.

- As an anti-inflammatory and antiseptic: apply to swellings, sunburn, rashes, ulcers, wounds, sores as a poultice or wash.
- For an eyewash: prepare an infusion for eye inflammations, conjunctivitis, and seasonal allergies.
- As a bitter digestive tonic to enhance digestion and improve liver function and bile flow: prepare a tincture or tea.
- To stop bleeding: take internally and apply externally.
- For allergies and sinus congestion: combine with nettles, plantain, and goldenrod as a tea or tincture for antihistamine properties.

- For athlete's foot or stubborn toenail infection: mix with other antiseptic herbs, such as oregano, as an antifungal footbath.
- For varicose veins: prepare a poultice with red raspberry.
- For strep, tonsillitis, thrush, and sore, bleeding gums: use a throat gargle with an infusion or tincture.
- For antidiarrheal effects and astringent, binding properties for loose bowel movements: use a tincture or strong infusion.
- For candida yeast infection and leukorrhea: prepare an infusion of calendula, thyme, and chamomile—using equal parts as a topical wash.

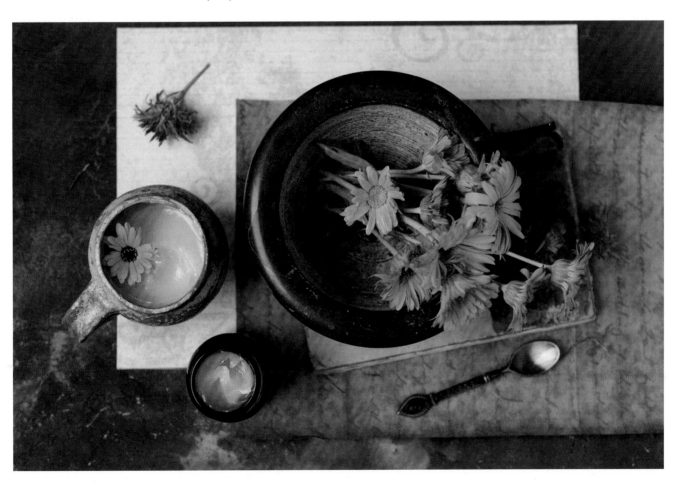

# Chamomile

Chamomile is an herb to know, use, and grow if you can. Consider it an important ingredient in your herbal medicine cabinet. It offers numerous gentle benefits for the whole body from digestive support, anxiety, and insomnia to pain and hormonal support.

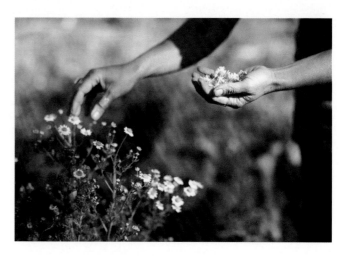

Many species of chamomile are used interchangeably for their medicinal action, including wild, German, and Roman chamomile. The German chamomile (also known as blue chamomile) contains higher concentrations of azulene.

Chamomile grows up to two feet in height with delicate wispy leaves (look for the leaves and the flower heads for accurate plant identification). Look closely at the flowers and flower center; the characteristic yellow center is surrounded by one row of white petals. Distinguish between the leaves of chamomile and pineapple weed, a shorter, smaller plant without petals (yet similar leaves). Feverfew has similar flower petals, yet with thicker, fuller leaves.

The flower heads are used medicinally and typically harvested days after opening throughout the spring and summer, ensuring the highest concentration of chemical constituents. The taste is bitter and is coupled with an aromatic scent characteristic of the plant.

**Constituents**: volatile oils (azulene, chamazulene, and bisabolol), flavonoids (apigenin, quercetin, apiin, rutin), coumarins, tannins, bitter glycosides. The essential oils azulene and chamazulene both offer strong antiseptic and anti-inflammatory properties for cramping and spasms of the digestive, reproductive, and urinary tracts. It also has antiallergic effects.

**Medicinal Actions**: relaxant, carminative, antispasmodic, anticatarrhal, antimicrobial, antiseptic, digestive bitter, wound healer, anti-inflammatory

**Applications**: infusion, tincture, poultice, infused oil, fomentation, cream, salve, honey, hair rinse, salve, wash, body care, capsules

Chamomile is a traditional children's remedy for colic, anxiousness, hyperactivity, and insomnia. Many a child has been coaxed into dream time with a small dose of chamomile tea or tincture. Chamomile offers adults dose-dependant support for tension, anxiety, and insomnia. Consider preparing an herbal tea as a bath for an infant with colic and fussiness, or for a young tot with restlessness or chronic stomachache. For a loved one who is showing the effects of long-term stress and worry, prepare a strong tea and ensure it is consumed in several cupfuls throughout the day. Chamomile is a non-habit-forming sedative of value for both long-term and occasional use.

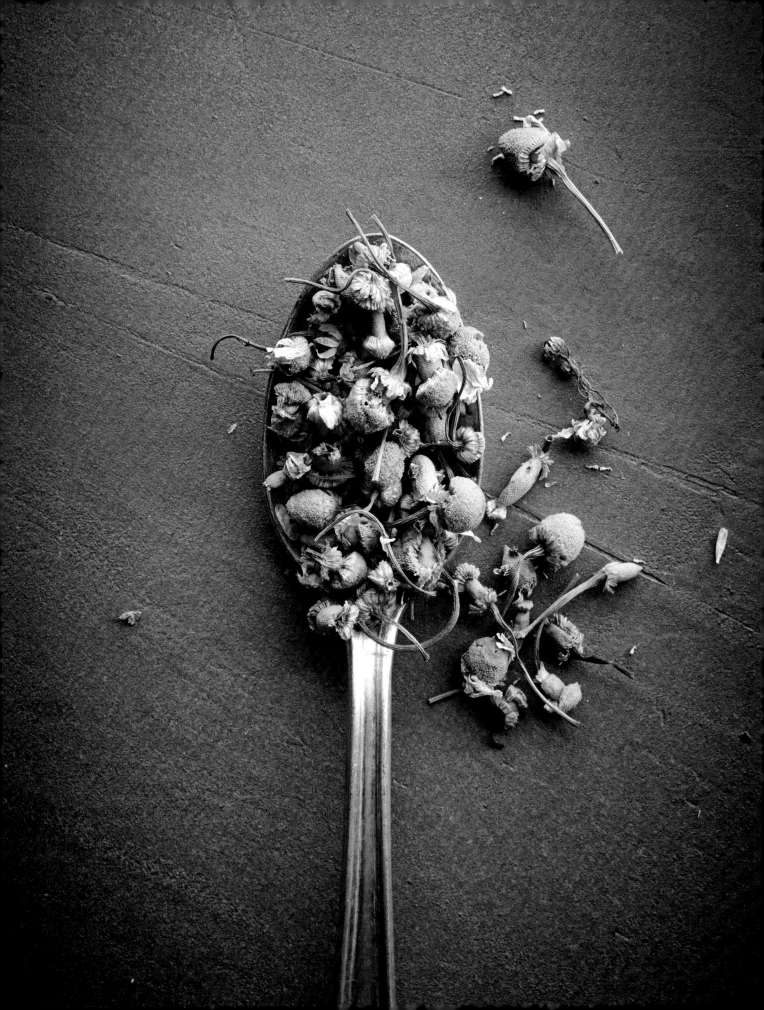

# Chickweed

Chickweed, one of the most common weeds, is found growing in all parts of the world. The French common name Stellaire refers to a constellation of the stars named after the heavens' brilliant stardust. Chickweed has also been called starweed and starwort because of its divided, tiny, white, star-shaped flower heads with ten tiny-rayed narrow petals. It is found nestled in the five green sepals surrounding the petals.

Look for a trailing plant with a tangled mat of delicate, lush green stems, and egg-shaped leaves formed into a point and placed on the stem in equal pairs (with or without a leaf stalk depending upon the species). For positive plant identification, look even closer and notice the tiny white tufts of fine hairs running vertically up one side of the stem only.

The herb is gathered from May through July in the northern hemisphere. The whole herb is used medicinally, and this delicate, tiny plant is a delicious edible green added into salads. It can be prepared fresh, steamed briefly (no more than five minutes), or dried and stored for future use. Some species are very furry, requiring brief cooking to make them more palatable.

**Constituents**: saponins, coumarins, triterpenoids, flavonoids, ascorbic acid. Chickweed is a nutritional powerhouse, providing vitamin C, rutin, vitamin A, vitamin D, folic acid, riboflavin, niacin, and thiamine, as well as the minerals calcium, potassium, manganese, zinc, iron, phosphorus, sodium, copper, and silica.

**Medicinal Use**: refrigerant, demulcent, vulnerary, alterative, anti-itch, emollient, mild laxative, antirheumatic

**Applications**: poultice, nutritive green in salads, infusion, infused oil, salve, herbal bath, skin wash, fomentation, juiced, tincture

Chickweed is viewed by herbalists as a refrigerant, an agent used to remove excess heat from the body. Think of it for relief from inflamed and hot, itchy skin. Chickweed's cooling anti-inflammatory actions make an ideal application for hot swellings, skin ulcers, infections, abscesses, eczema, cradle cap, diaper rash, sunburns, dry skin, and wound healing of all kinds. Any topical application will work, though I am fond of chickweed-infused oil, poultices, and salve for topical afflictions.

- Chickweed is a spring tonic and gentle cleanser with slight laxative properties, called a depurative or cleanser. Use the fresh juice of chickweed as a morning tonic and purifying blood cleanser for stubborn, itchy skin conditions.
- A galactogogue of benefit to increase lactation in breastfeeding mothers.
- Eyewash: prepare an infusion of chickweed for irritation and inflammation.
- Well-known Canadian herbalist and elder Terry Willard uses chickweed for its stomach-healing properties in circumstances where there is bleeding in the digestive tract or the lungs

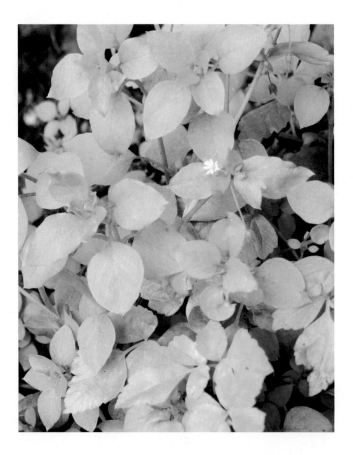

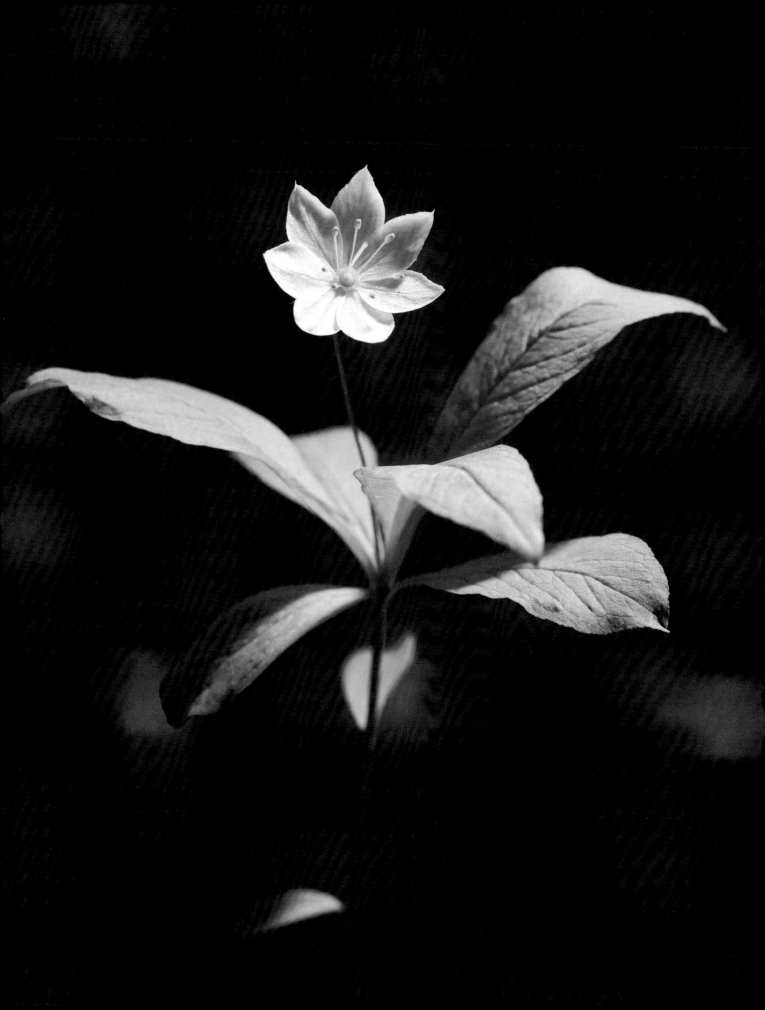

# Daisy

Daisy was once a popular medicinal herb; however, the invaluable lung tonic is not used today with the same frequency. The Latin name, *bellis*, translates to "beautiful," which is probably why the daisy is a symbol of purity and survival. Ironically, it is also considered an invasive weed; or perhaps it is one of nature's subtle reminders of perseverance. Many related plants share the common name "daisy." It has many synonyms: common daisy, lawn daisy or English daisy, the more descriptive bruise-wort, and occasionally woundwort (referring to the wound-healing properties of the plant). Both dried and fresh aerial plant parts (flower heads, stalks, and leaves) are used medicinally and can be picked between March and October.

**Constituents of flower**: organic acids; minerals; volatile oils; inulin; flavonoids—flavones, glycosides and aglycones (quercetin, apigenin, kaempferol, rutin)—tannins; malic, acetic, and oxalic acids; resin; wax

**Constituents of roots**: triterpenoid saponins (primarily in the roots) Kaempferol, one of the daisy's flavonoids, supplies antioxidant, anti-inflammatory, antimicrobial, and nerve-protective properties.

**Medicinal Actions of the whole plant**: mild astringent, demulcent, emollient, vulnerary, demulcent, antimicrobial, anticatarrhal, digestive tonic, liver and kidney tonic, antidiarrheal, anti-inflammatory, diaphoretic, febrifuge, anodyne, antispasmodic, antitussive and expectorant, antiarthritic, laxative

**Applications**: herbal vinegar, infusion, poultice, skin wash, tincture, bath. Consider this plant a blood cleanser useful for skin afflictions such as eczema when taken internally with other alterative herbs, such as burdock and nettle.

The astringent nature of the plant makes it useful for internal and external hemorrhage, inflammation of the digestive tract, and cramping. Prepare a tea and use as a mouth rinse, gargling for a sore throat and inflamed gums.

- For mouth ulcers: chew fresh leaves.
- As an insect repellent: prepare an infusion in a spray bottle and apply to the skin.
- For a cold, flu, or cough: use the tincture or infusion for its diaphoretic properties.
- For headaches: prepare a compress on the head.
- As a digestive tonic: the tea or tincture helps to increase the appetite and acts as a gentle bitter tonic.
- For menorrhagia or excessive menstrual flow: combine with other hormone balancers and astringent-rich plants.
- As an antispasmodic: apply topically for bruises, sprains, and symptoms of arthritis.
- As a compress: mix with plantain to offer support for acne and rashes.
- For a dry cough or bronchitis: prepare a gentle, soothing tea.
- For wound healing, rashes, skin inflammations, bruises, swollen feet, and ulcers: apply topically (poultice, skin wash).
- For perineum tearing during childbirth: prepare a poultice.

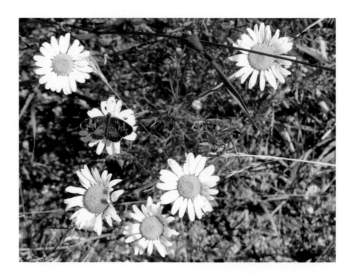

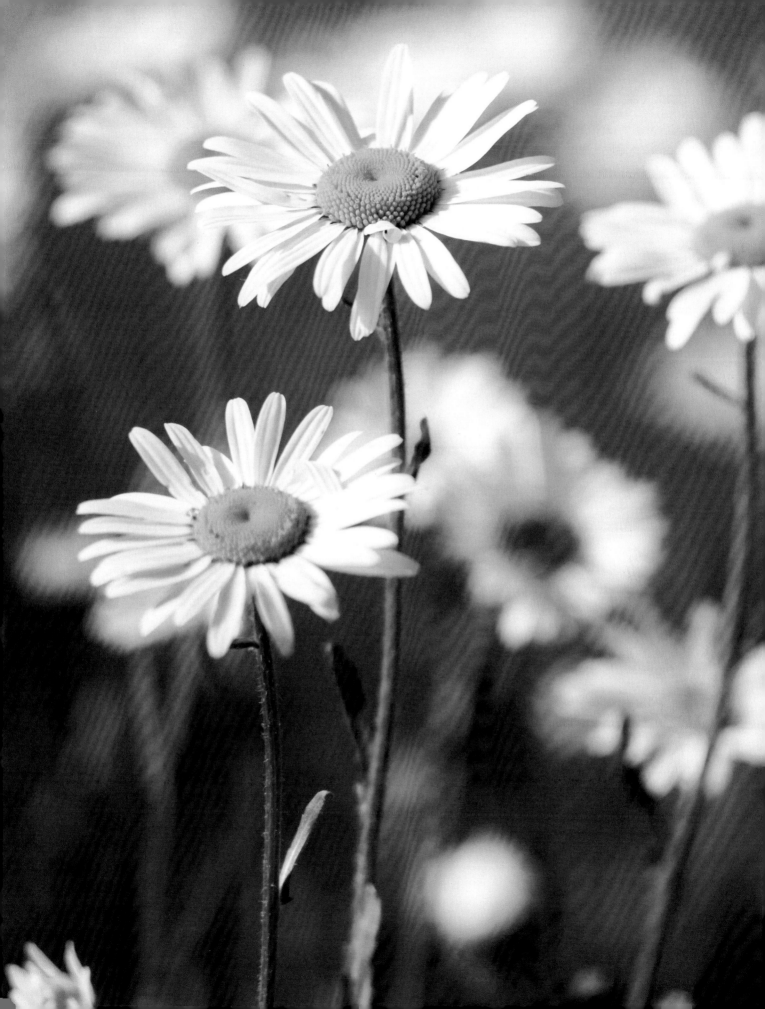

# Lavender

The word "lavender" comes from the Old French, *lavandre*, with the Latin root *lavare*, meaning "to wash." Historically, lavender has been used to wash laundry, imparting a fresh scent to the sudsy wash. There are over thirty-nine known species of lavender, such as *Lavandula vera* and *Lavandula angustifolia*, which can be used interchangeably. The leaf shape varies depending upon the species. The flowers appear as whorls on spikes, varying in color from light bluish tones to violet and dark purple.

**Constituents**: volatile oil, flavonoids, triterpenes, flavonoids, coumarins, saponins, tannins

**Medicinal Actions**: cholagogue, carminative, neuralgia, nervous system tonic, insect repellent, body care and cosmetic use

**Applications**: infusion, wash, tincture, infused oil, poultice, fomentation, honey, vinegar

Lavender's flowers are used medicinally. The aromatic scent of its flowers balances the nervous system. It is one of those herbs that help bring the body back into balance, reestablishing equilibrium. It can be used in the daytime for symptoms of uneasiness, agitation, and turbulent thoughts and as a gentle antidepressant to help brighten low spirits during intense stress and enhance feelings of calm and well-being. It is also known as a sedative herb, used at night for symptoms of sleeplessness, and as a carminative herb for heartburn, acid indigestion, and digestive upset.

Lavender is effective as a valuable antispasmodic for burning or shooting pain along nerves, painful joints, muscular cramping, or connective tissue discomfort. Apply herbs topically or soak in a bath with Epsom salt and lavender.

**First aid application**: The essential oil of lavender is my favorite first aid application for burns to prevent blistering from scalds and burns of all kinds. The analgesic properties take the pain out of the burn while the essential oil is antiseptic. If applied frequently enough at the onset of the event, it may prevent blistering altogether.

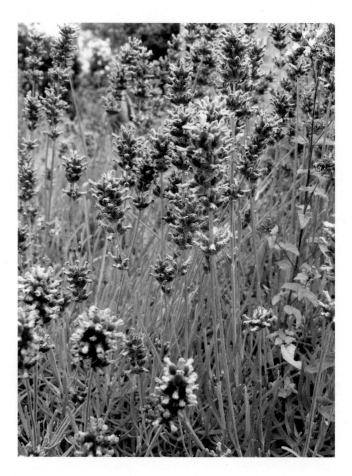

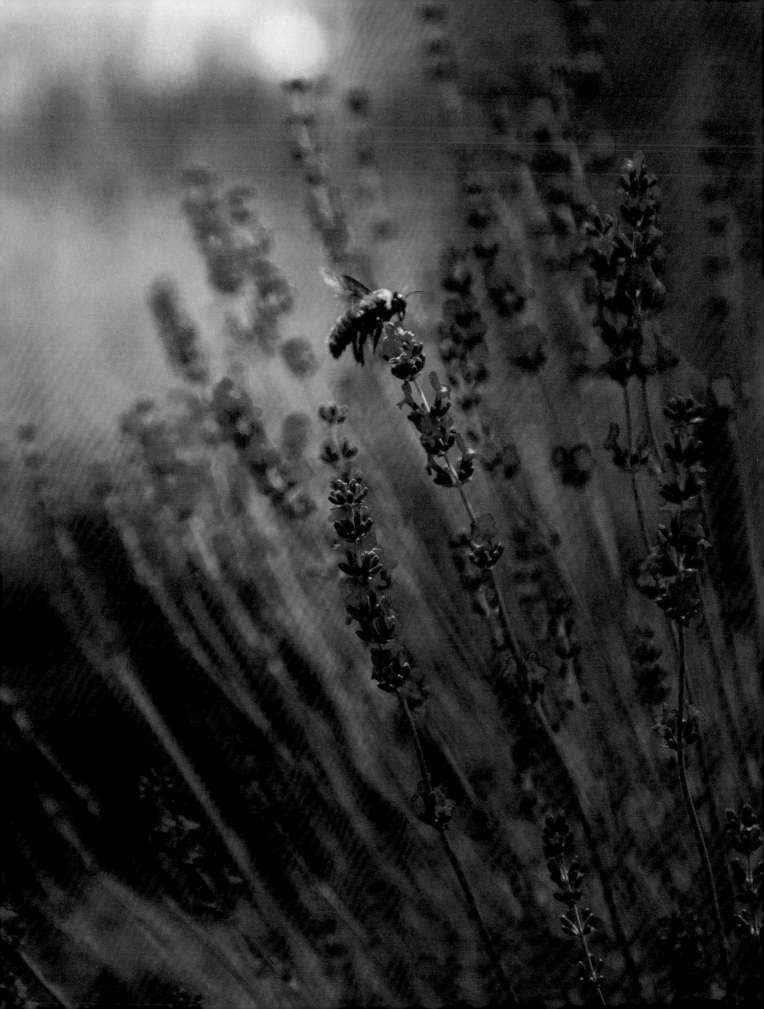

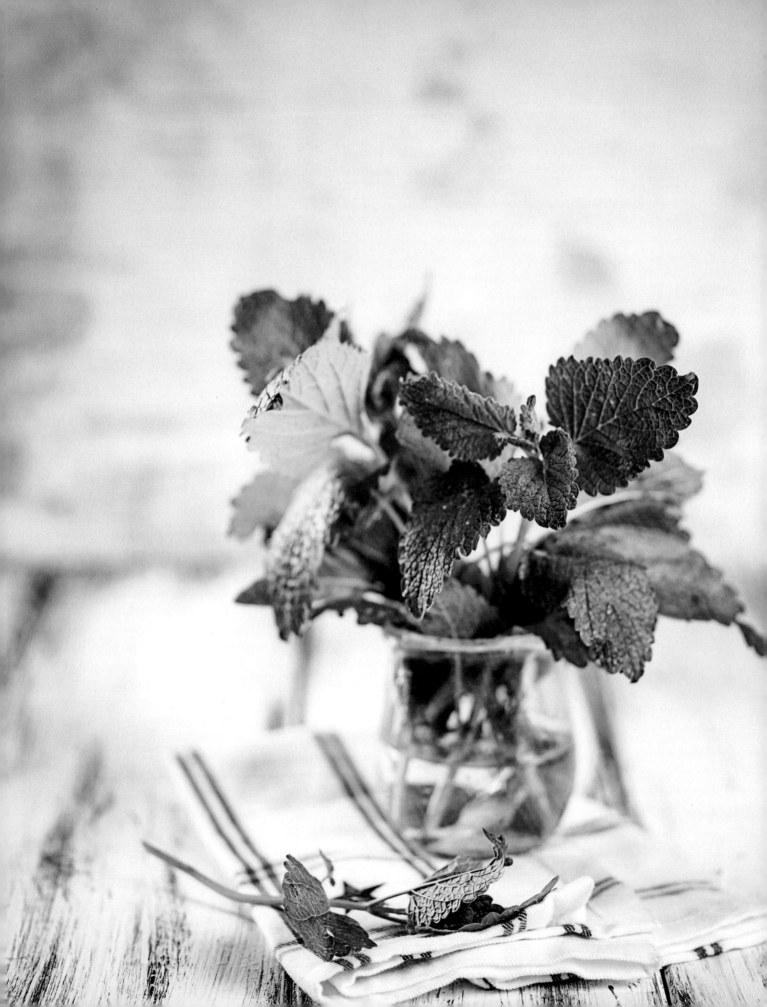

# Lemon Balm

The Greek word *melissa* refers to the honey or sweet nectar found in the flowers. Thus, lemon balm has been called "bee balm" and "the honey plant" as well as the descriptive term of "cure all." For centuries, lemon balm has been used to uplift the spirits and alleviate the blues, promoting a bright, cheerful disposition.

It is a perennial herb that likes full sun. For positive plant identification, notice the heart-shaped leaves, appearing opposite or at right angles to the previous leaf on a square stem. Lemon balm is easy to grow through planting seeds or spring stem cuttings. The aerial plant parts—including its leaves, stem, and flowers—are used medicinally.

**Chemical Constituents:** volatile oils, flavonoids, polyphenols (tannins, rosmarinic acid), triterpenes, bitter principles

**Medicinal Actions:** carminative, febrifuge, diaphoretic, sedative, antispasmodic, antiviral

**Applications:** infusion, essential oil, tincture, cream, oil, poultice, honey, vinegar, bath, salve, fomentation

The volatile oils can be immediately released by crushing the fresh flower or leaves with your hand (inhale the lemon scent). These constituents play a key role in the sedative properties. They have relaxing and antispasmodic effects for all digestive upsets, including a nervous stomach and associated cramping, overeating, gas, heartburn, and digestive upset. There are also benefits for painful menstruation and headaches. Lemon balm is a gentle, sedative herb to counter frequent worries, anxiety, and insomnia. It is good for sedating children who are high energy or those who are sensitive with frequent stomachaches. Traditionally, lemon balm was used to uplift the spirits when one feels blue. Brew a tea in a bath for a young child to encourage relaxation before bed.

With its antiviral and diaphoretic properties, lemon balm is great for flu and cold symptoms.

The antiviral properties are due to polyphenols filling receptor sites on cells, thus if the receptor site is filled, there is no room for the virus to attach. So think of it for all types of viral infections such as Epstein-Barr virus, mononucleosis, cold sores, and viral-related nerve pain. Apply topically to the lingering phantom nerve pain after a shingles outbreak, and apply a poultice for sciatica. The more concentrated essential oil of melissa also works well topically in salves for cold sores or related herpesviruses.

Excessive ingestion of lemon balm should be avoided by those with an underactive thyroid, as "it may decrease serum and pituitary levels of Thyroid Stimulating Hormone." This does however make an ideal herb for overactive/hyperactive thyroid conditions, reducing symptoms associated with the condition of nervousness, agitation, and generally feeling wired.

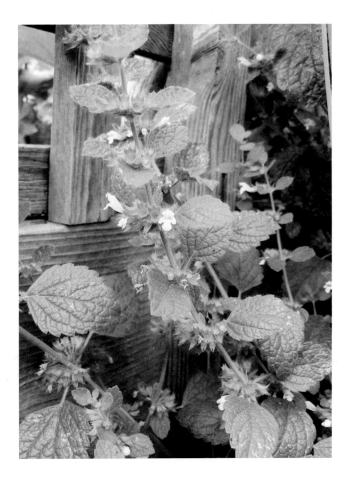

# Mint

With so many varieties of mint, one can dive deep into discovering the various subtle flavors. All can be used interchangeably, with the whole aerial plant (stem, leaves, and flowering tops) used medicinally. Mints are harvested in the summer or spring and have square stems, slightly ridged, serrated leaves, and are generally oval or round in shape; the flowers bloom throughout the summer with white, pink, or purple flowers.

Constituents: volatile oil (menthol, carvone, limonene, and others), flavonoids

In the case of spearmint, one of the volatile oils includes menthol, a cooling agent and local anesthetic. Recall the effects of mint-flavored toothpaste in the mouth? Menthol binds to receptors, which trigger a cooling sensation, beneficial for itching and decreasing the sensation of pain. Spearmint is slightly less cooling than peppermint.

Medicinal Actions: diaphoretic, antispasmodic, carminative, analgesic, decongestant, anti-inflammatory, weakly antiviral, digestive tonic

Applications: infusion, tincture, essential oil, salves, creams, poultice, fomentation, honey, syrup, vinegar

- As a digestive aid (for indigestion, nausea, gas, and bloating): prepare infusion or tincture or topically apply a diluted essential oil or poultice to the abdomen.
- For headaches: prepare an infusion, tincture, essential oil or poultice.
- For toothaches: prepare a topical poultice, tincture, or infusion.
- As a cold and flu remedy: ingest internally as a diaphoretic and use as a steam for congested sinuses.
- As a gentle antispasmodic and anti-cramp remedy: use the tincture, infusion, or poultice.

Spearmint gently supports the entire processes of digestion. The volatile oils in the plant are responsible for the characteristic scent of all mints and their carminative nature. It is used for settling the stomach, relaxing smooth muscles of the digestive tract, minimizing cramping, alleviating bloating and a gaseous stomach linked with overeating, colic and general acid indigestion, and settling an upset stomach related to worry and tension, nausea, and travel sickness.

All herbal tea blends created for immune-system support will benefit from the addition of spearmint due to its antiviral and diaphoretic nature, encouraging sweating and lowering an elevated fever and high temperature. The characteristic flavor is a welcome taste enhancer. It makes any medicinal tea more palatable, and the volatile oils—when inhaled—can disinfect and open the sinus passages in cases of congestion. Remember to contain the volatile oils by keeping a lid on the brewing tea until consumption.

Add spearmint tincture or a couple drops of essential oil into a lip balm for prevention from cold sores and the herpes simplex virus, or use it on an insect bite, or for itch relief from dermatitis. Known as a cooling, analgesic herb used for athletic stiffness. Apply as a poultice, oil, massage oil, herbal wash, or in a cream for topical relief.

The essential oil of spearmint, which is not the same as the dried herb, is much stronger. It can provide benefit for the pain of headaches and migraines when inhaled or diluted in a carrier oil, such as almond oil or grape-seed oil, and gently applied to the temples.

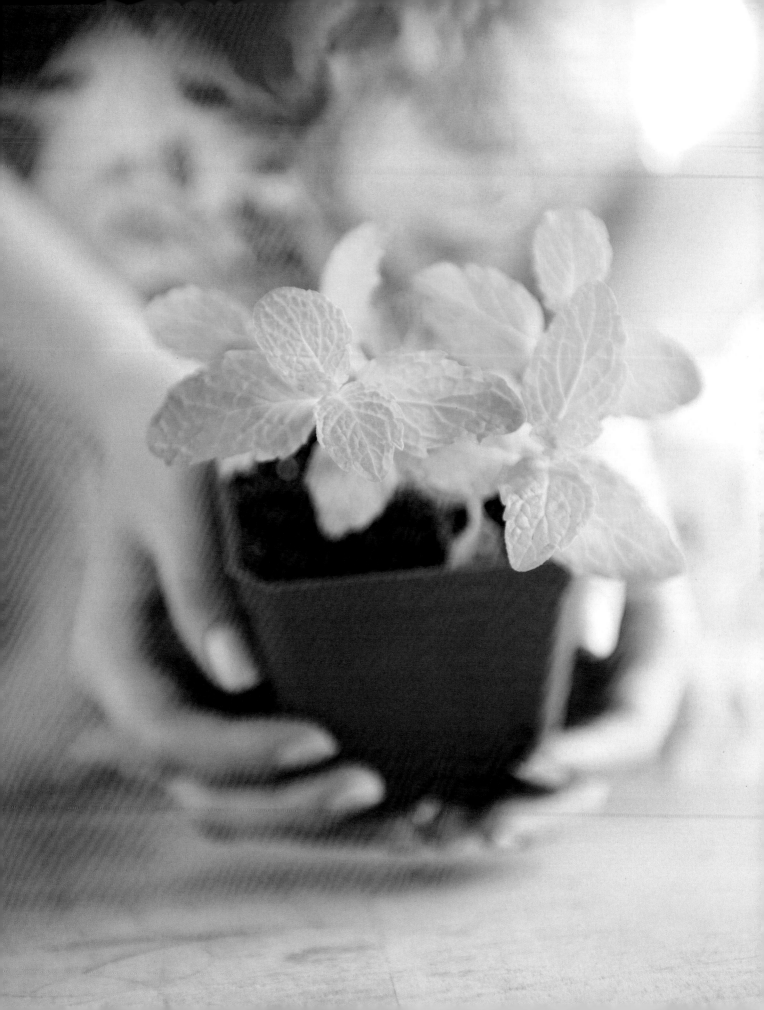

# Oregano

Oregano is a popular remedy on the market in the last couple of years and another example of Mother Nature's potent medicines. Perhaps most widely known for its antimicrobial properties, oregano can be used to address infections like *H. pylori* infections, candida, opportunistic parasitic infections, fungus such as athlete's foot, and respiratory and skin infections. Oregano is native to the Mediterranean and is recognized by its white and pink flowers and tiny green leaves. The leaves and seeds are used medicinally.

Used frequently as an immune tonic for labored and difficult breathing and symptoms of a cold and flu, the potency of this herb is not in question; however, it is important to be clear about the modes of application. The tea and tincture of oregano are available for ingestion in small dosages. The essential oil of oregano is very strong and needs to be extremely diluted in a base oil prior to topical use. Oregano, in correct administration, provides antibacterial properties against gram-positive and -negative bacteria, including salmonella, *Escherichia coli*, and staphylococcus, and many other growing risks of antibiotic-resistant infections. The chemical constituents carvacrol and thymol are most concentrated in the essential oil and are responsible for the antioxidant, antimicrobial, and antifungal actions. Oregano, prepared as an infusion or tincture, offers effective antiseptic support for urinary tract and lung infections as well as gum inflammation and indigestion. The volatile oils from a tea are carminative in nature, good for digestive upset and trapped abdominal gas.

**Constituents**: volatile oils containing phenols (carvacrol, thymol, pinene), phenolic acids (rosmarinic acids, caffeic acid), flavonoids, saponins, bitter principles

**Medicinal Actions**: antifungal, antibacterial, antioxidant, antispasmodic, antimicrobial, antiseptic, carminative, analgesic

**Applications**: infusion, tincture, liniment, poultice, fomentation, infused oil, vinegar, honey, salve, essential oil

Prepare a strong infusion as an antiseptic for a sore throat and gargle several times throughout the day. Ingest the tea for symptoms of a cold and drink to relieve an elevated fever. Keep the tea covered until ready for use and inhale the potent volatile oils to open up the sinus passages.

Use as a topical preparation, as an antispasmodic and pain-relief herb for general aches, muscle pains, rheumatism, and arthritis. Topically, the effect of oregano is rubefacient, sending fresh blood flow to localized tissues and working as an antiseptic wash for open wounds and sores.

Caution: May be irritating to the skin and mucous membranes for susceptible individuals—try on a small area with a reduced dose first. Avoid use during pregnancy.

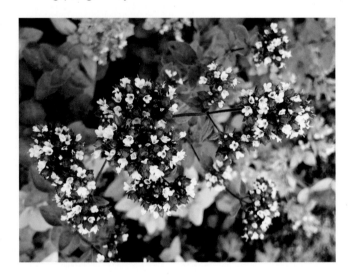

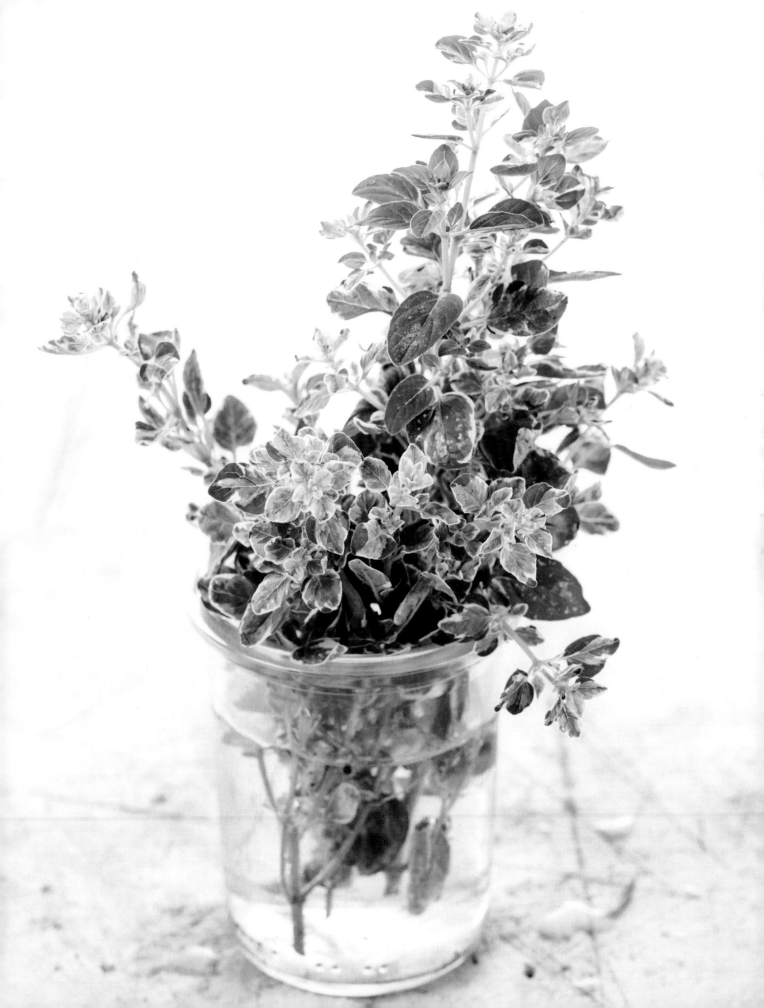

# Parsley

Parsley is a recognized food worldwide. Adding a delicious green flavor to foods, it is also considered an herbal medicine. There are many species. Italian parsley, common parsley, and rock parsley are all effective. The leaf is harvested in the summer months and used as a garnish in cooking. The root is used in fall. The whole plant's herb (leaves and stem), root, and seed are used medicinally. The root is considered an edible root vegetable and a liver tonic herb.

**Chemical Constituents**: volatile oil (apiol, myristicin, eugenol, thujene, pinene), vitamins C, E, flavonoids (apigenin, luteolin), iron and folic acid, coumarins
**Medicinal Actions**: diuretic, blood purifier, digestive tonic, galactagogue, emmenagogue, carminative, antiseptic, expectorant, anti-inflammatory
**Applications**: infusion, food, juiced, topical application, hair rinse

Parsley leaf is a chlorophyll-rich, nutritious food, remineralizing to the body. 100g of fresh parsley leaf contains 138mg calcium, 6.2mg iron, 50mg magnesium, 1.07mg zinc, 133mg vitamin C, 8424 IU vitamin A, and 1640 ug vitamin K. Parsley is a rich source of calcium and also contains trace amounts of zinc and boron, both of which assist in the metabolism and absorption of calcium. Parsley is an ideal green food addition to a diet with iron deficiency when the leaf is eaten raw, sprinkled over vegetables, added to stews, or blended into your favorite mixed greens.

As a spring tonic, parsley is cleansing and assists removal of waste matter and uric acid from the body. It is supportive to the liver and kidneys. Reach for its nutritious properties for arthritis, gout, and joint stiffness, and to provide essential nutrients and minerals for healthy hair and strong nails.

Parsley's diuretic effect is attributed to the flavonoid content and the volatile oils myristicin and apiole, which are of benefit for swollen ankles, for fluid retention related to premenstrual syndrome, and any condition relating to lack of urine flow. The whole plant can be used to encourage the release of fluid from body tissues, although the seed may be most effective.

It is considered a dose-dependent emmenagogue (an agent that regulates and promotes or brings on menstruation). Apiol, one of the numerous volatile oils, is responsible for this action. For this reason, do not use during pregnancy. After birth, however, reach for parsley to offer assistance with returning the uterus to its previous size and proportions. In addition, parsley poultices may assist with tender, engorged breasts and assist in drying up milk once breastfeeding has ended.

- For skin infections: prepare as an antiseptic topical application.
- For head lice: juice fresh parsley and use as a hair rinse.
- For gas, bloating, and indigestion: prepare a carminative tea.
- For natural breath-freshening properties: munch on leaves after eating.
- As a natural deodorant: consume the fresh leaves and prepare tea.

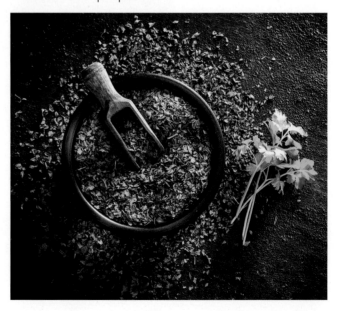

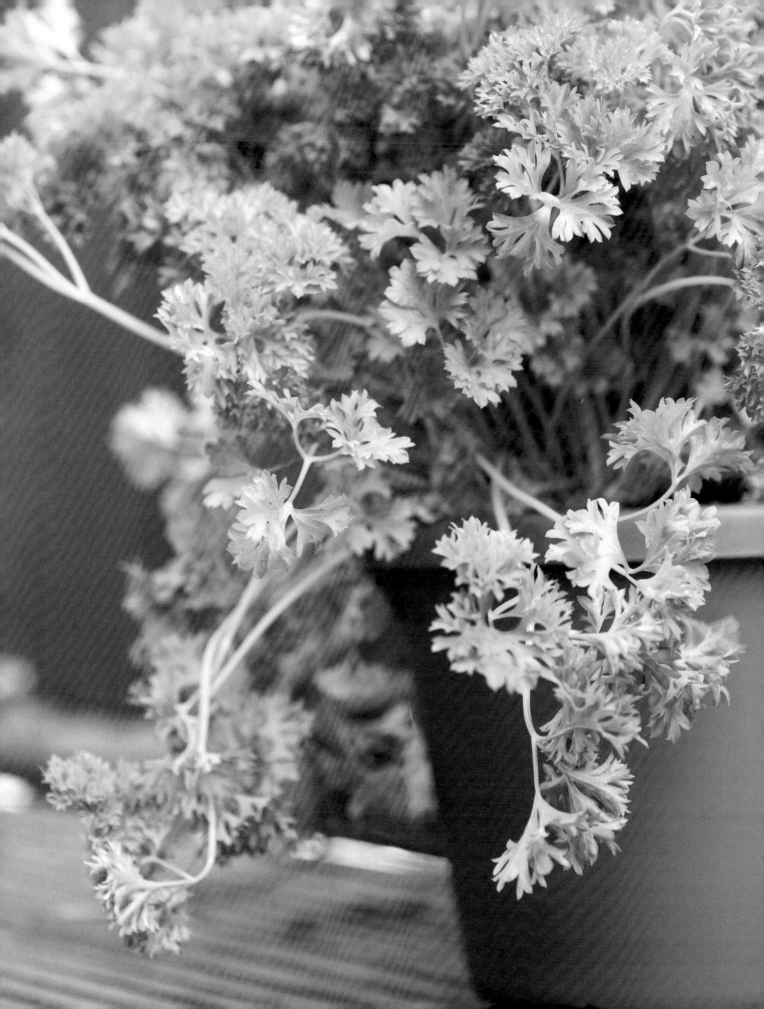

# Rosemary

Often thought of as a culinary herb, rosemary is more than just a garnish, and despite its name, rosemary has nothing to do with roses or a woman named Mary. Actually, the name stems from the Latin word *rosmarinus*, which means "dew of the sea," a reference to its light blue flowers and love for wet environments.

A member of the mint family, rosemary has been traditionally used in Mediterranean cuisine; you might recognize it doused in olive oil, sprinkled over chicken, and eventually lodged in between your two front teeth. Its anti-inflammatory effects and antioxidant properties promote health and wellness and provide many health benefits, which include improving digestion, helping prevent hair loss, reducing skin irritations, enhancing memory, promoting eye health, and perhaps even preventing brain aging.

Recorded uses of rosemary date back to 500 BC, when it was used by the ancient Romans and Greeks for its medicinal, culinary, and mystical properties. Roman gardens almost always had rosemary bushes, and many believed they grew only in the gardens of those who were righteous, while protecting people from evil spirits. Today, we also use rosemary as a means to protect us, but for health purposes rather than evil ghosts.

If you're a fan of English literature, Shakespeare's Juliet was buried with rosemary as an honor of her remembrance—many early Europeans were buried with sprigs of rosemary as a symbol that the dead would not be forgotten. To this day rosemary is used as a funeral flower, symbolizing remembrance and respect for those who have passed. But death isn't rosemary's only claim to fame; love and romance often look to rosemary as a fixture in weddings, courtships, and fidelity. However, I don't believe bringing home a sprig of rosemary would do much today to make your beloved swoon. Although maybe a potted rosemary plant would!

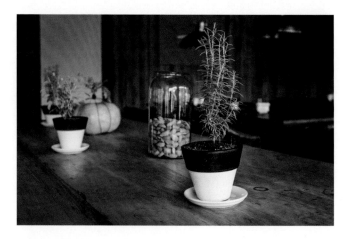

## Health Benefits

Rosemary's unique past shows the importance of this culinary herb, often overlooked not only in culture and tradition but also for its healing properties. When eating your favorite Mediterranean dishes, you might not be aware that the rosemary garnish is a good source of calcium, iron, potassium, magnesium, manganese, and vitamin B6, and recent research has discovered many potential health benefits related to memory and concentration, preventing hair loss, reducing stress, and improving digestion, just to name a few. After learning about the various health benefits of this herbal sprig, rosemary will never look or taste the same again.

### Improves Digestion

Approved for the treatment of digestion by Germany's Commission E, rosemary is used by many Europeans as a digestive aid, although there isn't a lot of scientific evidence to support this claim. It's important to note, however, that research has a long way to catch up with herbal medicine, and that shouldn't stop you from safely using herbs to improve your life and health. Thousands of years of tradition and anecdotal evidence should be noted. In this case, rosemary has a lot of history for its use in digestion, such as helping reduce gas, upset stomach, and indigestion.

## Improves Memory and Concentration

For thousands of years, one of the most popular uses for rosemary has been to improve memory. The Greeks would place rosemary sprigs in their hair while studying for tests, and it was often used as an aromatherapy for cognitive decline due to aging. Research from *Therapeutic Advances in Psychopharmacology* has found that the aroma of rosemary essential oil affects cognition and improves a person's concentration, accuracy, mood, and performance. Try it next time when you have a big meeting or need to study for a big exam—make sure to study with a few drops of the essential oil on your temples and wrists. The aroma of rosemary will trigger your memory recall and help you ace those big moments.

A different study tested the effects of rosemary on cognitive function in an elderly population and found that rosemary essential oil had a significant benefit for their performance and overall memory and improved the speed of retrieving memories. In fact, speed of memory is a predictor of cognitive function during aging, and rosemary was found to have a statistically significant effect.

## Fights Cancer

Numerous studies have found that rosemary can play a role in preventing diseases such as colorectal, breast, and ovarian cancer. Rosemary extract contains numerous polyphenols, such as carnosic acid, carnosol, and rosmarinic acid, all of which inhibit the proliferation of certain cancer cell lines.

A study published in *Bioscience, Biotechnology, and Biochemistry* found that rosemary is useful as an antitumor agent. And, interestingly, adding rosemary extract to ground beef can reduce the formation of cancer-causing agents that may develop while cooking. Make sure to take some rosemary extract to your next barbecue!

## Improves Hair

Historically, rosemary has been used to treat a variety of hair problems from hair loss to dandruff, making hair thicker and shinier, treating head lice, and even preventing graying of hair. When applied to the scalp, rosemary essential oil can help stimulate hair growth, and a 2015 study compared the effectiveness of rosemary oil to 2 percent minoxidil, otherwise known as Rogaine. The results showed that rosemary oil was as effective as Rogaine, and the patients in the rosemary group also experienced far fewer side effects compared to the minoxidil group. Both treatments seemed to produce significantly increased hair counts after six months of use. However, there is a big caveat. Rogaine users often use 5 percent minoxidil, rather than the 2 percent solution used in the study, thus skewing the results. However, it's good to know that rosemary has some effect on preventing hair loss.

A different study looked at rosemary extract for the treatment of hair loss from testosterone use. The study was conducted on mice that were injected with hormones to induce varying degrees of baldness. The results were varying and found that rosemary could be promising for hair growth.

More research looked into the effects of essential oils on baldness, specifically alopecia, a condition that leads to partial or complete absence of hair leading to baldness. The researchers looked into a mixture of essential oils, which included thyme, rosemary, lavender, and cedarwood. The mixture was massaged onto the scalp daily for seven months. They concluded that essential oils are a "safe and effective treatment for alopecia." While not a blockbuster conclusion, this is good enough reason to go out and buy yourself some essential oils for a nice scalp rub.

## Stress

Who doesn't need a daily dose of stress-lowering goodness? Used in aromatherapy combined with other oils, rosemary can lower cortisol levels, thereby lowering anxiety. If you're having a stressful day, take a few drops and place in the palms of your hands. Rub the oil between your hands and take a few deep breaths in of the essential oil aroma.

## Possible Side Effects, Contraindications, and Drug Interactions

Though generally considered safe, there have been occasional reports of allergic reactions to rosemary. Consuming excessively large amounts of rosemary leaves can cause serious side effects, including spasms, vomiting, pulmonary edema, and even coma. Pregnant and nursing women should not take rosemary as a supplement, but it is safe for them to eat as a spice in foods.

People with high blood pressure, ulcers, Crohn's disease, or ulcerative colitis should not take rosemary. Rosemary oil can be toxic if taken orally.

Rosemary may affect the blood's ability to clot, and could interfere with blood-thinning drugs such as Warfarin and Clopidogrel. Rosemary may also interfere with the action of ACE inhibitors taken for blood pressure. If you are diabetic and are taking drugs to help control your diabetes, use precaution when consuming rosemary, as it may alter blood sugar levels and interfere with those drugs.

## Rosemary Care Guide

Rosemary can be a tricky herb to grow indoors. The key to its survival is abundant sunlight and efficient watering practices. I've had many rosemary plants die in my hands, and it's not a fun road to discovery.

Rosemary is native to the Mediterranean, where there is plentiful sun, well-drained soil, and a lot of heat, along with moisture from the ocean air. Thus, it's no wonder that rosemary loves the sun but also needs enough moisture to keep it thriving. It's also important to note that growing rosemary outdoors in a garden is a completely different practice than growing it in containers. Below are instructions for container rosemary gardening.

**Lighting**: Rosemary needs full sun, indoors or outdoors. Make sure that if you are growing lavender indoors you have plenty of bright natural light.

**Water**: When inside a container, rosemary will need to be watered just enough. Yes, this is not a greatly detailed explanation, but here's the thing. Too much water is bad, because it can lead to root rot, but too little water can also spell death. Make sure to water the soil at least every two weeks, but also make sure to check that the soil is dry first. And because rosemary likes to absorb water from the air (remember its ocean origins) make sure to place rocks or pebbles on the drainage pan for a more moist environment, and sit the pot on top of the rocks.

It's important to remember that indoor air is drier than outside. Rosemary enjoys moist foliage, and it would be good to take a spray bottle with water and mist the foliage about once or twice per week.

**Soil**: Known as an "upside-down" plant, rosemary enjoys dry roots but moist foliage, and will want to absorb moisture from its leaves. When growing this plant in a container, you will need to have drainage holes and well-draining soil. Use cactus soil mix or something similar.

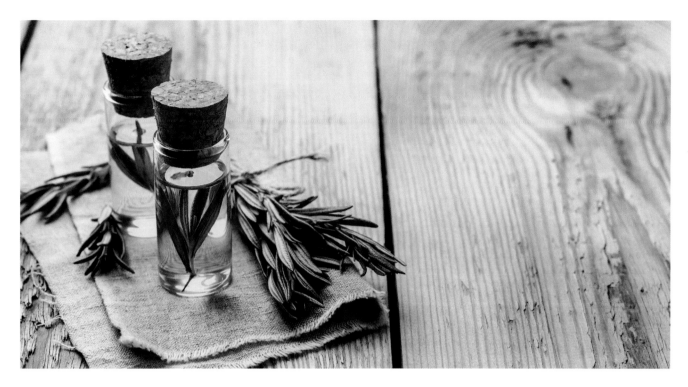

## Rosemary Oil

Rosemary oil is a great way to get all the important essences out of your rosemary plant for the ultimate healing benefits. Use as a moisturizer for your skin, a massage oil, or rub it into your scalp to stimulate hair growth.

### Ingredients:

Fresh rosemary
Mason jars
Olive oil or jojoba oil
1-ounce glass bottles with droppers

### Directions:

1. Pick your fresh rosemary, wash it, and let it completely dry. Cut enough to fill up a mason jar. Cutting and crushing the rosemary will bring out the aroma and various oils in the herb.

2. Fill up your mason jar with your freshly cut and clean rosemary.
3. Fill your jar with your oil of choice, completely covering the plant. I like to use olive oil or jojoba.
4. Place your jar on a windowsill that gets plenty of sun, for about a month.
5. After a month, strain your oil into a clean jar and throw away any pieces of the plant that have been separated during straining.
6. Fill your 1-ounce bottles with your rosemary oil and label the bottles!

If you keep your bottle closed tightly and out of direct sun, the oil should last you for up to six months.

# Sage

Sage is often used by healers and homeowners as a way to cleanse and heal spaces and to get rid of that weird smell in the kitchen. Sage is easily grown indoors, assuming there is plenty of sunlight around, and its health benefits abound. A relative of rosemary, the botanical name comes from the Latin word *salvere*, meaning "to be saved."

Used throughout the centuries, this herb has been beloved by the Romans, Charlemagne in France, the ancient Egyptians, the ancient Greeks, and the ancient Chinese. Should I forget an ancient culture that loved sage dearly, I truly apologize, but this plant is just too darn popular. Not to mention, sage also has a wide range of uses, from aiding digestion to cleaning ulcers and wounds; stopping bleeding; treating sprains or a hoarse voice; regulating women's menstrual cycles; improving memory; alleviating sore throats, coughs, and the common cold; and more.

Throughout the ages, sage has been considered somewhat of a panacea, being of utmost value in herbal medicine cabinets throughout history. Today, sage is often used for muscle aches, rheumatism, aromatherapy, increasing memory, mental clarity, and treating cognitive decline. Its tea is known as "thinker's tea" and even eases depression. To get the most out of the medicinally diverse plant, many ingest it by eating, drinking (as a tea), or making it into a tincture.

## Health Benefits

The many health properties of sage don't just come in the form of burning, but also from ingesting. Sage has anti-inflammatory and antiseptic properties; it also contains a wide array of volatile oils and can be used medicinally for a variety of ailments including muscle aches, rheumatism, depression, asthma, and even atherosclerosis.

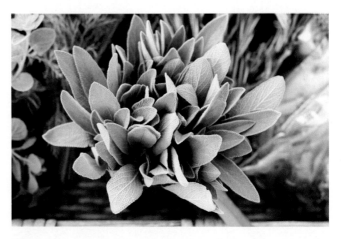

Sage also includes many vitamins and minerals, including vitamin K, vitamin A, folate, magnesium, manganese, calcium, folic acid, riboflavin, copper, vitamin C, and vitamin E.

## Improves Memory

One small study found sage to be a useful treatment in enhancing memory and cognition. This placebo-controlled, double-blind study showed significant improvement in word and cognitive recall immediately following and several hours after ingestion of sage compared to the placebo group. Those who were given the sage oil tablets were found to be significantly better at word recall than those who weren't. Spanish sage has been shown to be effective in enhancing the speed of memory and improving mood.

Other studies have shown sage to be effective in treating memory disorders and cognitive decline. Traditional Chinese medicine uses Chinese sage as a restorative of lost and declining mental function, such as Alzheimer's disease. Sage essential oil has been found to inhibit the enzyme acetyl cholinesterase by 46 percent. This enzyme is known to inactivate acetylcholine, which leads to Alzheimer's.

## Anti-Inflammatory Properties

More recently, research has shown that two plant-derived compounds from sage known as diterpenoids are potent anti-inflammatories and could help treat pain. The two compounds, known as carnosol and carnosic acid, are known to interfere with the pathways related to pain and inflammation in the body. This breakthrough could mean that nonaddictive sage is a safer approach to treating pain than most mainstream methods.

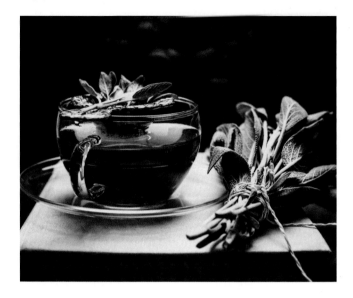

## Combats Diabetes

Cultures throughout the world have used sage to combat diabetes, and there's research to corroborate these methods. Studies on animals have shown many glucose-lowering effects. In one study, drinking sage tea twice a day resulted in an improved lipid profile without any side effects. And one study showed that sage extract had a hypoglycemic effect in diabetic animals, but more research is needed.

## Eases Symptoms of Menopause

For those experiencing hot flashes, you may want to add sage to your toolbox of aids. A study conducted in Switzerland found that a preparation of fresh sage reduced the number of hot flashes by 50 percent in four weeks and 64 percent in eight weeks in participants who experienced at least five hot flashes daily

## Possible Side Effects, Contraindications, and Drug Interactions

Generally recognized as safe by the Food and Drug Administration, sage is commonly found as a spice for food or used in seasonings. Some species of sage, however, contain a compound called thujone, which can affect the nervous system. Large amounts of ingestion or extended use can lead to vomiting, vertigo, restlessness, tremors, increased heart rate, and even kidney damage. Ingesting sage essential oil may be toxic.

Some possible drug interactions to be aware of include diabetic drugs, due to sage's ability to lower blood sugar. Antiseizure medications and sedative medications could also be interactive, as sage may cause drowsiness and sleepiness. If you are currently taking sedative medications, including clonazepam, lorazepam, phenobarbital, zolpidem, and others, please remain cautious.

## Sage Care Guide

If you want the most economical way to enjoy and use sage, grow it yourself. It's an easy plant to keep healthy due to the herb's hardy nature and drought-tolerant qualities. It also grows well in a wide range of temperatures and climates, and has a long growing season. You'll be harvesting this herb well into the fall, and best of all, sage will do great in containers! Sage is also special because it's one of the few herbs whose flavor intensifies as the leaves grow larger.

**Lighting**: Sage needs lots of light, so make sure it's placed in a part of the house with full sun.

**Water**: This hardy and drought-tolerant plant will do best if you let the soil dry in between watering. Never let it sit in soggy soil (but do water when the soil gets fully dry) and you'll do just fine.

**Temperature**: Sage will do well indoors as long as it's kept away from cold drafts.

**Soil**: Make sure your sage lives in well-draining soil that's sandy or loamy.

# Sunflower

Found in open fields and along roadsides, from the southern regions of Chile and Peru all the way through Mexico and into North America, this sunny plant has earned the nickname "marigold of Peru" and has the Latin name *helianthus* (derived from the Greek words *"helios"* meaning sun and *"anthos"* meaning flower). This happy plant brings a smile to those who see it. Every part of the plant can be used. Sunflowers are considered a sacred plant in many cultures. The Incas' and Aztecs' respect for this plant is found preserved in artwork around historical sites with depictions of women carrying the sunflower in their hands as an offering of gratitude to the sun gods. The entire plant (seeds, flowers, leaf, stem, and roots) has a use. The seeds and leaves are used most often in herbal medicine preparations.

**Chemical Constituents**: Black-seeded variety of the sunflower seeds contain polyunsaturated fatty acids, resulting in a high-quality expressed oil and protein. 100g of dried sunflower seeds deliver 8.6g of dietary fiber, 78mg of calcium, 5.25mg of iron, 325mg of magnesium, 645mg of potassium, 5mg of zinc, 8.33mg of niacin B3, 1.48mg of thiamine B1, 1.345mg of vitamin B6, 227 ug folate, 35.17mg of vitamin E, 18.52g of monounsaturated fatty acids, and 23.13g polyunsaturated fatty acids—sunflower seeds are a superfood.

**Medicinal Actions of seeds**: diuretic, expectorant, antiseptic, antitussive, diaphoretic; used for colds, chest congestion, and as a stop-smoking aid

**Medicinal Actions of leaf**: astringent

**Applications**: infusion, food, poultice, infused oil, syrup; decoction of the seed for a demulcent cough remedy

- For a lung tonic, elevated fever, or for expectorating congestion in the lungs: prepare an infusion or topical poultice from the leaf and seed, or a decoction from the seed.
- To relieve diarrhea or for a diuretic: prepare an infusion from the leaf.

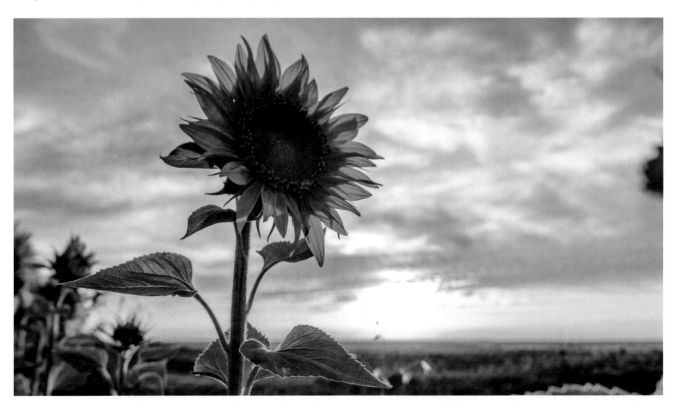

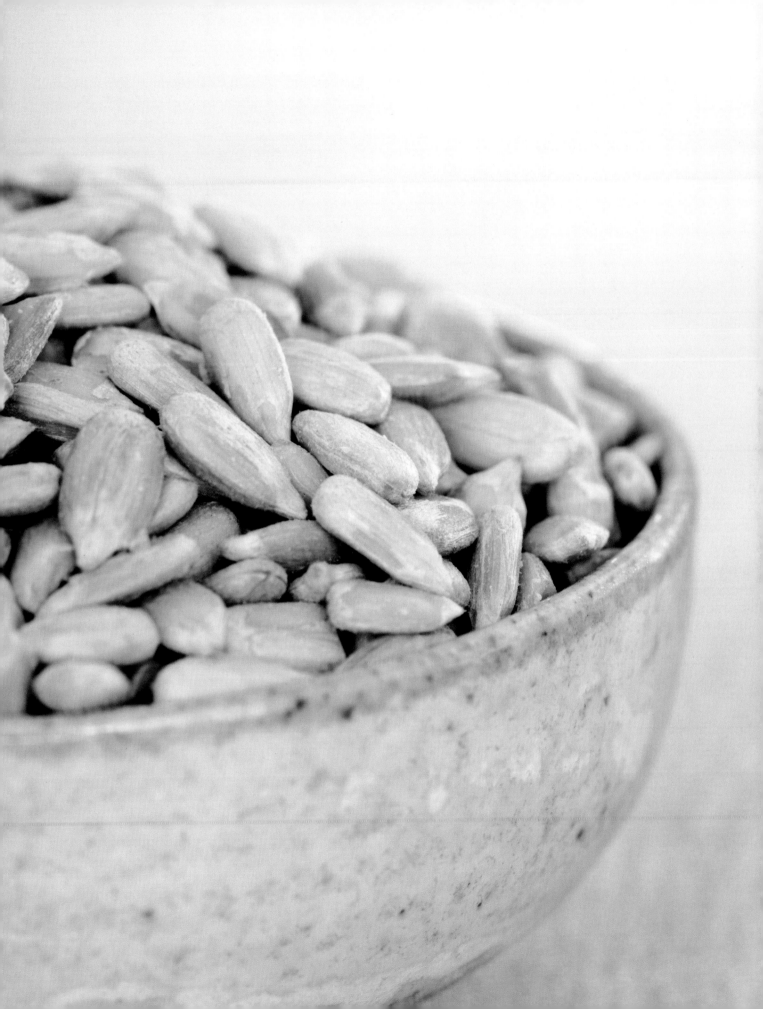

# Thyme

The name thyme is derived from the Latin name *thymus*, traced back to the Greek name *thymos*, meaning spirited. Thyme is a much-respected herb associated with bravery and strength, historically gifted to soldiers heading to battle. Dried thyme bundles can be burned to impart a sense of courage while unleashing the strong, smoky, antiseptic nature of thyme. Historically, thyme was added to foods as a seasoning spice, an ingredient in liqueurs, and was used to both prevent and assist in overthrowing food poisoning. It has a long history of use during the times of the plague to ward off illness. Harvest leaves in the morning, before the plant flowers in the summer.

**Constituents**: volatile oils (thymol, carvacrol), tannins, flavonoids, triterpenoid saponins, resins

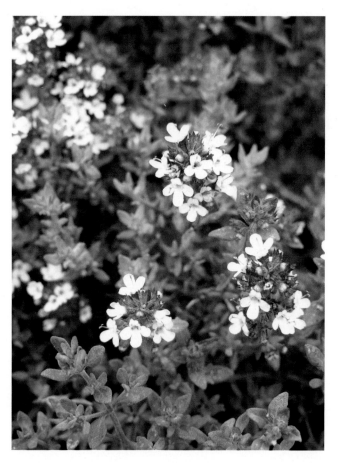

**Medicinal Actions**: antiseptic, antibacterial, antiviral, antioxidant, antifungal, expectorant, anti-candida, vermifuge, carminative, antitussive, antispasmodic, diaphoretic, rubefacient

**Applications**: infusion, infused oil, essential oil, tincture, fomentation, poultice, honey, syrup, steam

This infection-fighting plant is packed full of volatile oils, which contribute to its antiseptic properties: the thymol and carvacrol are disinfectant to the mucous membranes of the lungs and kidneys as they are excreted from the body. Thyme offers valuable antimicrobial support for gut infections, including food poisoning, and those unwanted yet common childhood parasites (such as pinworms and threadworms).

In addition to the antibacterial and antiviral properties, thyme is an expectorant herb: it loosens thick, sticky phlegm and creates a productive cough for removal of copious amounts of mucous. It is known especially for combating a dry cough with raw mucous membranes, as it produces a protective covering over the dry membranes and assists the productivity of the cough. It is useful for asthma, bronchitis, and breathing issues. Consider this a useful antiviral and diaphoretic herb for a cold or flu. Create a syrup of rose hips, yarrow, and mint as a "flu therapy on a spoon" or use thyme in an herbal steam for congestion using the two teaspoons of herb of thyme and two to three drops of lemon essential oil in a basin of boiling water. Its antispasmodic properties make this an ideal home remedy for sporadic convulsive coughs, thickened mucus, and inflammation of the bronchial tubes in cases of bronchitis. It also provides benefit topically for aching joints and muscle spasms related to rheumatism and arthritis.

The highly astringent nature, due to the tannin content, makes thyme an option for diarrhea, especially related to foreign bacteria in the gut, and a topical antiseptic for cuts.

Thyme is both a bitter and carminative herb for supporting digestion: prepare an herbal vinegar, tea, or tincture for symptoms of diarrhea, gastritis, colic, and gas. Its bitter nature is used to stimulate digestion and support liver function.

- For skin fungus, viral infections (warts and shingles), and antiseptic wound care: prepare a disinfectant skin wash.
- For tight muscles, athletic injuries and rheumatic issues such as arthritis and inflammation: use a poultice, liniment, or topical applications.
- For strep throat and candida infections of the mouth: prepare an infusion and use as a gargle.

- For ear infections: prepare an infused oil and use for ear drops or poultice.
- For sinus congestion, asthma, allergies, and colds: prepare an infusion and use as a steam inhalation.
- For leukorrhea or candida fungal infection: prepare as an herbal wash.
- For mastitis: combine with plantain and prepare as a poultice.
- For cold and flu symptoms, congestion, and body aches: prepare an infusion as a steam or herbal bath.

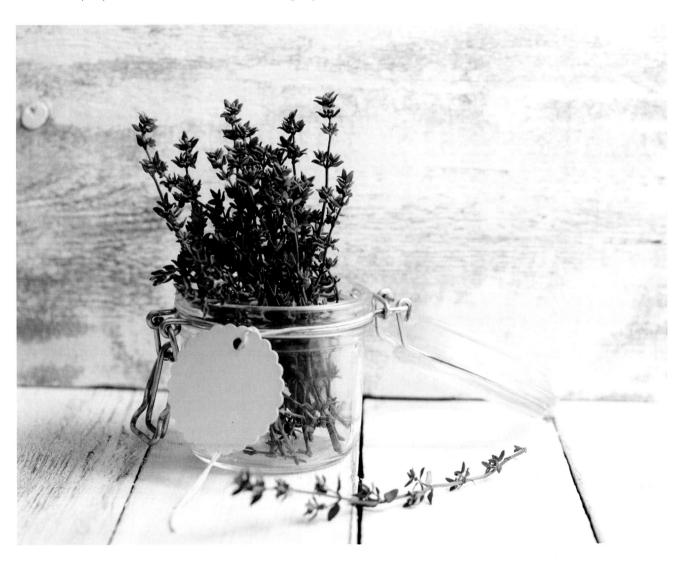

# Watercress

The pungent, peppery flavor reminds us that this plant is also found in the mustard family. The Latin name is derived from the words nasus tortus, meaning a convulsed nose, of course referring to the slightly pungent, spicy mustard scent and flavor of the leafy greens. The whole herb is used medicinally.

Be certain to wash this tender herb well before ingestion. I personally use a vegetable wash to soak the plant and to ensure that the only thing being ingested is the watercress.

**Constituents**: flavonoids (quercetin), sulfur compounds, glucosinolates, isothiocyanates, carotenoids, lutein, iodine

Watercress is a valuable tonic to build the blood. Consider combining with carrots and spinach for enhanced mineral content. For every 100g of plant material, there are 43mg of vitamin C, 120g of calcium, 330ml potassium, and 3,191 IU of vitamin A.

**Medicinal Actions**: antiseptic expectorant, cholagogue, antioxidant and nutritive, lung tonic

**Applications**: nutritious food, fresh juice, broth, infusion

Known as a detoxifying and body-purifying spring tonic, watercress is packed full of vitamins and minerals. It has been said to cleanse the blood and strengthen the body. Typically, it is used in the spring to remove toxins accumulated during the winter months and for mild constipation. An alkaline tonic for acidic conditions such as arthritis, gout, and rheumatism, it is also used to improve the appetite, warm the stomach, nourish the entire body, and to stimulate liver and gallbladder function. Use as a food, tea, or tincture.

Being a member of the cabbage family, watercress also contains glucosinolates and high amounts of antioxidant nutrients, making this food a useful immune and possible anticancer nutrient. From laboratory and in vitro studies, animal models to some human research, studies indicate that isothiocyanates in cruciferous vegetables can inhibit cancer development by activating the ability of phase II liver enzymes (such as glutathione S transferases) to detoxify. They can also stimulate apoptosis (selective cancer cell death), and may inactivate nitrosamine carcinogens in mice studies by inhibiting specific cytochrome P450 enzymes. Finally, they may assist in the regulation of normally uncontrolled growth of cancer cells.

As a lung tonic, watercress can be used as a food staple to strengthen the lungs, removing congestion and excess phlegm, for bronchitis or regular smoking.

- For spider bites: prepare a poultice from steamed watercress.
- A relief for hemorrhoids: prepare a poultice from steamed watercress.
- For skin spots and freckles: the fresh watercress juice can be applied directly on spots, wrinkles, and freckles.
- A topical application for eczema: apply as juice or poultice.

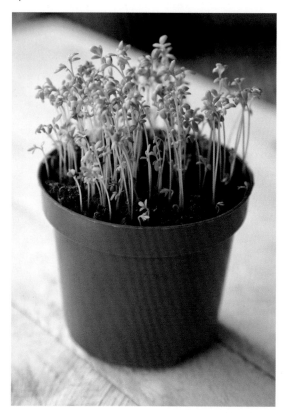

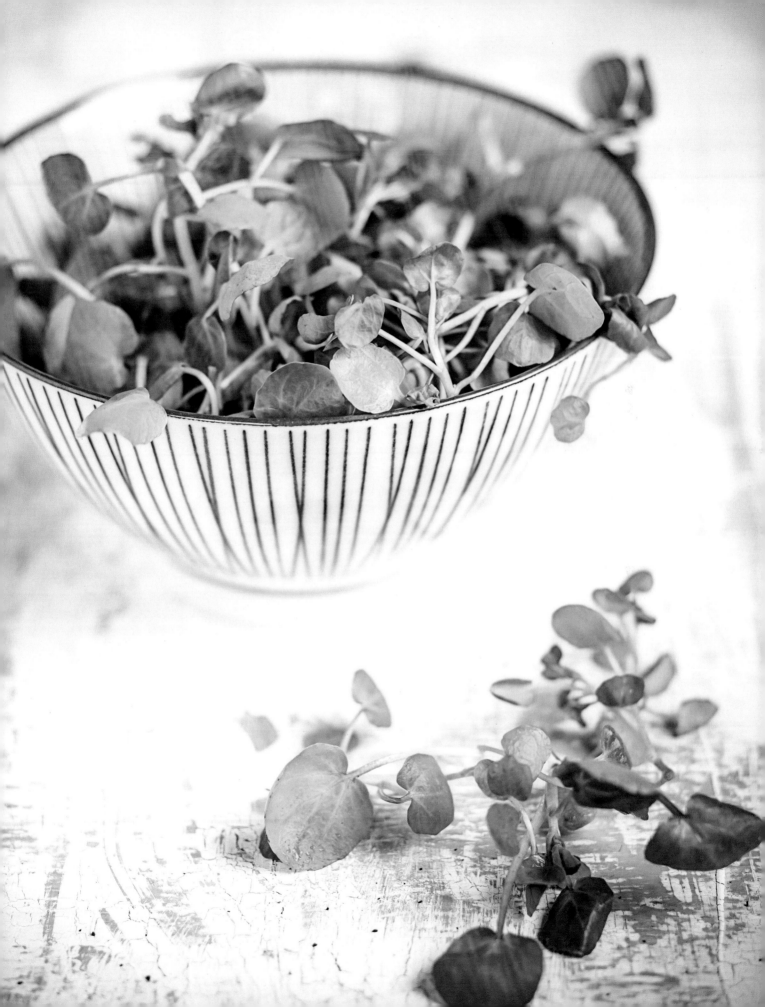

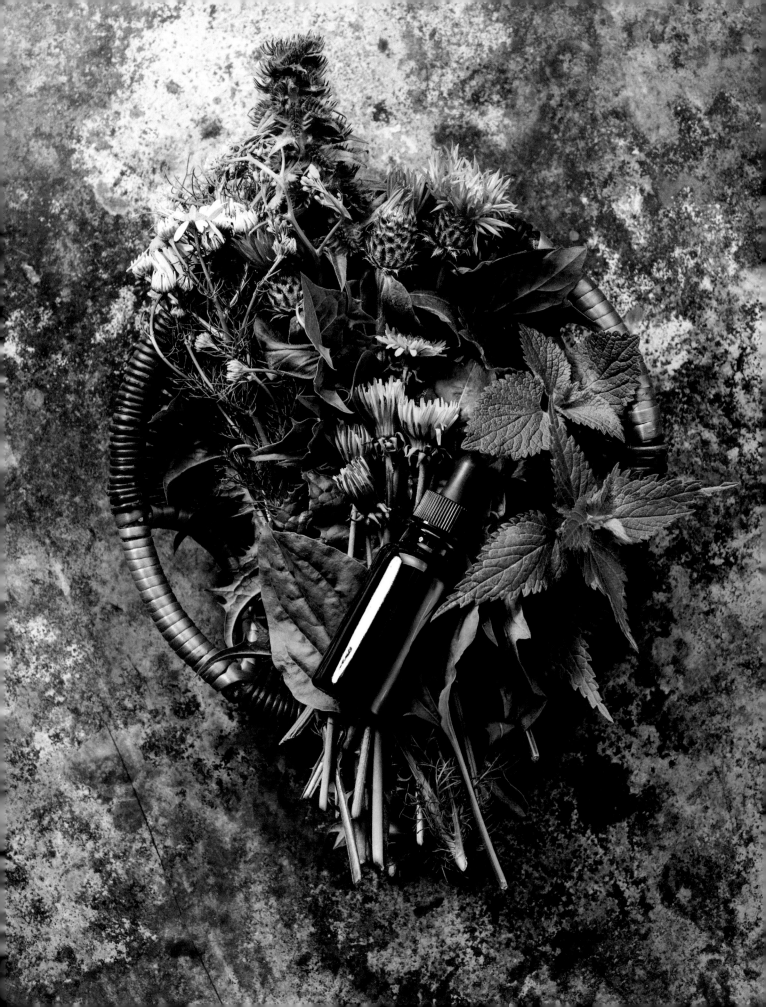

# Edible Wild Plants

## Beech

**Description:** Beech trees are large forest trees. They have smooth, light gray bark, very dark leaves, and clusters of prickly seedpods.

**Location:** Beech trees prefer to grow in moist, forested areas. These trees are found in the temperate zone in the eastern United States.

**Edible Parts and Preparing:** Eat mature beechnuts by breaking the thin shells with your fingers and removing the sweet, white kernel found inside. These nuts can also be used as a substitute for coffee by roasting them until the kernel turns hard and golden brown. Mash up the kernel and boil or steep in hot water.

**Benefits:** The leaves can be boiled to create a poultice to help relieve headaches. Beechnuts are high in folate, though overconsumption can be toxic.

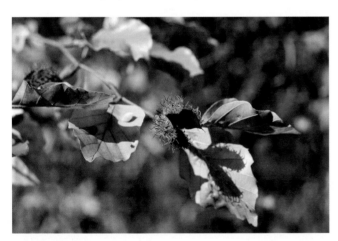

## Burdock

**Description:** Burdock has wavy-edged, arrow-shaped leaves. Its flowers grow in burrlike clusters and are purple or pink. The roots are large and fleshy.

**Location:** This plant prefers to grow in open waste areas during the spring and summer. It can be found in the Temperate Zone in the north.

**Edible Parts and Preparing:** The tender leaves growing on the stalks can be eaten raw or cooked. The roots can be boiled or baked.

**Benefits:** Burdock root is full of antioxidants, may interfere with cancer cell growth, detoxifies the blood, and may help treat acne when applied topically.

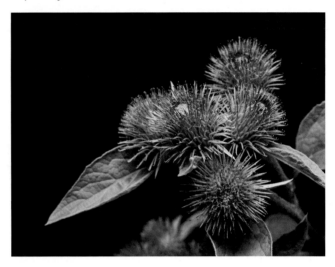

## Chicory

**Description:** This is quite a tall plant, with clusters of leaves at the base of the stem and very few leaves on the stem itself. The flowers are sky blue in color and open only on sunny days. It produces a milky juice.

**Location:** Chicory grows in fields, waste areas, and alongside roads. It grows primarily as a weed all throughout the country. Don't harvest from areas likely to be contaminated with pesticides, herbicides, or car exhaust.

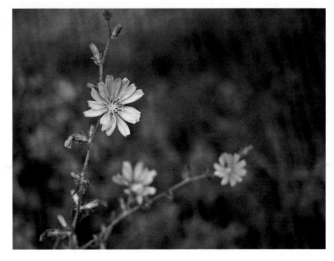

**Edible Parts and Preparing:** The entire plant is edible. The young leaves can be eaten in a salad. The leaves and roots may also be boiled as you would regular vegetables. Roast the roots until they are dark brown, mash them up, and use them as a substitute for coffee.

**Benefits:** Chicory is a good source of the prebiotic fiber inulin, which contributes to gut health. It also has manganese and B6, which are linked to brain health.

## Dandelion

**Description:** These plants have jagged leaves and grow close to the ground. They have bright yellow flowers.

**Location:** Dandelions grow in almost any open, sunny space in the United States.

**Edible Parts and Preparing:** All parts of this plant are edible. The leaves can be eaten raw or cooked and the roots boiled. Roasted and ground roots can make a good substitute for coffee.

**Other Uses:** The white juice in the flower stem can be used as glue.

Benefits: Dandelions are a good antioxidant, a natural diuretic, and may help in detoxifying the liver.

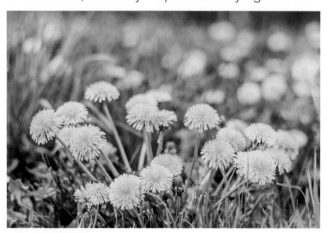

## Elderberry

**Description:** This shrub has many stems containing opposite, compound leaves. Its flower is white, fragrant, and grows in large clusters. Its fruits are berry-shaped and are typically dark blue or black.

**Location:** Found in open, wet areas near rivers, ditches, and lakes, the elderberry grows mainly in the eastern states.

**Edible Parts and Preparing:** The flowers can be soaked in water for eight hours and then the liquid can be drunk. The fruit is also edible but don't eat any other parts of the plant—they are poisonous.

**Benefits:** Elderberry fruit is a powerful immune system booster.

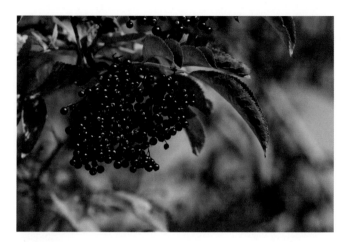

## Nettle

**Description:** Nettle plants grow several feet high and have small flowers. The stems, leafstalks, and undersides of the leaves all contain fine, hairlike bristles that cause a stinging sensation on the skin.

**Location:** This plant grows in moist areas near streams or on the edges of forests. It can be found throughout the United States.

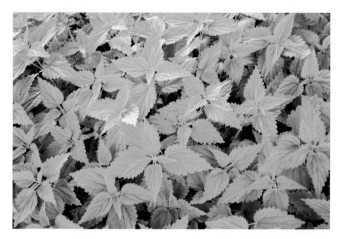

**Edible Parts and Preparing:** The young shoots and leaves are edible. To eat, boil the plant for 10 to 15 minutes.

**Benefits:** Helps relieve the pain and inflammation associated with arthritis, alleviates seasonal allergies, balances blood sugar, may reduce growth of noncancerous enlarged prostate.

## Self-Heal

**Description:** This plant is related to mint and has very small tubular lavender flowers.

**Location:** It grows in moist soil across the United States.

**Edible Parts and Preparing:** The leaves can be eaten raw, boiled, or dried and used as a tea. The flowers are also edible.

**Benefits:** Self-heal is a digestive aid, anti-inflammatory, lymphatic stimulant and diuretic, antiviral (especially good for alleviating cold sores), and immune system booster.

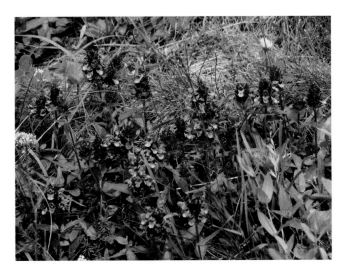

## Thistle

**Description:** This plant may grow very high and has long-pointed, prickly leaves.

**Location:** Thistle grows in woods and fields all over the country.

**Edible Parts and Preparing:** Peel the stalks, cut them into smaller sections, and boil them to consume. The root may be eaten raw or cooked. Tea can be made from the crushed seeds or the leaves.

**Benefits:** The silymarin in milk thistle helps to detoxify the liver. It helps to lower cholesterol, aids in weight loss, and boosts the immune system. Used topically, it may have an antiaging effect on the skin.

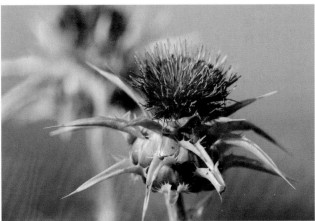

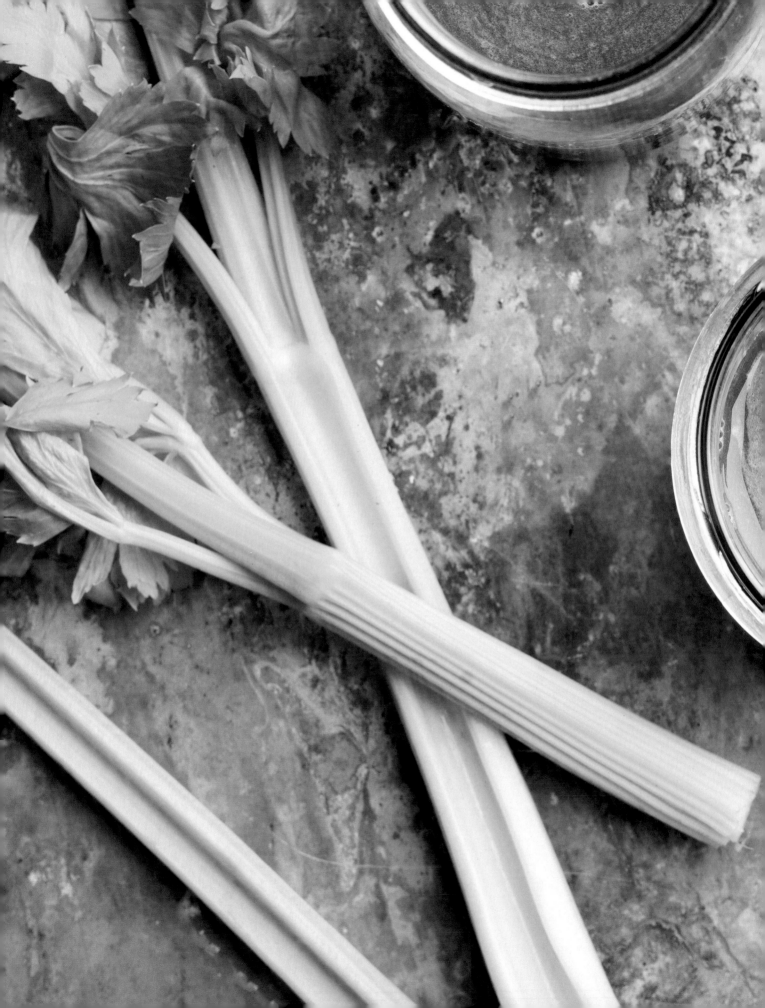

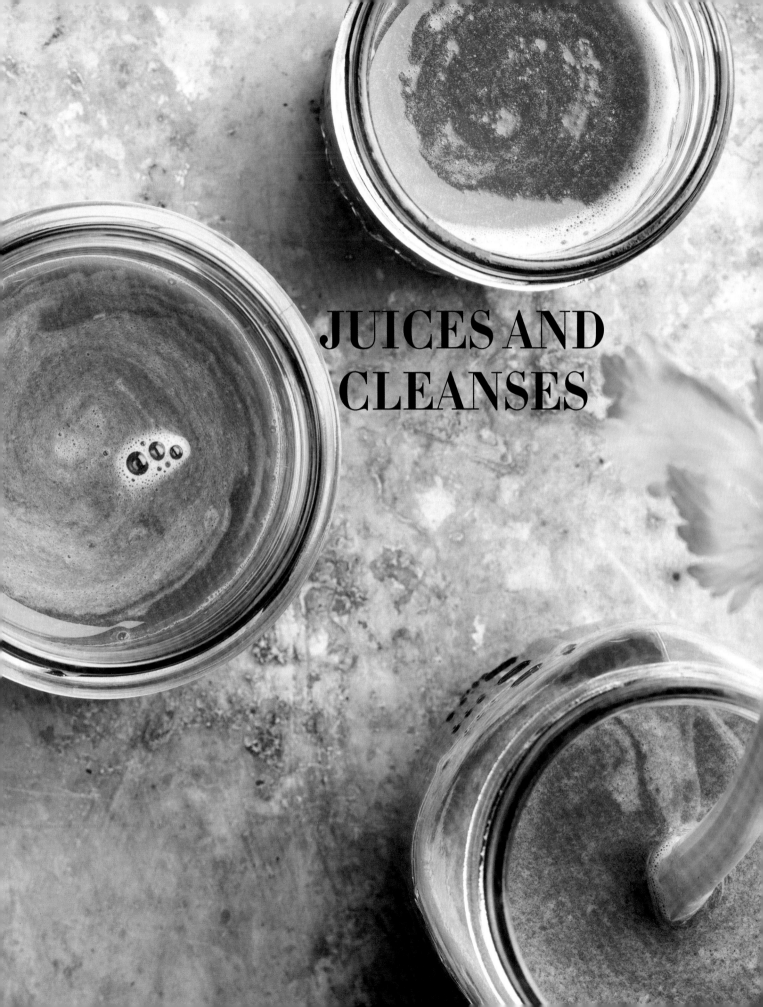

JUICES AND
CLEANSES

# The Truth about Toxins

Toxins are all over the place. To completely avoid them is both impractical and impossible. Shampoos, perfumes, plastic water bottles, pesticides in food. . . . Wherever you turn there's a myriad of chemicals waiting to enter your body. The result is that this unnatural way of living throws a far bigger toxic toll on us than our organs were meant to handle.

The problem is not that our detoxifying organs can't do their job well, but that they're given far too much work and they can't completely keep up! This is the moment when all those itches, aches, and discomforts start appearing, externalizing the fact that toxins have set camp in our bodies.

## Toxic Overload

Do you always feel like something is wrong in your body yet you can't pinpoint the cause? Do you feel lousy or unbalanced in any way more often than you would like to? If you feel anything but splendid most of the time, your body could be waving its hands high in the air, trying to tell you that it's overwhelmed by your highly toxic lifestyle. (Even if you don't suspect you have a highly toxic lifestyle. By the way, most people do.)

### Such symptoms may include:
- Bad digestion
- Chronic fatigue
- Headaches
- Mood swings and depression
- Coated tongue
- Irritable bowel
- Yellow spots on your skin
- Overheating and excessive perspiration
- Acne
- Fat around the waist
- Weak immune system
- Low metabolism
- High cholesterol
- Allergies and rashes
- High blood pressure
- Intolerance to alcohol and medicines
- Heartburn
- Dark circles under your eyes

These are just a few of the problems that an excess of toxins in your body could be causing, and that juicing regularly could start relieving. The list is really much, much longer, as any and all of your symptoms could potentially be caused by too many toxins.

## The Liver: General of the Body's Army

The liver is one of your hardest-working organs, second perhaps only to the heart. Its role is to decide what is beneficial and can stay, and also what will cause damage and is inadmissible. It is no coincidence that Chinese medicine describes it as the general of the body's army. This organ is multitasking for you day in and day out, evaluating everything that enters your bloodstream with an eagle eye, and transforming it into a different biochemical form so that the body can use it as nourishment, get rid of it, or store it as fat in the exact places where you want it the least. This is done by filtering the blood like a mega-sophisticated kitchen sieve, singling out the unwanted toxins, and helping them make a discreet exit when you sweat or visit the bathroom. Despite kicking ass at what it does, there are several factors that can make your liver less efficient at managing its job.

## The Culture of Overeating

Can you imagine never giving your car a rest, never taking it to maintenance or changing its parts, and just making it go, go, go? It's pretty obvious that the machine in question would soon start having problems, and eventually burn out. That is, if it doesn't explode first! In *The FastDiet*, Dr. Michael Mosley compares the compulsive way we eat, without giving our digestive systems a second's rest, with digging our foot deep in the accelerator pedal of a car all the time. It's strange that most people would never treat their toys and gadgets this way, yet find it acceptable to put that kind of burden on their own bodies. And it's even wilder that they believe their bodies will keep working just fine, without any complaints, despite the unfriendly treatment!

Think about how many times a day you eat a full-on meal, or nibble here and there. Be honest. If you're like most people, the answer is many times a day whether you're hungry or not. As a result of this food obsession, our energy is hyper-focused on the sole mission of digesting food. When we give our digestive systems a rest from solid foods, our energy can be invested in more important endeavors, such as resting, detoxifying, and repairing. Our liver can stop stressing about all the new toxins coming in, and catch up with all the stored ones from past excesses. This is one of the reasons why replacing food with juices during a cleanse is so important. Another reason is that the fruits and vegetables used in large amounts when juicing are packed with antioxidants that help protect the liver from the free-radical attack caused by too many toxins and poor nutrition.

## The Free Radicals Attack

Free radicals are not just the bad boys most people think they are. They actually assist the liver in getting rid of toxins. Unfortunately, they also attack healthy cells, turning them into free radicals themselves. In turn, these attack new healthy cells, and the cascading effect begins. The body, wise as always, has a backup plan for this problem: it produces its own antioxidant enzymes that protect the healthy cells against free radicals. But when there are too many free radicals drifting around, as a result of too many toxins that need to be cleared out of the body, we are eventually unable to maintain this delicate balance.

Detox diets halt the inflow of toxins at least for a while, allowing for a more efficient release of stored toxins. On top of this, the superior nutrition in juicing gives your body the extra antioxidants it needs to balance out all the free radicals produced as a result of our chaotic lifestyles. Are you starting to understand why juices are such detoxifying rock stars?

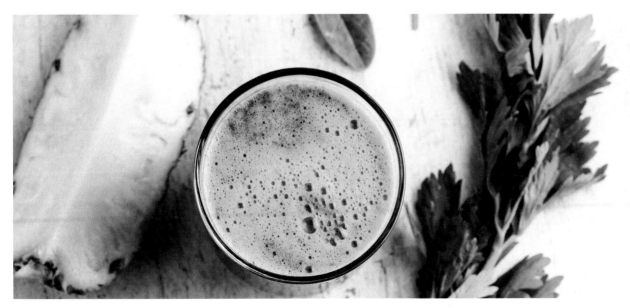

# The Power of Juicing

Drinking juices regularly is like taking the most potent multivitamins you could ever get your hands on. All the wonderful properties that make fruits and veggies the nutritional powerhouses they are are trapped in the fiber, and you get only a small fraction of them by chewing your food. When you juice them, on the other hand, you unlock all this nutrition out of the fiber and send it shooting straight into your bloodstream. You could never dream of getting those high doses of nutrients just by eating whole foods unless you were in a veggie-eating contest and ate till you passed out. Under better conditions the body probably wouldn't need the high levels of nutrition that juicing provides. But we don't live under better conditions, so our bodies could definitely use a hand.

## How Juicing Helps the Body Detoxify

As discussed, when you juice you give your body a break from the daily grind, and your energy can finally stop focusing on never-ending digestion, and start being invested in other repair work. One of the jobs it can now concentrate on more efficiently is ridding itself of stored waste. But there is more.

## Hard-Core Nutrition

Juicing also helps the body detoxify itself more efficiently by giving it superior nutrition. The high doses of nutrients we get from these drinks are wonderful cleansing agents, as they nourish and stimulate our detoxifying organs, making sure they're healthy and strong. The juices themselves don't clean our bodies. They just help our cleansing organs do a better job at it.

When they get a little bit of help, these organs start flushing stored toxins out of the body in bigger quantities and at a faster pace than when left on their own, or even worse, when being fed a Standard American Diet (very appropriately called SAD). At the same time, getting rid of those toxins helps the body start absorbing nutrients more efficiently, as there is less waste blocking it from doing so. And this makes your organs even healthier and better at detoxifying. This is the replenishing cycle that takes place in your body when you start juicing. Don't you love it?

Even if you keep eating three meals a day and don't go for a full-on cleanse, adding detox juices to your diet will help your body work more efficiently. As an added bonus, they will help you feel fuller and leave less space for unwholesome foods. Eating processed food without nutrition and full of toxins does the exact opposite. Every time we eat a meal taken out of the Standard American Diet's catalog, we get little or no nutrition (hence, weaken our organs), and feast on toxins instead. When you do this, you are begging for trouble.

## Juices vs. Smoothies

The difference between juices and smoothies is not rocket science. In short, juices are devoid of all the fiber in the fruits and veggies, whereas smoothies contain all the fiber. But which one is best? The answer is they both have pros and cons.

Juices may spike your sugar levels a little, because the fiber is not there to anchor all those natural sugars. However, this can be avoided by drinking greener juices with fewer sweet fruits and veggies in them. The fact that juices go directly to your bloodstream without any distractions has a super health shot effect on the body. You can actually feel your cells vibrating with vitality and joy when you drink them. Try it, and you'll see what I mean.

Smoothies, on the other hand, take more time to get into your bloodstream, as the fiber still needs

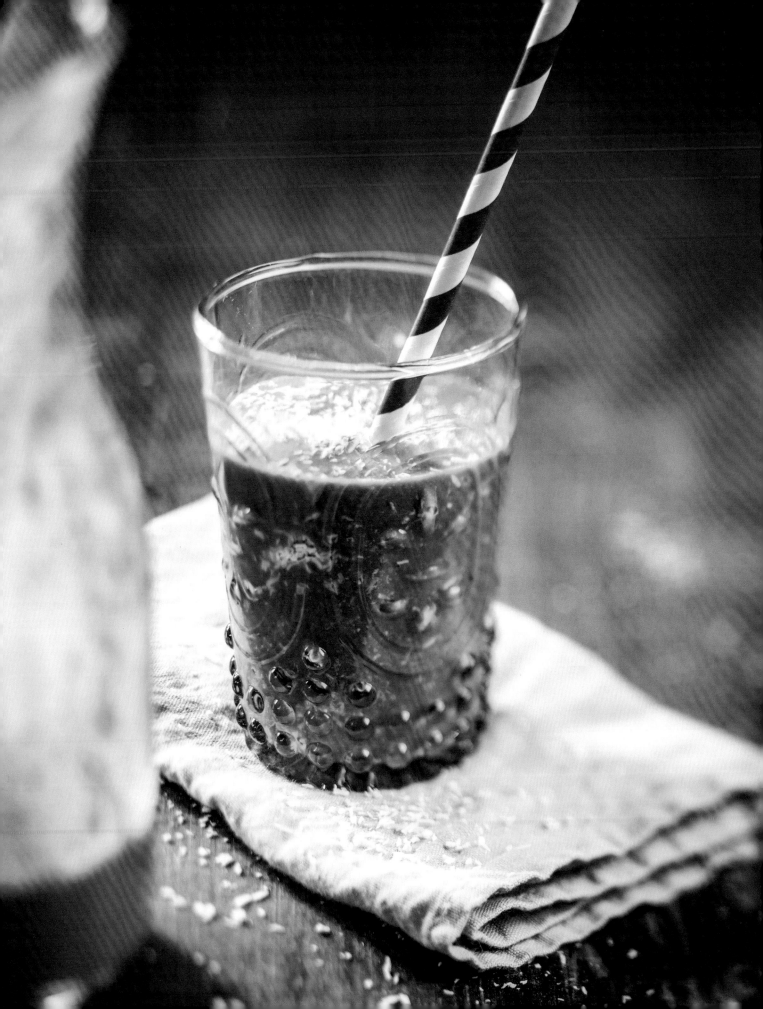

to be digested, delaying the process. You also use smaller amounts of fruits and veggies (hence, less nutrients) in a smoothie, as the bulk of the fiber would make you feel too full if you added more. Of course, this is a pro if fullness is what you're looking for. All things considered, I prefer to drink juices more often than smoothies, as I get larger amounts of nutrients that way, and they give my body a break from digesting. If you have the time (and the juicer), try to make this your first choice most of the time.

If you have only a blender, however, or if you are always in a rush, smoothies are still a great way of including more fruits and vegetables in your daily routine, and of improving your health by unlocking more nutrients out of the fiber. Just make sure you don't use frozen fruits or veggies too often, as they weaken your digestion (if possible, avoid them completely, or thaw before using), and that you drink them on an empty stomach, and wait at least an hour before you eat something else. Most of the juices in this book can be easily turned into smoothies by adding a little water, green tea, or almond milk to them.

## Does Detox Juicing Have Lasting Effects?

Some nutritionists are against detox diets because they consider them a fad, and a quick fix without lasting effects. I partially agree with this. Detox juicing won't completely change your life if you do it just once and then dive right back into smoking, drinking cocktails every day at happy hour, and having doughnuts for breakfast and pizza for lunch. But if done right, juice cleanses can be a gigantic step toward better health, and greater awareness of your body, how it works, and what you put in it.

To get lasting effects that will be noticeable, you need to accompany your periodic cleanses with a change in diet, and, if possible, a change of lifestyle too. Changing your diet, by the way, is not as hard

as you may imagine. Excess eating and cravings are usually the effect of poor nutrition. You may be giving your body large amounts of food every day, but if those foods don't contain what your body needs, it will keep asking for more. Once you start eliminating stored toxins out of your system and your starving cells get a taste of real nourishment, your body will become more efficient at letting you know exactly what it needs.

In fact, one of the great things about juicing is that it is highly addictive. Hooray for that! Once your cells know what they were missing out on, they will never get enough of this royal treatment. Can you imagine how different the world would be if we all had this kind of addiction?

## What Happens After a Detox?

Even if you go back to total food and lifestyle chaos after your cleanse, and only juice and eat healthy once in a blue moon, I do believe that some detoxifying every now and then is by far better than nothing. By bringing your organs back to balance ever so slightly, your body will carry less of a toxic burden for a while, be more efficient at absorbing nutrients, and start working more efficiently than if you never gave it proper maintenance.

But of course, we encourage you to keep drinking these nutrient-rich juices on a regular basis, and to make wholesome food choices for the rest of your life. Doing this will be totally worth your effort.

## Ten Reasons to Do a Juice Cleanse

1. You have been eating the Standard American Diet for far too long!
2. You want to know what your body really wants.
3. Your digestive system needs a much-needed vacation from all that overeating.
4. You want to look younger for longer, and to feel it too.

5. It's spring, and you feel the urge to do an internal house cleanse.
6. You want to get rid of your compulsive cravings, and get new, healthier ones in their place.
7. You want to feel amazing for the first time in a very long time, and get rid of annoying physical, mental, and emotional symptoms.
8. You want your clothes to fit better.
9. You want to navigate more smoothly through the physical and emotional toxins in your daily life.
10. You're feeling adventurous and want to try new fruits and veggies every day.

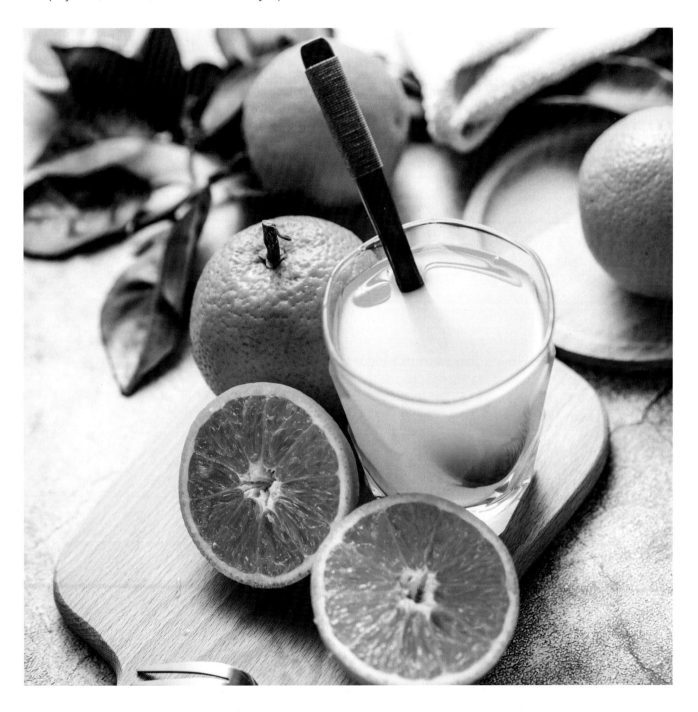

# Detox Juicing 101

There are many different opinions as to what the best way of doing a juice cleanse is. Some people go on for several weeks drinking only water or only juice, and avoiding all solid foods. And there are those who do both juices and food at the same time.

Then there is the question of time. I have friends who have gone up to three weeks just juicing. They say they stopped feeling hungry by the third day, and had more energy and mental clarity than ever before. Most people, however, prefer doing this for shorter periods of time.

Our approach tends to be of the gentler kind, and we run away from anything radical. When it comes to juicing, we truly believe that the most important thing is that you actually do it! Cleansing in a way that will leave you starved and grumpy, and will be a huge (too huge) test on your willpower, won't do. What's the point of choosing the most life-changing diet if you'll cheat or quit by the second day? We want you to succeed, and to enjoy the ride while you're at it.

## How Often and For How Long Should You Do a Cleanse?

I personally like adding one daily juice to my regular daily meals. Usually, I take this as a snack, or a prebreakfast or predinner appetizer. If I'm too full from overeating the previous day, or feel a bit undigested, I'll replace dinner or breakfast with a juice, as well.

I also like doing one-day juice fasts every now and then, particularly when the seasons change, or during a new moon. When I do this, I only drink juices and eat no other food. On that day, I have at least three or four juices. I have no problem maintaining these one-day cleanses, as they go quickly enough and I know I can eat whatever I want the following day. I have a very fast metabolism, and

feel too weak, and get cold extremities and strong headaches if I fast for longer than that, or if I do it too often. Everybody is different, so you should try different approaches and see what works best for you.

If, after trying, you find that a three-day program works wonders for you, it could be a good idea to do it once a month, or once every change of season, depending on your lifestyle and the state of your health. Seven- or fourteen-day programs can be practiced once or twice a year for optimal results.

Spring is an ideal time to do a cleanse. It is no coincidence that we feel moved to do a spring cleaning of our homes every year. The liver is more active during this season, and cleaning our surroundings is just an outward expression of what's going on at this time of year inside our bodies. So go ahead and cleanse away when you see the first flowers blooming in your garden or hear the first birds chirping.

## To Eat or Not to Eat?

Try to always stay on the safe side, and if you don't feel well, stop, increase the amount of food, or decrease the amount of juices. Every body is unique, and you should honor your particular constitution. If you're more of a free spirit and want to create your own detox programs using our recipes, follow these guidelines to have a pleasant detox experience:

- For three-day programs, replace breakfast and dinner with a juice, and have two juice snacks during the day as well. Eat a regular lunch.
- For seven-day programs, we recommend you replace breakfast and dinner with a juice on the first, fourth, and seventh day, and have a big, healthy lunch. Have two juice snacks throughout the day, when you feel hungry. During the other days replace dinner with a juice (choose one of the greener kinds) and

have a healthy breakfast and lunch. Again, don't forget to snack on green juices if you get hungry.

- For a fourteen-day detox, we advise that you replace two meals with a juice on the first day, one meal with a juice on the second day, and eat your regular three meals on the third day. However, you should snack on one or two green juices, as always, even on the day when you eat three regular meals. Repeat this process several times, until you complete the fourteen days.

As you can see, in all programs we encourage you to have one or two juices as snacks between meals if you feel hungry. If you do this, pick the ones with less fruit and more veggies in general. Try to use this time to start listening to your body closer, and realize when you're actually hungry, as opposed to thirsty, anxious, or bored. Why do you want to eat a particular thing at a certain time? What feelings triggered that craving? What are you trying to avoid, or what space are you trying to fill with that food? Cleansing is a great opportunity to reconnect with your inner guide, and perhaps dig deeper into your relationship with food, with your body, and with your emotions. If done with awareness, cleanses can impact your life at deeper levels than you would expect.

## Is it Safe to Do a Cleanse?

Cleansing is a fun and natural way of pressing the reset button on your body's healing mechanisms. Wise men and women all around the world have been practicing fasting (both with and without juicing) for centuries as a regular way to bring balance back to their bodies, minds, and even souls.

We recommend juicing as a way to enhance your life and health. However, we are not medical practitioners, and talk only from our own lifelong experience with juicing. As with any other lifestyle and dietary changes, you should consult a physician before starting a detox program, especially if:

- You have any serious or chronic health concerns.
- You have an eating disorder.
- You are taking medications.
- You are pregnant, trying to get pregnant, or nursing.
- You feel there is any other reason that may put you at risk. Use common sense to evaluate this.

Even if you're healthy, we don't recommend you follow these programs for longer than fourteen days, unless you are under strict supervision from a doctor. You may, however, keep adding a juice or two to your daily routine after you finish a cleanse, or even replace a meal with one or two juices every now and then if you feel your body needs it. If you're about to have a naughty snack between meals, you can't go wrong by replacing it with a juice.

## Side Effects of Juicing

When you go through a cleanse, you release toxins stored in your colon, liver, lungs, bladder, sinuses, skin, kidneys, and fatty tissue. The more toxins you've accumulated throughout the years by having a lousy diet and a sloppy lifestyle, the more you will have to release. This may cause a few unpleasant symptoms that you would probably be happier without. Any discomfort caused by toxicity, such as bloating, phlegm, or acne, may become stronger at first, before it starts getting better.

Experiencing this toxic hump is natural, as the stored waste needs to be released back into your bloodstream before it can exit your body. At the end of the day this downside is nothing compared to the many upsides you will get from sweeping those little buggers out of your body once and for all. Just be patient and you will soon start seeing the light at the end of the tunnel.

If symptoms arrive, drink lots of water to flush them out of your system quickly. If they are too strong or persist, consider stopping the cleanse and trying a milder version of it in the future.

It may also be the case that you experience no negative symptoms whatsoever, so don't take this potential scenario too seriously. We just feel that for the sake of honesty, it's better to warn you that this may not be a complete walk in the park for everyone.

To avoid a tough ride, make sure you begin slowly, especially if you don't have the most "kosher" of diets. Start getting acquainted with a higher daily dose of fruits and veggies little by little. Be slow but sure like the turtle, and build your detox practice one juice at a time.

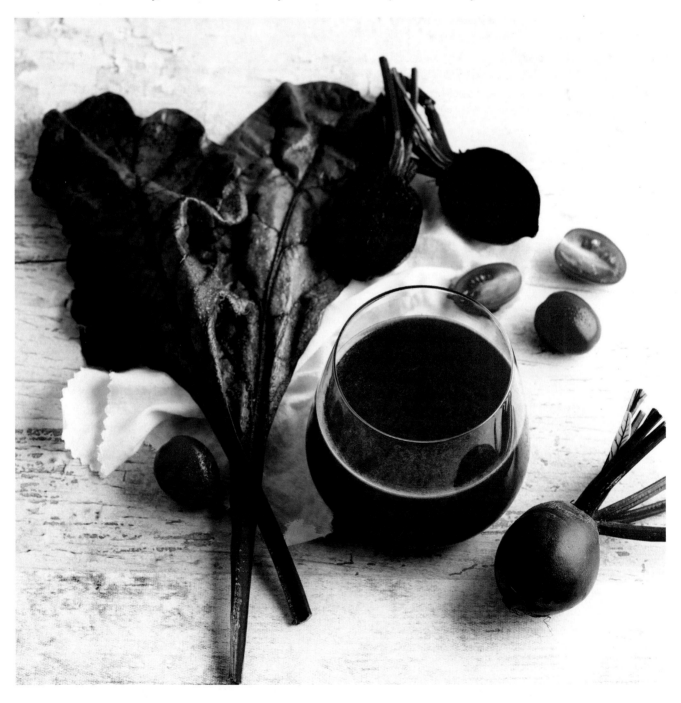

# Juice Recipes

### Red Hot Love
- Yields 2 cups
- 1 small peeled grapefruit
- 1 medium beet
- 3 carrots
- Small chunk ginger

### Beet and Sweet
- Yields 2 cups
- 1 small beet
- 1 peeled orange
- 4 carrots
- ½ lemon

### Green Delight
- Yields 2 cups
- 6 leaves lacinato (dinosaur) kale
- ½ bunch parsley
- ½ Italian cucumber
- 1 green apple
- ½ lime

### Peachy and Tangy
- Yields 2 cups
- 6 carrots
- 2 pitted peaches
- 1 large bell pepper
- Small chunk ginger

### Pear and Grape Joy
- Yields 2 cups
- 3 stalks celery
- ½ green pepper
- 1 cup grapes
- ½ Italian cucumber
- ½ pear

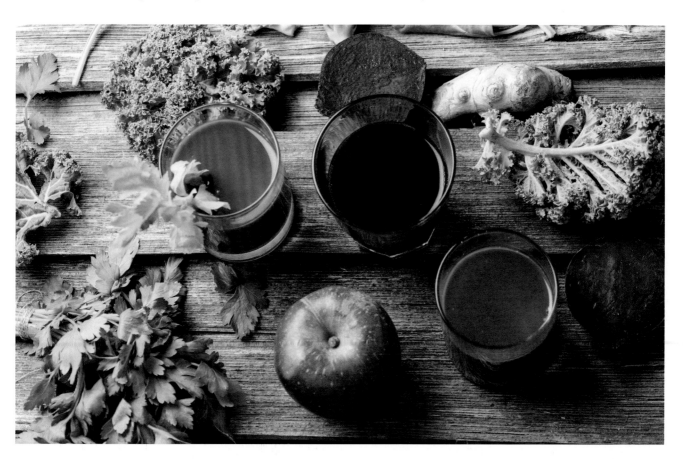

## Green & Clean

- Yields 2 cups
- 3 stalks fennel, ¼ fennel root included
- 6 leaves lacinato (dinosaur) kale
- 1 cup grapes
- ½ pear
- ½ green apple

## Crown Me Queen

- Yields 2 cups
- 3 broccoli crowns
- ½ pear
- ½ green pepper
- ½ Italian cucumber
- ½ lime

## Potato & Tomato Spice

- Yields 2 cups
- 1 sweet potato, unpeeled
- 4 carrots
- 3 Roma tomatoes
- ½ lemon
- Pinch of cayenne pepper

## Rocking the Roots

- Yields 6 cups
- 3 medium to large size red beets
- 2 sweet potatoes
- 1 lemon
- 10 carrots
- Small chunk ginger
- Small chunk turmeric

## Green Apple Glee

- Yields 3 cups
- 1½ bunch watercress
- 2 apples
- 1 cup green grapes
- 1 English cucumber
- ½ lime

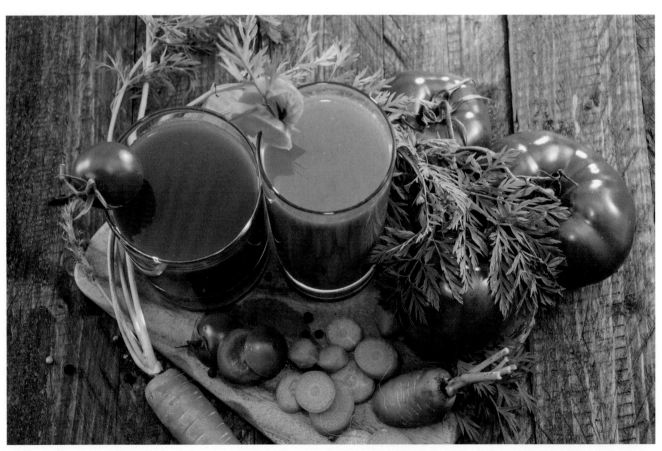

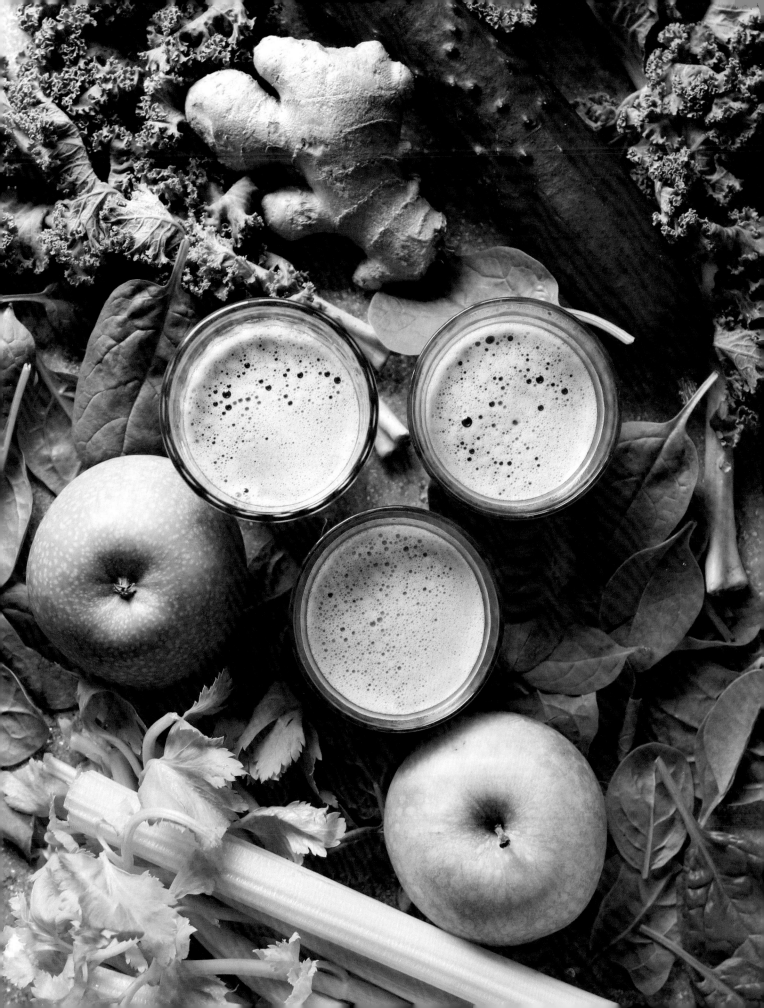

## Cherry Tasty

- Yields 3 cups
- 4 celery sticks
- 4 carrots
- 2 parsnips
- 1 lemon
- ½ lime
- 20 cherry tomatoes
- Small chunk ginger
- Pinch of cayenne pepper

## Seriously Detox

- Yields 7 cups
- 10 stalks celery
- 10 cups spinach
- 1 large Italian cucumber
- 1 brunch parsley
- 4 apples
- 2 lemons
- Small chunk ginger
- Small chunk turmeric

## Pine for Me

- Yields 8 cups
- 1½ lemons
- 10 stalks lacinato (dinosaur) kale
- ½ bunch parsley
- 4 Persian cucumbers
- 10 cups spinach
- 1 small whole peeled pineapple
- Small chunk ginger
- Small chunk turmeric

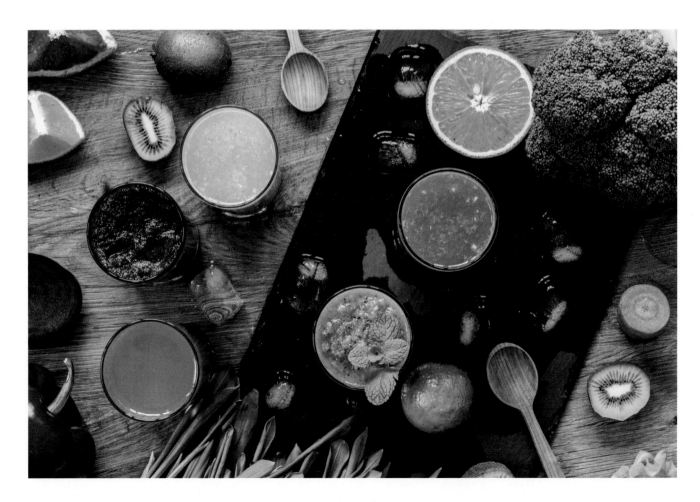

## Spa Day at Home

- Yields 3 cups
- 4 carrots
- 3 parsnips
- 4 celery
- 1½ yellow apples
- ½ lime
- ⅔ bunch parsley
- 1 cup green grapes

## Ultimate Cleanser

- Yields 4 cups
- 1 lime
- 1 lemon
- 2 celery stalks
- 3 large Roma tomatoes
- 1 large cucumber
- 4 stalks curly kale
- 1 bell pepper
- Small chunk ginger
- Small chunk turmeric
- Handful of mint

## Deep Kiwi Green

- Yields 3½ cups
- 4 stalks of Swiss chard
- 2 endives
- 4 kiwi
- 1 cup green grapes
- 1 lemon
- 1 English cucumber
- 1 pear

## Cool as a Cucumber

- Yields 2½ cups
- 2 peeled oranges
- 2–3 stalks kale
- ½ bunch fresh dill
- 1 English cucumber
- 1 cup green grapes
- Small chunk ginger

## Youth Glow

- Yields 2½ cups
- 1 bunch cilantro
- 4 cups packed spinach
- 1 whole lime
- 1 cup green grapes
- 2 kiwis
- 4 Persian cucumbers

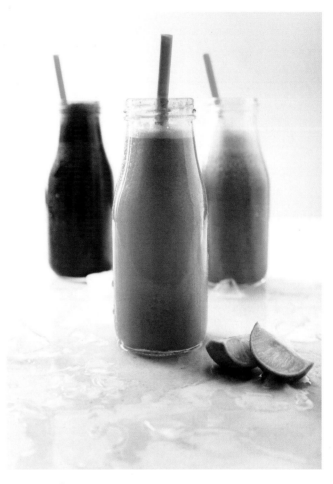

## Spicy Charm

- Yields 3 cups
- 4 cups spinach
- 1 Italian cucumber
- ½ bunch parsley
- 1 pear
- 2 small apples
- Small chunk ginger
- Small chunk turmeric
- ½ jalapeño pepper without the seeds

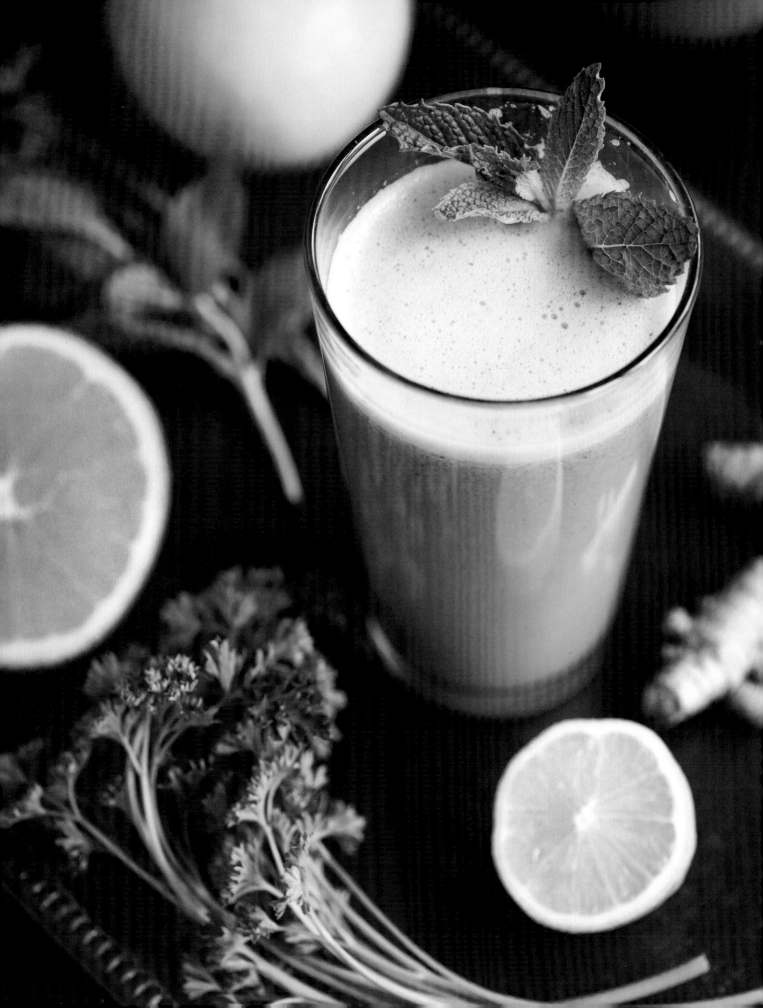

## Mint Condition

- Yields 3 cups
- 2 pitted peaches
- 1 cup green grapes
- 6 cups spinach
- 1 Italian cucumber
- 3 stalks celery
- ½ lime
- Handful of mint
- Small chunk ginger

## Kale to the Rescue

- Yields 3 cups
- 15 strawberries
- ¼ fennel
- 5 Persian cucumbers
- 4 curly kale without stem
- ½ parsley
- 1 lemon
- Handful of mint
- Small chunk ginger

## Gingerly Recovery

- 1 cup white grapes
- 2 Persian cucumbers
- 1 small lemon
- 10 stalks lacinato (dinosaur) kale
- ½ bunch parsley
- 1 cup spinach
- Small chunk ginger
- ½ cup unsweetened coconut water

## Butter Me Up

- Yields 2 cups
- ½ English cucumber
- 1 head of butter lettuce
- ½ bunch parsley
- 5 Campari tomatoes
- 1 whole lemon
- Small chunk ginger

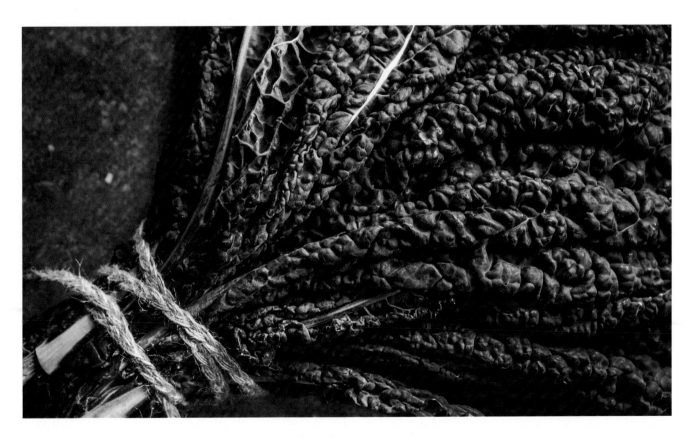

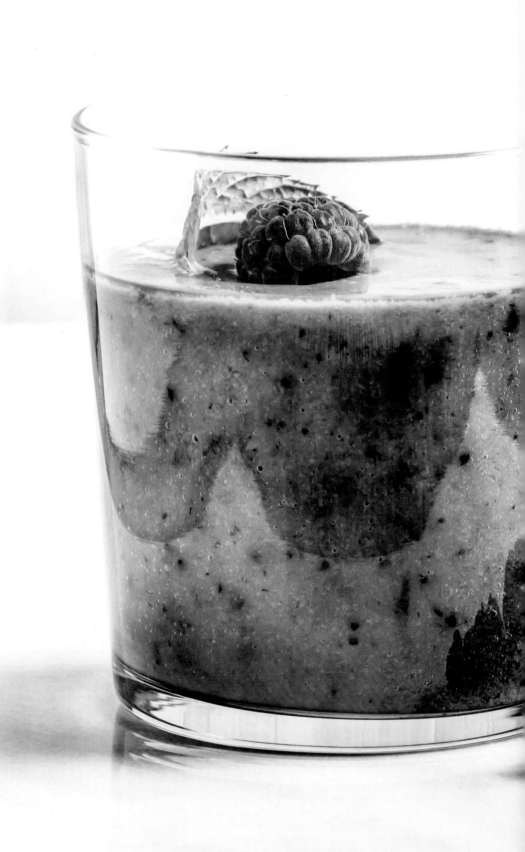

# SMOOTHIES

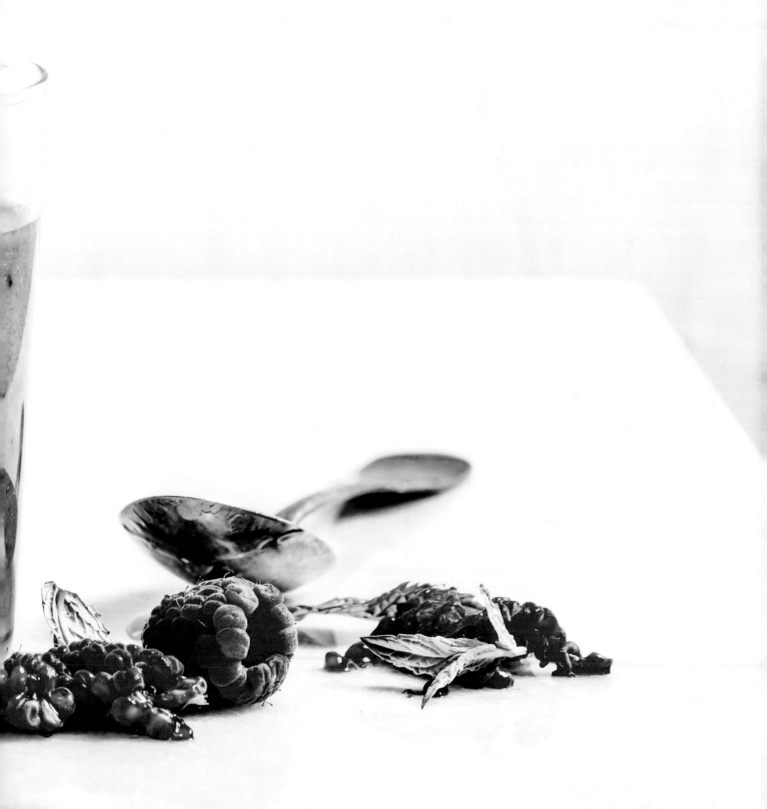

# Benefits of Smoothies

Smoothies are a great way to pack a lot of fiber and nutrients into a single beverage. They're quick to make, are easily customizable, effectively hydrate your body, and are delicious to boot!

## Mango Cream

Bananas are rich in dopamine, which means they can enhance our mood while the dopamine's anti-oxidant properties provide protection from cancer development. This tropical blend has a smooth and creamy texture and subtle mango fragrance.

### Ingredients:
½ banana
½ cup carrot juice
½ cup frozen mango
½ cup frozen green tea cubes
2 tablespoons hulled hemp seed
1 teaspoon probiotic powder

### Directions:
1. Combine all ingredients in a high-power blender or food processor and blend until smooth.
2. Drink immediately. Serves 2

## Banana Ginger Dream

Researchers found that eating bananas increases body concentration of the sleep-regulating molecule melatonin within two hours of consumption. Creamy and sweet, this smoothie tastes like candied ginger with a little bit of fresh ginger heat.

### Ingredients:
½ frozen banana
½ cup orange juice
½ cup frozen peaches
½ cup frozen green tea cubes
2 tablespoons fresh ginger root
2 tablespoons protein powder

### Directions:
1. Combine all ingredients in a high-power blender or food processor and blend until smooth.
2. Drink immediately. Serves 2

## Vanilla Bean Banana

Melatonin is a molecule that our bodies produce to help regulate our sleep cycles. However, it also provides protection against some neurodegenerative diseases and cancers. Researchers have found that pineapple, oranges, and banana are rich sources of this protective molecule. Light and creamy, this smoothie has subtle banana and vanilla flavors.

### Ingredients:
1 vanilla bean
½ frozen banana
½ cup orange juice
½ cup fresh pineapple
½ cup frozen green tea cubes
2 tablespoons protein powder

### Directions:
1. Combine all ingredients in a high-power blender or food processor and blend until smooth.
2. Drink immediately. Serves 2

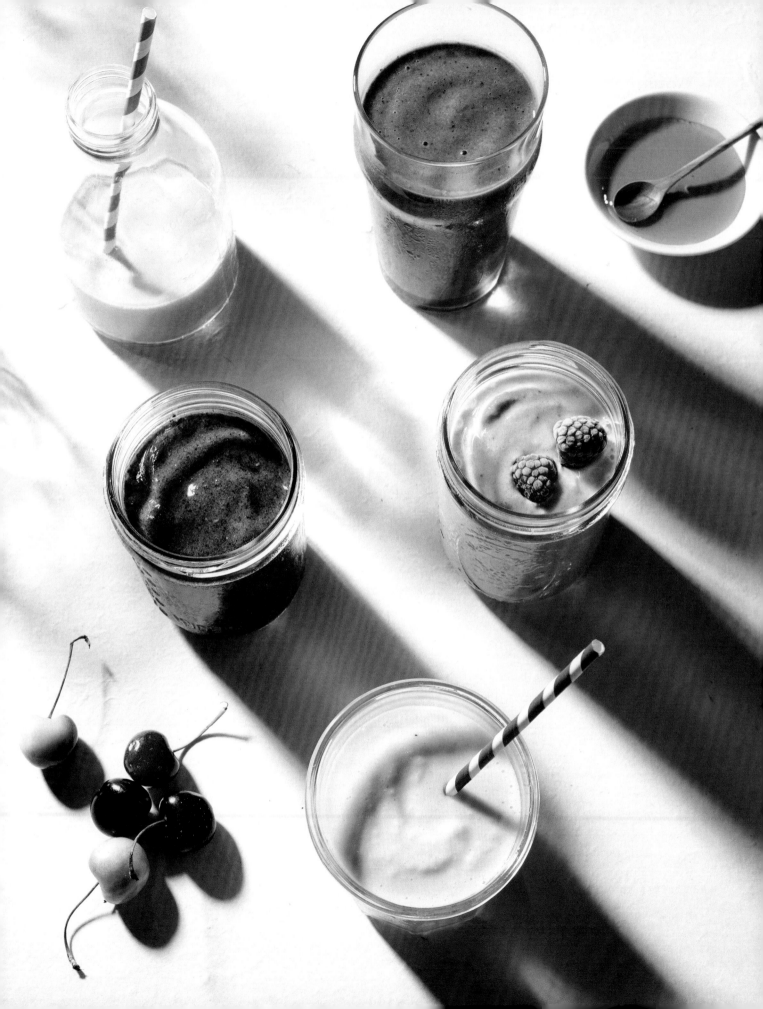

# Watermelon Raspberry Cooler

Watermelon is rich in carotenoids, which reduce the risk of lung cancer development.

Tart and sweet, this watermelon and raspberry combination is balanced by tangy cranberry juice.

## Ingredients:

1 cup frozen green tea cubes
½ cup frozen red raspberries
½ cup watermelon
¼ cup cranberry juice
2 tablespoons chia seeds

## Directions:

1. Combine all ingredients in a high-power blender or food processor and blend until smooth.
2. Drink immediately. Serves 2

# Kumquat Berry Cherry

Cranberries and cranberry juice have been shown to reduce growth of cancer cells via their antioxidative and anti-inflammatory properties. This tart and intense smoothie has a cranberry and citrus base with a bit of sweet berry flavor.

## Ingredients:

2 kumquats
½ cup tart cherry juice
½ cup frozen strawberries
½ cup frozen green tea cubes
¼ cup cranberry juice
2 tablespoons chia seed
1 tablespoon fresh rosemary

## Directions:

1. Combine all ingredients in a high-power blender or food processor and blend until smooth.
2. Drink immediately. Serves 2

# Berry Citrus Cream

Strawberries contain anti-inflammatory phenolics that can be absorbed by our intestines when metabolized by probiotics such as those in cultured coconut milk. This thick and rich strawberry smoothie is sweet and creamy with a heady vanilla fragrance and notes of tart citrus.

## Ingredients:

½ cup vanilla flavored cultured coconut milk
½ cup orange juice
½ cup frozen strawberries
½ cup frozen green tea cubes
2 tablespoons chia seed

## Directions:

1. Combine all ingredients in a high-power blender or food processor and blend until smooth.
2. Drink immediately. Serves 1

# Grapefruit Rosemary

Nobiletin is one of the bioflavonoids found in citrus fruits such as lemons, oranges, tangerines, and grapefruits. Nobiletin has anti-inflammatory and anti-cancer actions and the potential to suppress metastasis of breast cancer. This frosty blend has a perfect balance of citrus with a hint of bitterness from the grapefruit and rosemary. The flavor and fragrance are energizing, making this an excellent morning blend.

## Ingredients:

1 cup grapefruit
½ cup cherries
½ cup orange juice
½ cup frozen green tea cubes
2 tablespoons hulled hemp seed
1 tablespoon fresh rosemary

## Directions:

1. Combine all ingredients in a high-power blender or food processor and blend until smooth.
2. Drink immediately. Serves 2

## Cocoa Pom

Cocoa contains catechins that provide protection against stroke and other neurological damage. Cocoa is rich in procyanidins, theobromine, epicatechin, and catechins. This rich, chocolate smoothie is a healthy alternative to a sweet dessert.

### Ingredients:
½ cup frozen banana
½ cup orange wedges
½ cup frozen green tea cubes
½ cup pomegranate juice
2 tablespoons unsweetened cocoa powder
2 tablespoons protein powder

### Directions:
1. Combine all ingredients in a high-power blender or food processor and blend until smooth.
2. Drink immediately. Serves 2

## Blood Orange and Blackberry

Blood oranges contain concentrated amounts of tangeretin, a natural plant compound that triggers apoptosis in cancer cells. This blackberry and blood orange blend has bold citrus flavor and fragrance complemented by lime essence.

### Ingredients:
1 lime wedge
½ cup frozen blackberries
½ cup blood orange
½ cup frozen green tea cubes
½ cup green tea
2 tablespoons hulled hemp seed

### Directions:
1. Combine all ingredients in a high-power blender or food processor and blend until smooth.
2. Drink immediately. Serves 1

## Golden Berry Apple

Apples are rich in phenolic acids that inhibit cancer by reducing the growth of cancer and even reversing it, thereby reducing the risk for development of invasive cancers. This simple combination has sweet blueberry and apple flavor and nutrient-rich plant fiber.

### Ingredients:
½ apple
1 cup frozen wild blueberries
½ cup unfiltered apple juice
2 tablespoons hulled hemp seed
½ teaspoon turmeric powder

### Directions:
1. Combine all ingredients in a high-power blender or food processor and blend until smooth.
2. Drink immediately. Serves 2

## Grapefruit and Green Tea

Grapefruit provides kaempferol, which protects against cardiovascular disease and metastatic cancer growth. Light, cool, and creamy, this peach and green tea smoothie has a refreshing hint of tart grapefruit.

### Ingredients:
¼ cup grapefruit
½ cup frozen peaches
½ cup frozen green tea cubes
½ cup filtered water
2 tablespoons protein powder

### Directions:
1. Combine all ingredients in a high-power blender or food processor and blend until smooth.
2. Drink immediately. Serves 1

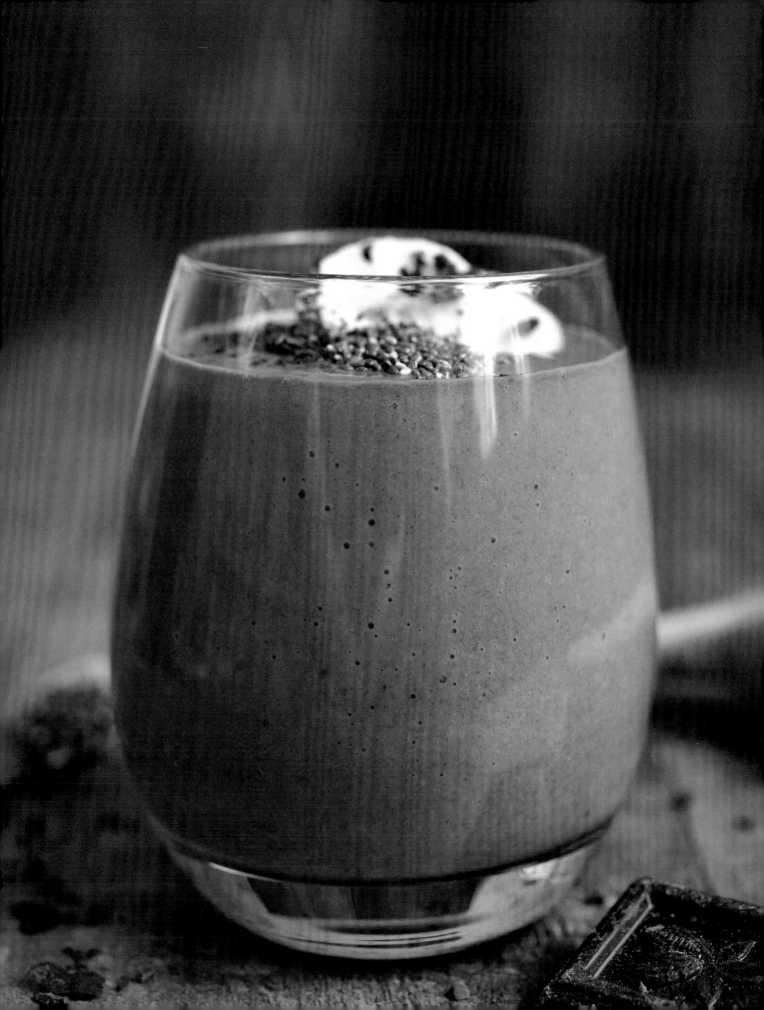

## Mexican Cocoa

Cayenne pepper contains capsaicin that has the ability to induce apoptosis of cancer cells. Cocoa, cinnamon, and cayenne flavors add depth to this rich and creamy combination of banana, hemp, and almond milk.

### Ingredients:
1 frozen banana
½ cup almond milk
2 tablespoons hulled hemp seed
1 tablespoon unsweetened cocoa powder
1 teaspoon cinnamon
Pinch of cayenne pepper

### Directions:
1. Combine all ingredients in a high-power blender or food processor and blend until smooth.
2. Drink immediately. Serves 1

## EGCG Power

The green tea polyphenol known as epigallocate-chin gallate (EGCG) has been found to have anti-neoplastic activity against cancer cells, particularly breast cancer cells. This slightly sweet, fruity combination is light and refreshing and rich in protein.

### Ingredients:
1 cup frozen green tea cubes
½ cup pomegranate juice
½ cup watermelon
½ cup pineapple
2 tablespoons chia seed

### Directions:
1. Combine all ingredients in a high-power blender or food processor and blend until smooth.
2. Drink immediately. Serves 2

## Cucumber Pom Mint

Cucurbitacin is a naturally occurring triterpenoid in cucumber that induces apoptosis (cancer cell destruction) and blocks the cell cycle progression of various cancers. This light smoothie has fresh cucumber, mint, and pomegranate flavors.

### Ingredients:
1 lime wedge
½ cup frozen cucumber
½ cup frozen mint tea cubes
½ cup pomegranate juice
2 tablespoons hulled hemp seed

### Directions:
1. Combine all ingredients in a high-power blender or food processor and blend until smooth.
2. Drink immediately. Serves 1

## Tart Peach Cream

Peaches contain numerous phytochemicals that protect against cancer by effecting signaling pathways that modulate cancer development. This creamy peach and coconut smoothie has an edge of cranberry tartness.

### Ingredients:
½ cup cultured coconut milk
½ cup cranberry juice
½ cup frozen peaches
½ cup frozen green tea cubes
2 tablespoons chia seed

### Directions:
1. Combine all ingredients in a high-power blender or food processor and blend until smooth.
2. Drink immediately. Serves 1

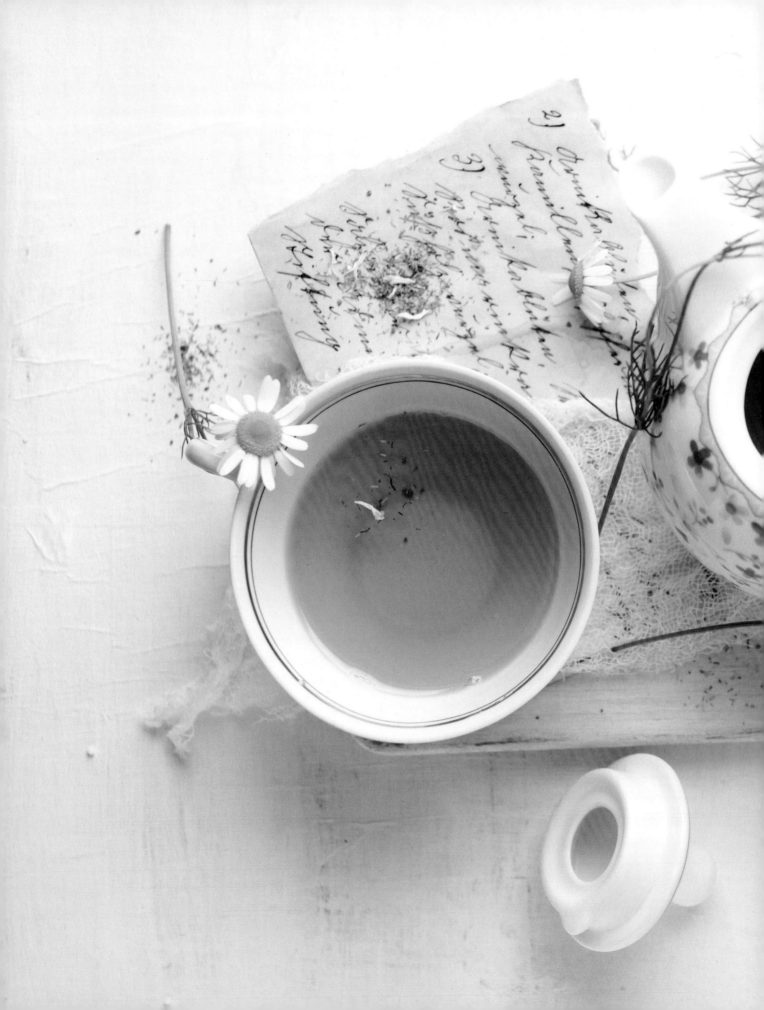

# TEAS AND ELIXIRS

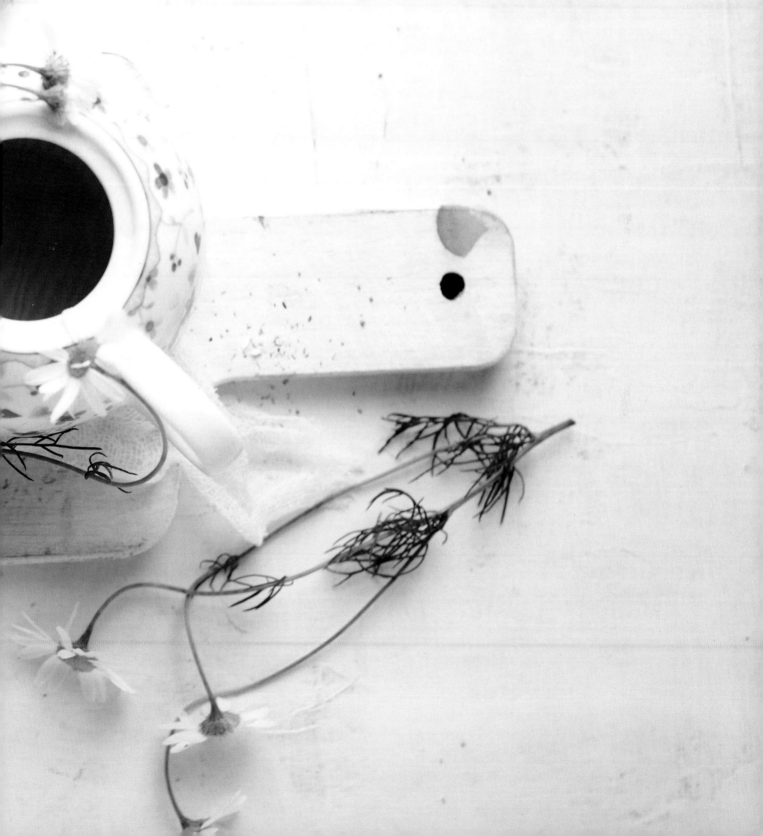

# Tea

Fun, creativity, reward, health—after the hard work of growing and gathering, it is time to put our herbs into action. This is our opportunity to be in our kitchens spending time bettering our health and creating powerful and delicious medicines for our family, friends, and selves.

On the following pages, you will find information, instructions, and recipes that will delight your senses, heal your ailments, and inspire you to further your own experimentation, creativity, and research.

The world is full of methods and recipes for herbal products. Never feel limited. Here we include many ideas for you to build upon.

## Herbal Infusion

Herbal infusions can be made a few different ways. Tea bags provide convenience when on the go. There are various kinds of contraptions—from tea balls to tea-steeping spoons—that can be used for this process. To get the most out of an herb for pleasure and medicine, the preferred method is working with loose herbs and steeping (which is a more common term for infusing) for a long period of time; for certain herbs, overnight is best. Infusions are used for the extraction of vitamins, minerals, and volatile oils, which are naturally occurring delicate oils of the flowers or leaves. The parts of the herbs used are usually the leaves and flowers, opposed to the roots or bark, which are more suitable to a decoction (see page 10) process.

## Instructions for Infusion

### Fresh Herb Infusion

Take a handful of fresh, chopped herbs, and place it in a quart jar (or use half the amount of herb if you plan on making a pint of infusion). Pour boiling water to fill to the top. Cover and let steep for at least 15 minutes and up to 8 hours. A nice added step here—and with all infusions—would be to place the jar in the sun, for sun tea, or under the moon, for moon tea!

### Dry Herb Infusion

If using dry herbs, put about half the amount into the jar, and follow the same instructions. There are herbs that are great for infusing as simples (by definition one herb), and the combinations of herbs

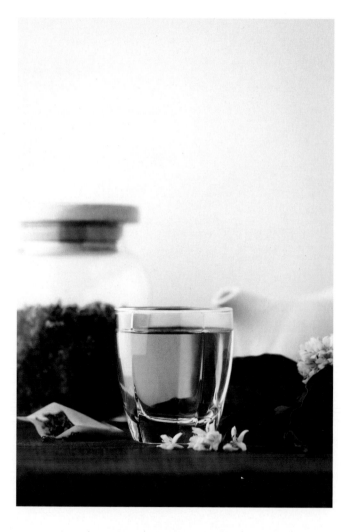

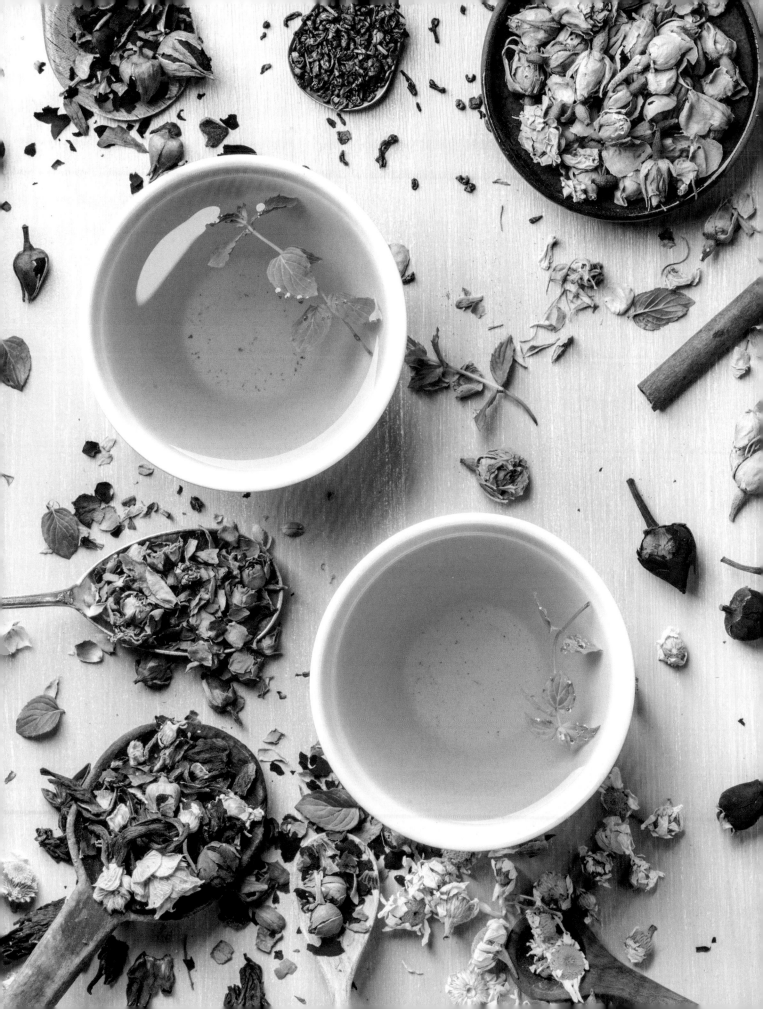

together are endless. Some are better fresh, and some dried. You can make infusions that are highly medicinal, or that are more for taste and pleasure. And they can be beautiful!

## Straining

After your herbs have been infused for the requisite amount of time, you can strain the leaves or residue out of the liquid by pouring through a strainer. This process can be made even more enjoyable by choosing or purchasing a strainer that in itself is a beautiful object.

## Using

If you are a fan of having your cup of tea hot when you drink it, you can either steep it for a little while, getting partial medicinal value, or you can reheat your infusion that has been steeping for up to 8 hours. You can also add sweetener or juice at any time! Here are some recipes to play around with. Have fun with this section—mix and match if you so desire—you'll start to feel the benefit of drinking these infusions every day.

## Vitamin C Flower Power Blend

**Ingredients:**
1 part rose hips
1 part hibiscus
2 parts lemon balm
1 part dandelion blossoms
½ part roses (whole buds or petals)

This blend will be a vibrant pink, with a very nice flavor, and is great for when you're under the weather or your immunity is low. Rose hips and hibiscus are both loaded with vitamin C, dandelion flowers will help build the blood, and also have many vitamins and nutrients, while the lemon balm is calming to the nervous system, and roses add beauty and flavor.

## Super Green Vitamin/Mineral Blend

**Ingredients:**
2 parts nettles
2 parts comfrey
1 part raspberry leaf
1 part yellow dock root
½ part peppermint (optional according to personal taste)

This is a blend that should definitely be steeped for as long as possible, especially because the nettle contains chlorophyll that takes a while to completely release all its goodness. This blend contains the entire spectrum of vitamins and minerals, making it a wonderful medicine for those struggling with low energy. Over time, this blend will build iron levels, help with magnesium and calcium deficiencies, and increase overall strength. Adding a little blackstrap molasses will add some nice sweetness, and more iron richness. The peppermint may not be right for some, and is mostly added to this blend for flavor. Without it, the taste is more earthy and rich.

## Relaxation Blend

**Ingredients:**
2 parts chamomile
1 part california poppy
1 part passion flower
½ part lavender
½ part oat tops

This is a beautiful blossom tea to promote relaxation and sleep. Depending on your energy level, this may be a blend to drink throughout the day to ease anxiety, or it may be perfect for the end of a busy day, or for those having trouble sleeping, or who often wake in the night.

## Wellness Blend

**Ingredients:**

2 parts astragalus
2 parts elder blossom
2 parts echinacea flowers and/or leaves
1 part tulsi (holy basil)
½ part yarrow
½ part rose hips

Deeply strengthening to the immune system, this blend is helpful when struggling with a cold or flu. It contains vitamin C and many vitamins and minerals that provide a deep immune tonic and stimulating properties. It is slightly diaphoretic, helping the body deal with fever. Add lemon and honey for added benefits and flavor!

## Energizing Blend

**Ingredients:**

2 parts lemongrass
1 part peppermint
½ part ginseng
½ part eleuthero

This blend is a nice invigorating tea to bring clarity and alertness to one's day. A possible alternative to caffeine, it provides a deep energy, with no crash.

## Healthy Gut/Digestion Blend

**Ingredients:**

1 part fennel seed
1 part chamomile
1 part ginger
½ part peppermint
¼ part orange peel

This blend is most effective when drunk along with meals. Stimulates and soothes the digestive tract for all-around smoother digestion.

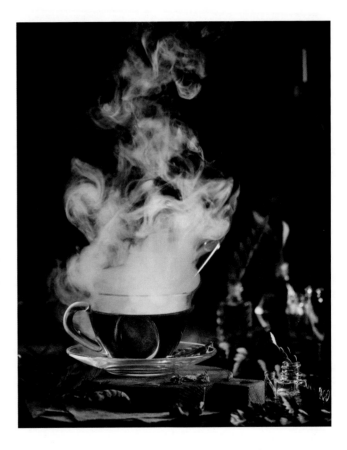

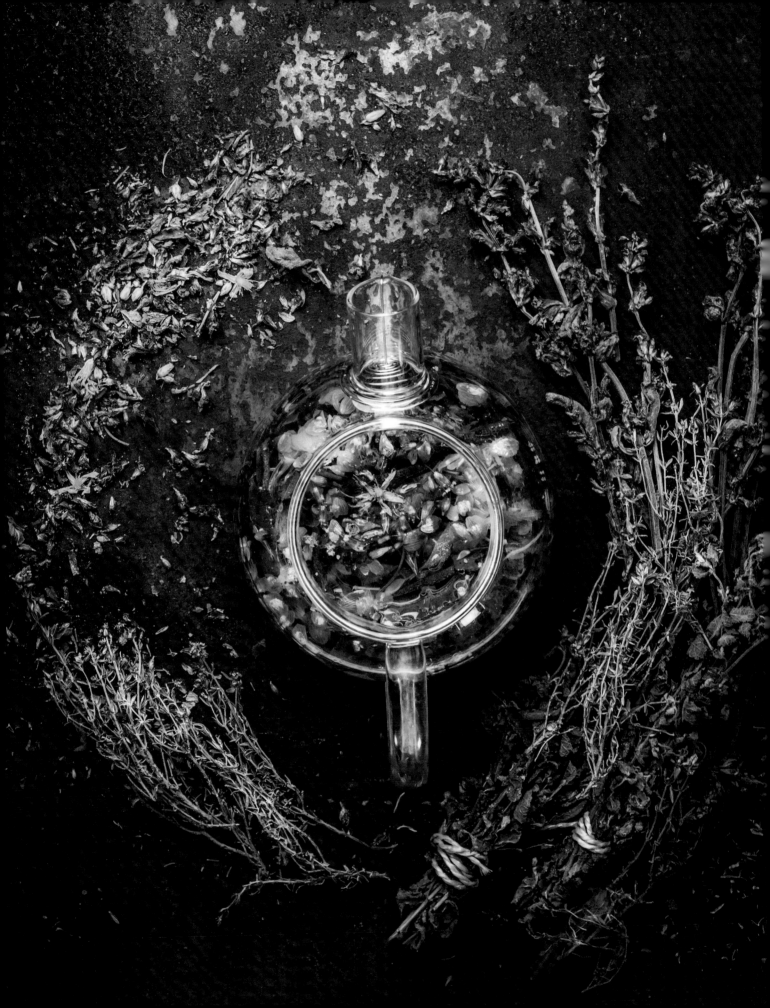

# Elixirs

## Lemongrass Ginger Thyme Elixir

This homemade herbal hot drink is easy to make, and all the ingredients can easily be found in your local grocery store. It is also packed with nutrients that your body will love. If you like to grow your own herbs, you can put them to good use with this recipe. This is a lovely after-dinner drink to help with digestion and doesn't contain any caffeine. It re-steeps well at least once. It is virtually impossible for any packaged herbal tea bag to taste this fresh! After making your homemade herbal drinks with fresh ingredients, I bet you'll never go back to herbal tea bags.

*Yields 1 serving*

### Ingredients:
1 tablespoon fresh mint
1 teaspoon fresh lemongrass
1 teaspoon fresh thyme
½ teaspoon grated ginger
¼ teaspoon fennel seeds
1–1¼ cups boiling water
Optional: ½ teaspoon raw honey, or to taste

### Directions:
1. Crush your herbs in a mortar and pestle for extra flavor.
2. Put all your ingredients in your teapot, then pour the hot water over it and steep 5–6 minutes. This tea re-steeps really nicely for a second time; leave it on for 7–8 minutes for a strong flavor.

## Starstruck Multi-Herb Elixir

This homemade herbal tea is slightly sweetened with honey, cinnamon, and star anise. You can find this star-shaped, one-of-a-kind spice in regular grocery stores or order it online. The flavor of this tea is three-fold: herbal, sweet, and spicy, and it is perfect for an afternoon of relaxation, reading, or contemplating.

*Yields 2 servings*

### Ingredients:
1 teaspoon fresh rosemary
1 teaspoon fresh thyme
½ teaspoon fresh oregano
1 teaspoon fresh basil
1 star anise
Zest of ½ medium orange
1 cinnamon stick
1 teaspoon raw honey
2 ½ cups hot water (195–205°F)

### Directions:
1. Crush your herbs in a mortar and pestle for extra flavor.
2. Add herbs and other ingredients to the teapot, then pour the hot water over it and steep for 5–6 minutes. If you prefer a stronger flavor, you can skip the honey or use only two cups of hot water. This tea also re-steeps nicely for a second time; leave it on for 7–8 minutes for a strong flavor.

## Lavender and Orange Zest Dream Elixir

This delicious lavender tea is a wonderful healing and calming nightcap. Lavender is known for reducing anxiety, calming emotional stress, and improving sleep. You can buy dried lavender at most grocery stories, and as long as you stock fennel seeds and the occasional orange, you can make this tea regularly. This is the perfect hot drink before bed, with just a touch of sweetness from pure maple syrup infused with the citrus flavor from your orange.

*Yields 1 serving*

### Ingredients:
1 teaspoon pure maple syrup
1 tablespoon fennel seeds
1 teaspoon lavender
Zest of ½ medium orange
1½ cups hot water (195–205°F)

### Directions:
1. Add all ingredients to teapot and steep for 5 minutes. You can re-steep this tea a second time for 7–8 minutes.

## Herbal Apple Cider and Honey Elixir

Apple cider vinegar and honey are made for each other. Curious what happens when you add herbs to the mixture? This hot herbal elixir is delicious and full of healing powers for better digestion. It also helps to relieve a sore throat and has been said by many to aid weight loss to boot.

*Yields 2 servings*

### Ingredients:
⅛ cup fresh rosemary
¼ cup fresh mint
⅛ cup fresh thyme
⅛ cup fresh lemongrass
1 tablespoon raw honey
2 tablespoons raw, unfiltered apple cider vinegar
2 cups hot water (195–205°F)

### Directions:
1. Crush your herbs in a mortar and pestle for extra flavor.
2. Add herbs and other ingredients to the teapot, then pour the hot water over it and steep for 5–6 minutes.

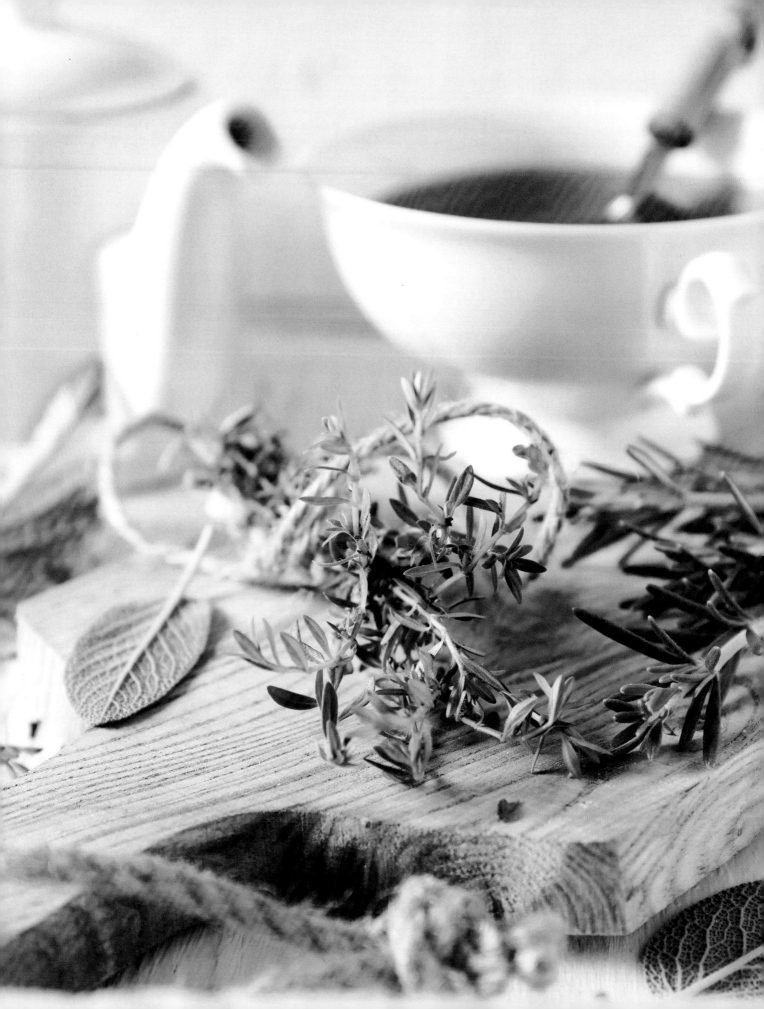

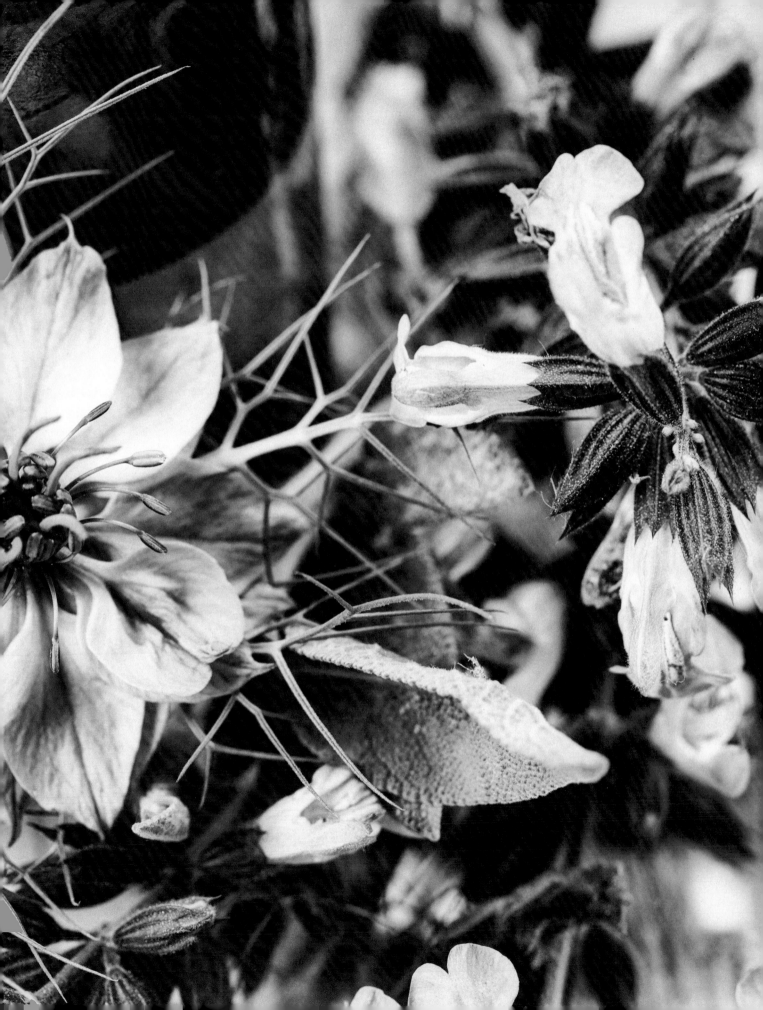

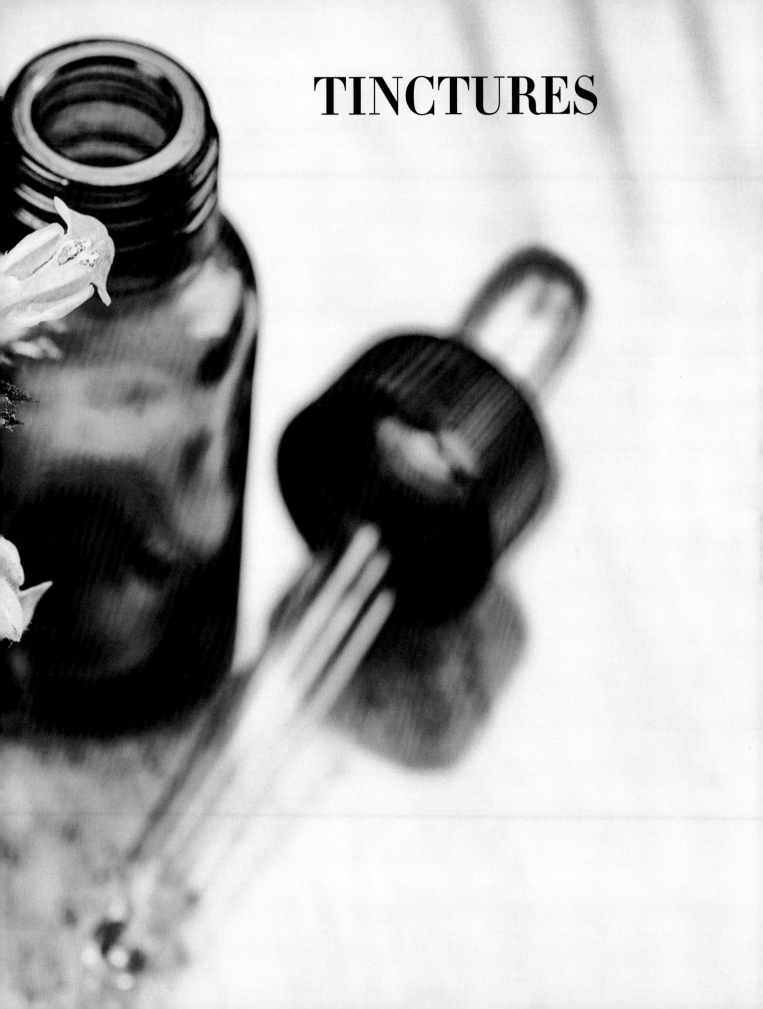

# TINCTURES

Tinctures are a way of soaking plants in a suitable solvent, generally a proportion of water and alcohol. Alcohol is the best solvent to extract chemical constituents from the plants and provides the longest shelf life of any preparation.

Herbalists most refer to alcohol and water-based preparations as "tinctures," but they can also mean products made with apple cider vinegar or vegetable glycerine. While not as strong, vinegar of glycerine can be considered for those with alcohol sensitivities, young children, those with liver issues, and/or those on numerous medications, or those avoiding alcohol for religious reasons or pregnancy.

Tinctures can be prepared using dried or fresh plant matter. When using fresh herbs, one needs to take into consideration the amount of moisture already contained in the fresh plant material in order to ensure a long shelf life and prevent spoilage. When making tinctures at home, gin, brandy, or vodka (or Everclear, if accessible) may be used as a menstruum.

### The simplest tincturing process is the Traditional Folk Directions:

1. Select your herbs of choice—fresh or dried plant material is just fine—and chop or shred finely. Do not use powdered.
2. Place herbs in a clean glass jar with a secure lid and a neck large enough to fit your hand for ease of cleaning.
3. Pour vodka over the herbs to cover entirely, adding 2 inches more above the plant material, as the herbs should be completely covered.
4. Secure the lid and shake daily; use this time to infuse the herbs with intention.
5. Soak 4 to 6 weeks, strain, and use your medicine. Adult dosage of most tinctures: 3–5 ml taken 3 times daily, diluted in hot water, and taken before meals.

## Hormonal Balance
### Ingredients:
2 parts vitex (chaste berry)
1 part red raspberry leaf
1 part wild yam
½ part American ginseng menstruum

## High Mineral Vinegar Tincture
### Ingredients:
2 parts nettle
1 part horsetail
1 part red raspberry leaf
1 part red clover
1 part cleaned and humanely sourced bones and/or egg shells

## Spicy Immunity Vinegar Tincture
### Ingredients:
1 part ginger—fresh and grated
1 part chili peppers
1 part horseradish—fresh and grated
1 part garlic—fresh, chopped or whole
1 part onions
⅓ part astragalus
¼ part fresh parsley
½ part honey

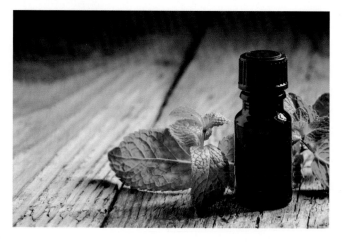

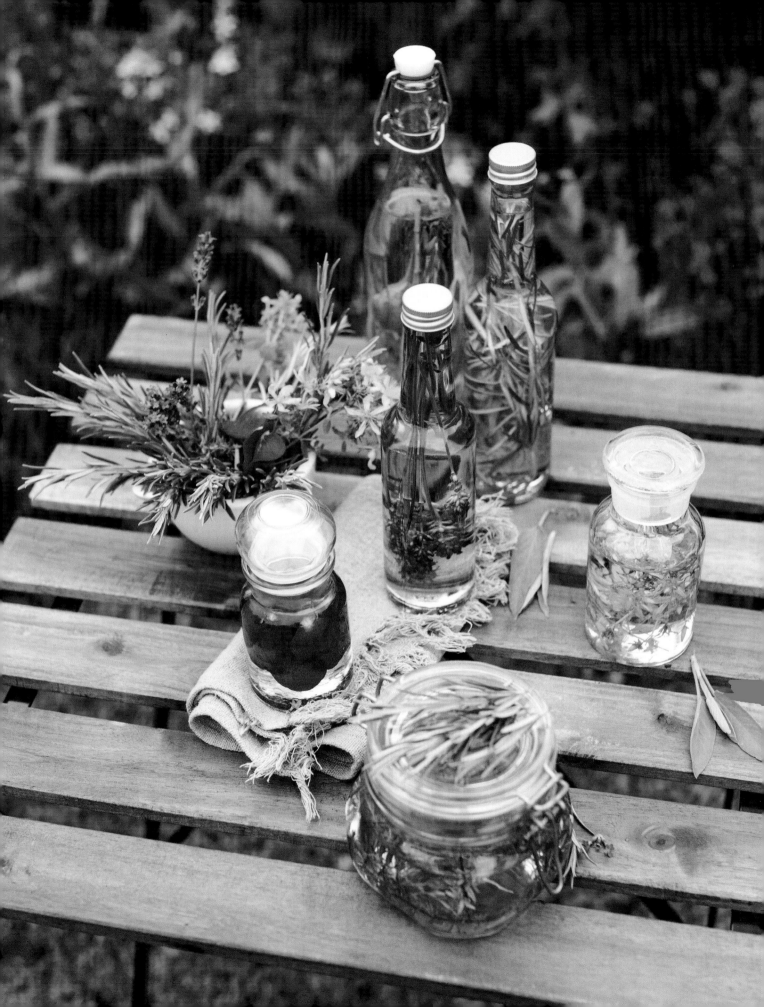

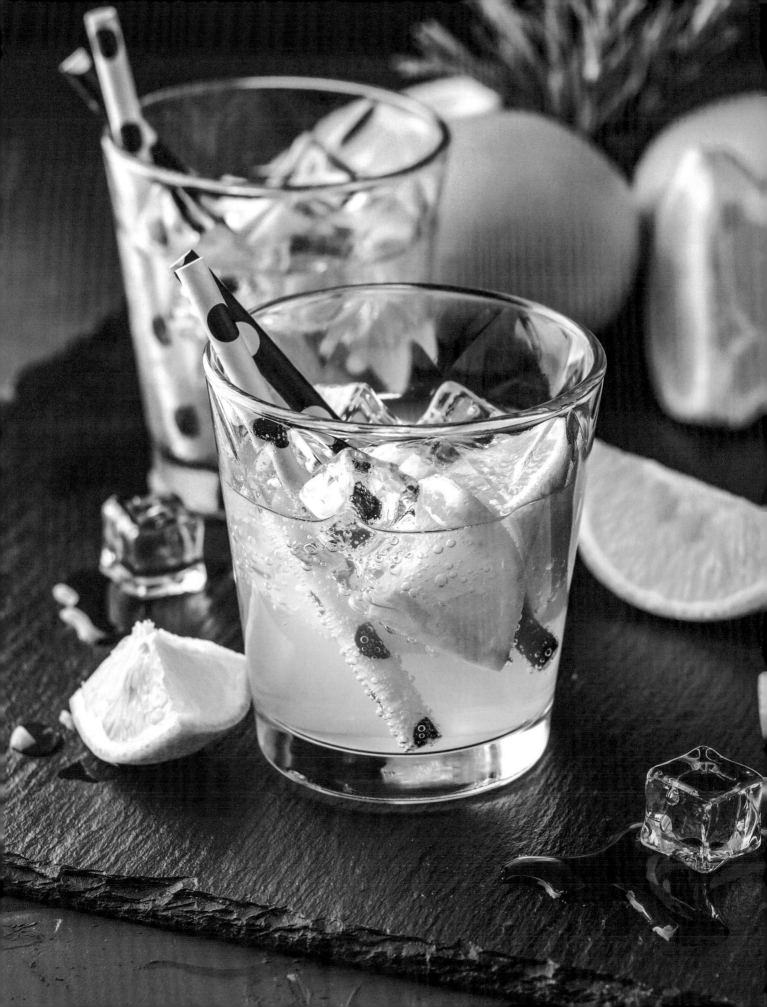

# TONICS AND SHOTS

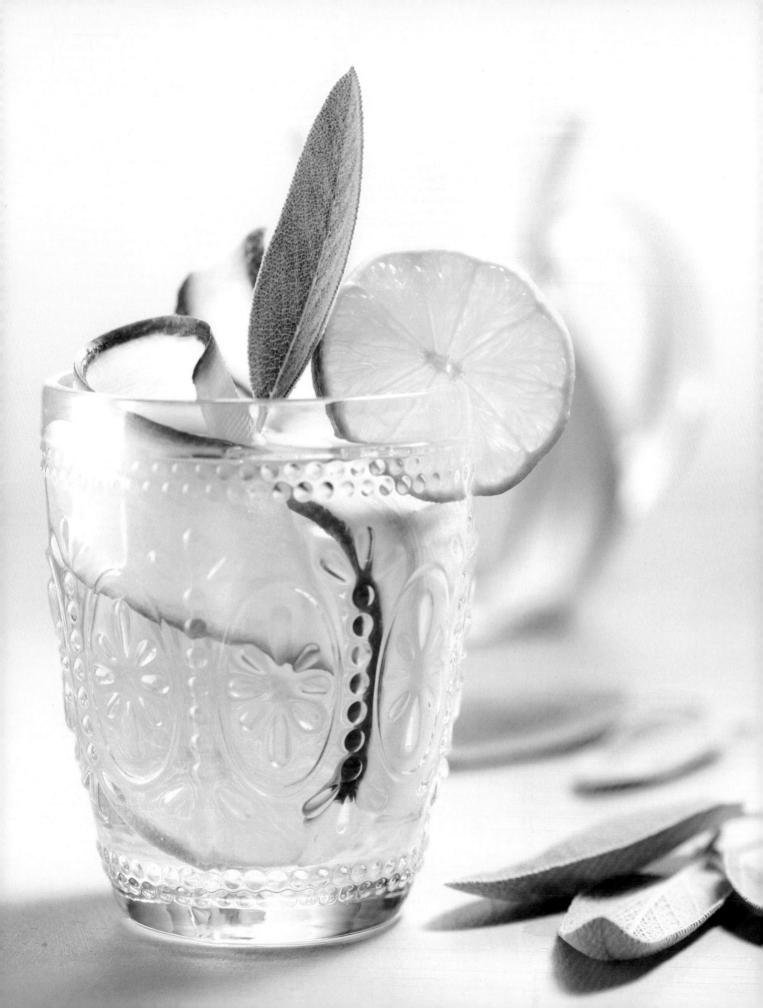

In this chapter, you learn how to make tonics and health shots using minimal equipment and in as little as two minutes—or however fast you can wash, mix, chop, slice, or grate a few ingredients! Some recipes require a bit of wait time while your ingredients marinate, but for most, you won't even need to get out your blender or juicer to whip up these delicious magic potions.

The way we define health tonics—sometimes also called immunity tonics or herbal tonics—is simple: concentrated caffeine-free, nutrient-rich drinks made through the steeping of any combination of herbs, spices, select fruits, oils, vinegar, and vegetable roots. You consume these health tonics chilled and in quantities of one or two shots. You would usually want to accompany a shot with a small snack if your tonic is strong. I like to drink my tonic after a workout or yoga and follow with some water and maybe a few salty nuts.

Health tonics have tons of benefits. They can help reduce inflammation, improve digestion, calm the nervous system, act as an energizing boost, and enhance your immune system. Because the nutritional information of these tonics is nearly negligible as far as calories are concerned, we have not included that information in this section. But rest assured, they are packed with nutrition!

The quantity produced by all of these recipes is only slightly more than the liquid base you use. Some tonic recipes you'll find online or in other books ask that you let the drinks sit in a cold, dark cabinet for a month before they are ready to consume. We did not have the patience to wait that long, and we are guessing that you don't either. So the "marinating" time for the tonics in this book is between one to two hours. Please take note of steep time in each recipe and consume it within a week.

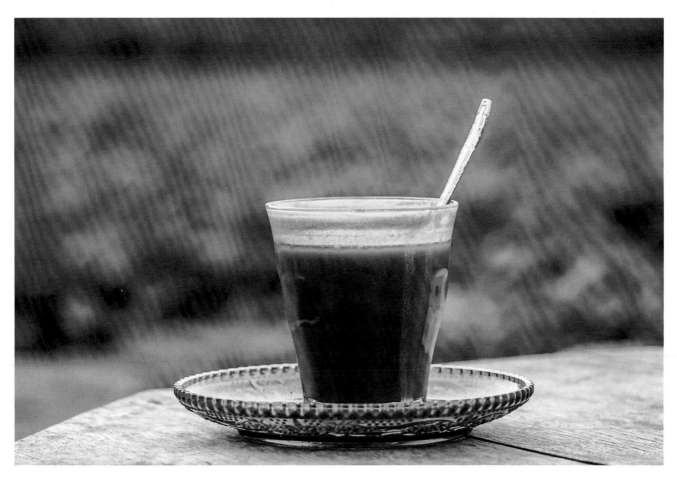

# Cool Tonics

## Sunshine Coconut, Ginger, and Turmeric Tonic

After making this delicious, refreshing, and zingy tonic, you might just be in heaven! The coconut water that I use religiously is C$_2$O. Get an unsweetened coconut water with just coconut water as the ingredient, and with low sugar content, which indicates that the juice is from a young coconut. You'll be loving this tonic on hot summer days. It's also a perfect refreshing drink to serve friends by the pool or at a health-conscious party!

### Ingredients:

4 cups unsweetened coconut water
¼ cup fresh ginger slices
¼ cup fresh turmeric slices
2 teaspoons fresh lemongrass, finely chopped
8 cardamom pods, crushed
1 lime, thinly sliced
3–4 pinches cayenne pepper

### Directions:

1. Add all ingredients into a glass jar with an airtight lid and place in the refrigerator. Set your timer for an hour, but don't let it steep for more than 75 minutes. I find that any more and it gets a little too spicy!
2. After the timer goes off, strain your tonic into another container and either serve it with fresh mint or by itself, or place back in the fridge to consume at a later time. Be sure to keep it either in a mason jar with a tight lid or any other glass container that is airtight. You can keep it in the fridge for up to a week.

## Refreshing Galangal Cider

Galangal root, also referred to as Siamese ginger or Thai ginger, has fabulous health potency, and while it looks and belongs to a similar family as ginger and turmeric and other similar roots, the taste is very distinct. I would describe it as bitter but also refreshing. You can find galangal in Asian grocery stores as well as some regular grocers. This root is better sliced than grated, and it makes a most hydrating tonic that wakes up all your senses. This tonic can be a wonderful refreshing drink any time of day.

### Ingredients:

20 grams galangal, thinly sliced
⅛ cup fresh mint
1 teaspoon fresh thyme
Zest of ½ blood orange (or other orange)
2 tablespoons raw, unfiltered apple cider vinegar
1 cinnamon stick, chopped into a few pieces
2 teaspoons raw honey dissolved first in
    2 teaspoons hot water
2 cups filtered water
Optional: frozen 5–6 Tie Guan Yin Oolong tea cubes

### Directions:

1. Add all ingredients into a glass jar with an airtight lid and place in the refrigerator. Set your timer for an hour, or at the most, 75 minutes. After the timer goes off, strain it all out into another container and either serve it or store back in the fridge to consume at a later time. Be sure to keep it either in a mason jar with a tight lid or any other glass container that is airtight. You can keep it in the fridge for up to a week.
2. You can also make oolong galangal iced tea. If you have Tie Guan Yin, which is a fabulous and common oolong tea, you can steep a cup of it, then pour it out into your ice cube tray. After it freezes, add your oolong ice cubes to the container with your Galangal Cider, and let it sit in the fridge for another hour. Serve cold and enjoy!

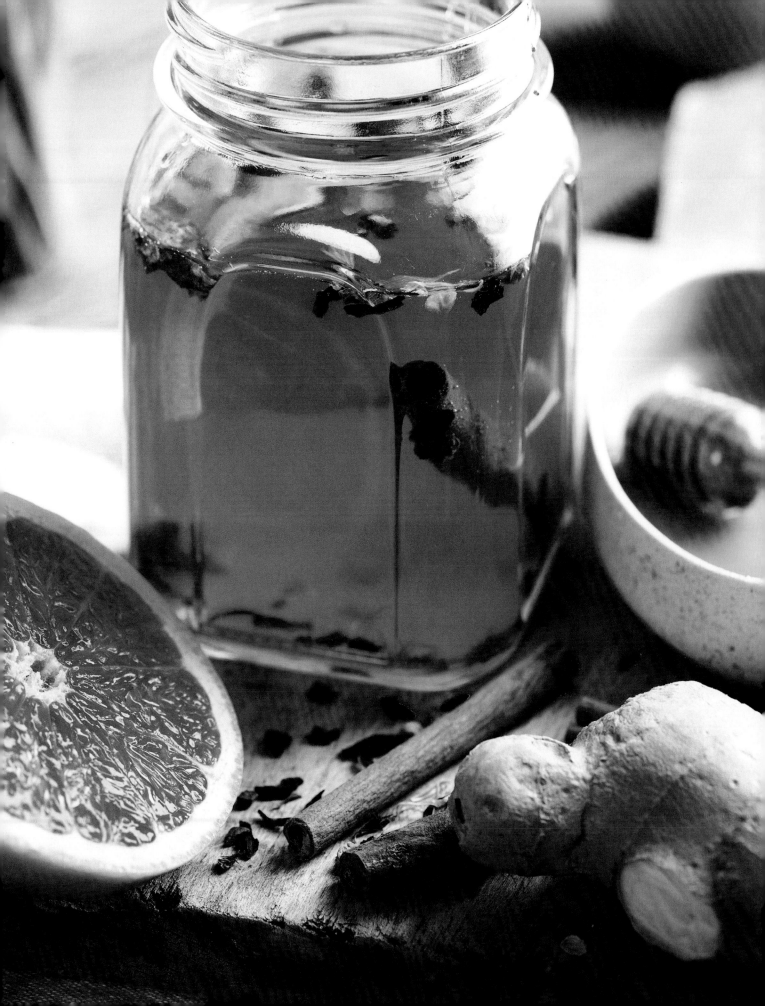

## Spicy Pomegranate and Coconut Tonic

This delicious, rejuvenating, and stimulating tonic has it all. There's a touch of sourness from pomegranate, the aroma from basil and oregano, a kick from the spicy jalapeño and ginger . . . and when they mix with the coconut water, it delivers the perfect tonic.

### Ingredients:

⅓ cup pomegranate seeds, crushed
½ fresh jalapeño pepper, seeded and minced
⅛ cup ginger slices
⅓ to ½ lemon, sliced
⅛ cup fresh oregano and mint leaves
2 cups unsweetened coconut water

### Directions:

1. Add all ingredients into your glass jar and let it steep in the fridge for 1 hour. Set your timer for an hour, or, at most, 75 minutes.

2. After the timer goes off, strain it all out into another container and either serve it or place back in the fridge to consume at a later time. Be sure to keep it either in a mason jar with a tight lid or any other glass container that is airtight. You can keep it in the fridge for up to a week.

## Cooling Peppermint Herb Tonic

Lemongrass, which is mainly used in Thai cooking, has a most energizing scent. It makes a fabulous tonic in this recipe along with fresh herbs, orange slices, turmeric, apple cider vinegar, and a touch of peppermint.

### Ingredients:

2 cups filtered water
1 tablespoon fresh thyme, crushed
⅛ cup chopped fresh dill, crushed
⅛ cup turmeric, thinly sliced
⅛ cup chopped cilantro, crushed
⅛ cup lemongrass, chopped
½ orange, thinly sliced
7–8 drops peppermint oil
1 tablespoon pure maple syrup

### Directions:

1. Slice up the unpeeled orange. Add all ingredients into your glass container. Steep it in the fridge for an hour, or, at the most, 75 minutes.

2. Strain it all out into another container and either serve it or place back in the fridge to consume at a later time. Be sure to keep it either in a mason jar with a tight lid or any other glass container that is airtight. You can keep it in the fridge for up to a week.

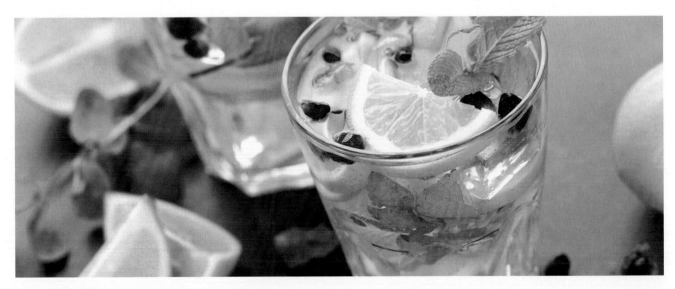

## Golden Yellow Spicy Garlic Tonic

This tonic requires a little more prep time, as you'll need your juicer to juice the orange and a lemon, but the extra effort is totally worth it. Think of it as a juice and tonic fusion with spicy garlic and ginger. The citrus flavor of fresh-squeezed juice and the amazing benefits of apple cider vinegar will deliver loads of goodies to your body. This is one of my favorites!

### Ingredients:

Fresh juice of 1 peeled orange
Fresh juice of 1 lemon
1 cup filtered water
2 tablespoons raw honey
3 cloves garlic, pressed
2 tablespoons thinly sliced or grated ginger
1 cinnamon stick, crushed
⅛ cup raw, unfiltered apple cider vinegar

### Directions:

1. Add all ingredients into your glass container. Steep it in the fridge for an hour, or at the most, 75 minutes.
2. Strain it all out into another container and either serve it or place back in the fridge to consume at a later time. Be sure to keep it either in a mason jar with a tight lid or any other glass container that is airtight. You can keep it in the fridge for up to a week.

## Berry Good Hydrating Tonic

For hot summer days, make yourself this delicious healing tonic with fresh berries, ginger, sage, and cucumber. It will help you cool down, hydrate, and consume some healing nutrients.

### Ingredients:

½ cup blueberries, crushed
4 strawberries, crushed
1 tablespoon minced ginger
5 leaves of sage, stems removed, crushed
20 Thai basil leaves, crushed
1 Persian cucumber, diced
4 cups filtered water
Optional: 1 tablespoon raw honey dissolved in 1 tablespoon hot water
Optional: 2 slices of lime

### Directions:

1. Add all ingredients to a glass jar and refrigerate for one hour. Strain. The berries soak up a lot of water, even if they were crushed, so gently press on the strainer to release all the juice.
2. If the tonic too strong, add a little honey. This tonic tastes best chilled, so feel free to add ice cubes. You can keep it in the fridge for up to a week.

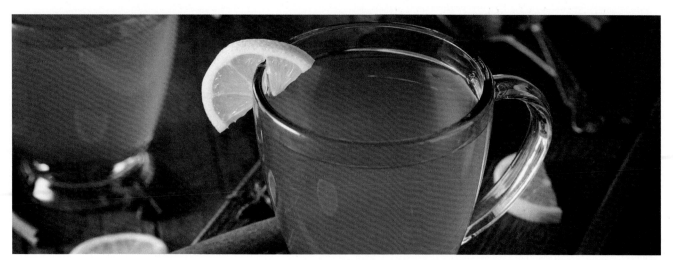

## Farnoosh's Magic Potion Tonic Recipe

Apple cider vinegar (ACV) is the most popular type of vinegar in the natural health community and is claimed to have enormous health benefits, some of which are well proven by science. You may hear of "ACV with the mother," which is the same as raw, unfiltered ACV and simply refers to the strands of proteins and enzymes and healthy bacteria that show up in unfiltered apple cider. That's what gives it the slightly murky appearance when you shake the bottle. You want this kind of raw, unfiltered ACV for maximum health benefits.

With this recipe, in addition to our raw, unfiltered ACV, I decided to throw in a few other highly potent ingredients such as garlic, ginger, turmeric, cayenne pepper, raw honey, and lemons. Below you'll find the preparation instructions to make what I call my Magic Potion Tonic Recipe as well as suggestions on how and when to consume it.

### Ingredients for Phase 1:
9–10 cloves garlic, peeled
3 unpeeled lemons
1–1 ½ cups fresh ginger root
¾–1 cup fresh turmeric root

### NOTE:
If you can't find fresh turmeric root, you can substitute 1 tablespoon turmeric powder dissolved in 1 tablespoon of hot water. You can do the same with ground ginger rather than fresh ginger root. I do recommend going for the fresh roots of both if at all possible.

### Directions for Phase 1:
1. Juice everything in your juicer. It's best to use a masticating slow juicer that completely juices the ingredients.

Next, you'll need the following ingredients:

### Ingredients for Phase 2:
2 tablespoons raw honey
1–1 ¼ cups raw, unfiltered apple cider vinegar
1 teaspoon cayenne pepper
Optional: 3–4 drops rosemary essential oil

### Directions for Phase 2:
1. Dissolve your honey in 2 tablespoons of hot water. Then add that and remaining Phase 2 ingredients into your juice made in Phase 1.
2. Stir everything for one minute. Store in an airtight glass container for up to two weeks in the refrigerator.
3. Take 1–2 tablespoons of your magic potion daily on an empty stomach and without diluting it. Immediately after, drink 16–24 oz. of filtered water. Then eat your breakfast. Be sure to eat within 15–20 minutes of drinking the potion, or you may feel nauseous. If you're not ready for a full meal just yet, have a few salty nuts with some water.

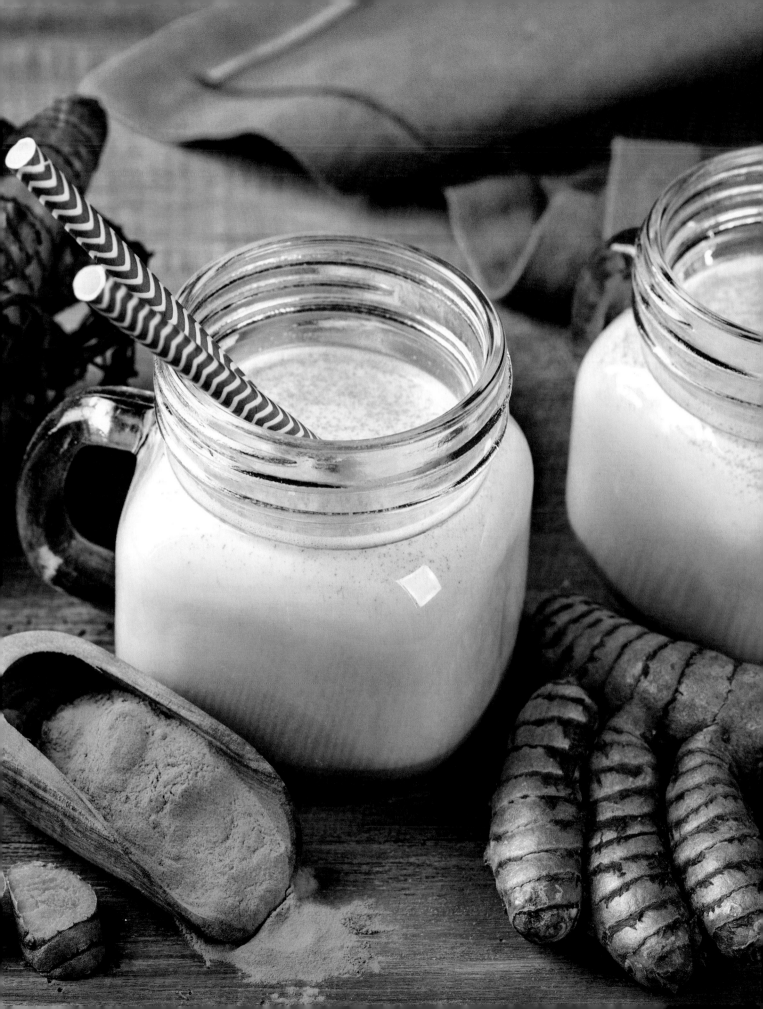

# Health Shots

## Anti-Inflammatory Spicy Wake-Me-Up Shot

This cold, latte-like drink can be whipped up in two minutes. It is perfect for mornings when you don't have a lot of time. You most likely already have turmeric powder, cayenne pepper, and ginger powder in your spice cabinet. I love this wake-me-up for the anti-inflammatory benefits of the spices. Plus, it's delicious! I've found that these spice powders dissolve best in hot water, but you don't want to raise the temperature of your cold milk either, so use no more than two tablespoons to dissolve the powders, let it sit for a minute to cool slightly, then add your cold nut milk. This is a spicy drink with a warming aftereffect. It will help your muscles release inflammation and it can also be great for any digestion issues or act as a quick detox before the start of your day.

### Ingredients:

½ teaspoon turmeric powder
¼ teaspoon ginger powder
⅛ teaspoon cayenne pepper
½ cup almond or cashew milk

### Directions:

1. Dissolve all ingredients in 1–2 tablespoons of hot water. Allow to cool for 1 minute.
2. Add cold almond or cashew milk. Mix and drink it up.

## Trace Minerals Nightcap Shot

Do you get your trace minerals? Our bodies need tiny amounts of minerals such as iron, zinc, selenium, fluoride, chromium, copper, iodine, and magnesium on a daily basis. A versatile and healthy diet can and often does contain most of these minerals, but then again, how often do we have days when life happens and we can't prioritize complete, healthy meals? While getting your trace minerals from a natural food source is the best option, what's most important is that you get them one way or another on a daily basis. Supplements are one way to get them, but my preferred method is in powder form so that your body can absorb it as quickly and efficiently as possible.

For the past three years, I've kept a bottle of Mezotrace in my cupboard, and every night, before bed, I make my soothing presleep nightcap. What I love about Mezotrace is that it tastes delicious when mixed with just a little nut milk. While taste buds can vary, I can say that my neighbor agrees, too. She not only loves it, but after taking this for a week, her splitting headaches disappeared. I'm not promising that Mezotrace is a cure-all, but if you're low on your trace minerals, this can be a quick fix and an easy, healing drink to incorporate into your daily habits. You don't have to stick with Mezotrace brand either. You can search other brands that offer these essential minerals in powdered form for your healing nightcap!

### Ingredients:

½ teaspoon Mezotrace or your choice of powdered minerals
½ cup almond or cashew milk, or even water

### Directions:

1. Mix until powder is dissolved, and drink.

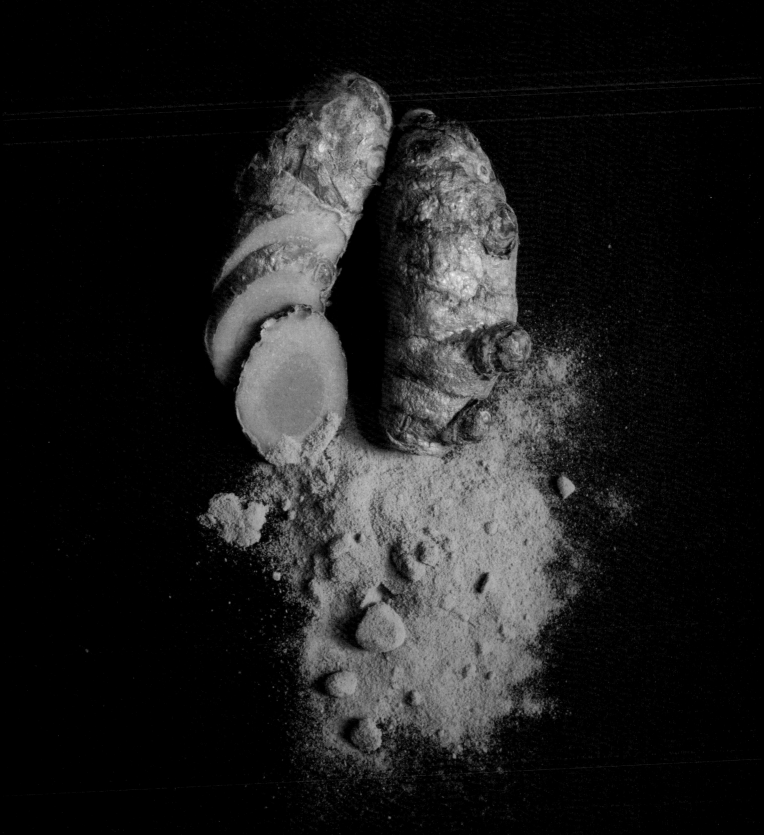

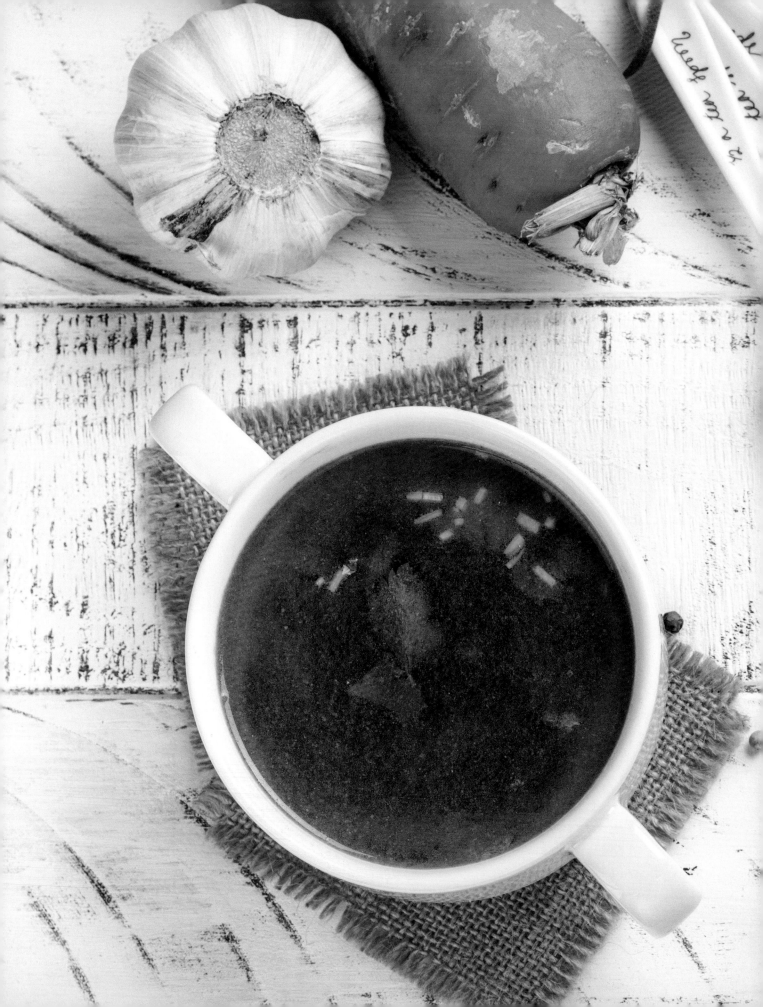

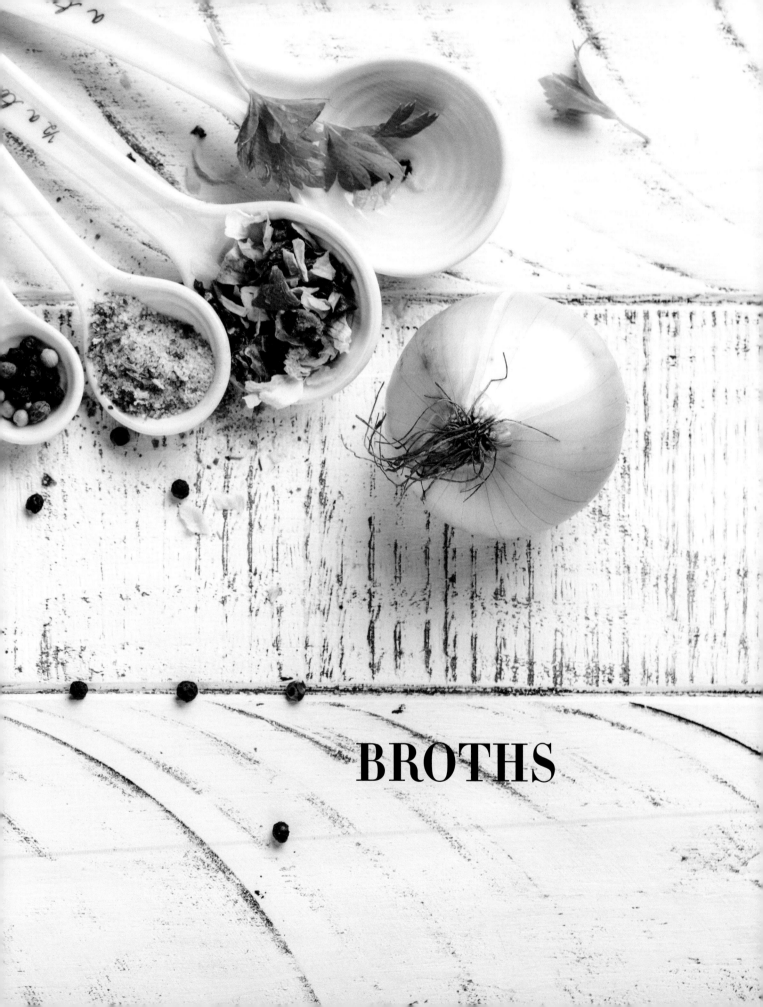

# BROTHS

The recipes to follow use a mix of fresh ingredients, leftovers, and scraps. That is one of the best things about broths—you can use ingredients that would typically go in the trash. Take a look at the things you often discard while cooking—things like chicken bones, meat scraps, onion peels, potato peels, vegetable pulps, and corn cobs (but only ones you have cut the corn from, not gnawed on!). These things can go into your next broth. Experiment.

## Vitamins and Minerals in Bone Broth

Among the many health benefits of bone broth is the mineral content of this slow-cooked nourishing liquid. Minerals like calcium, magnesium, phosphorous, and potassium are released over the course of several hours as the bone softens and breaks down in the simmering heat. While the precise amount of these minerals in each batch of broth can differ depending on how long the broth is cooked for, whether the bones are organic and grass-fed or not, how healthy the animal was,

and other mitigating factors, the estimated mineral content in broth is a welcome addition to an already healthy practice of consuming broth regularly in your diet.

## Inflammatory Disorders

Inflammation, when functioning properly in the body, is a good thing. It is the body's way of responding to dangerous attacks and bringing in resources to fix or rid the body of these hazards. When an individual experiences trauma, physical injury, burns, or even small nuisances like splinters in the skin or dust in the eye, inflammation is the response that makes the area swell, feel hot, get red, and feel painful. The immune system then sends white blood cells to clear out or destroy the problem. Situations like these, when stimuli hurt or damage the body and then inflammation kicks in to repair the affected areas, is called an innate response. It is a generic reaction to foreign agents or stimuli.

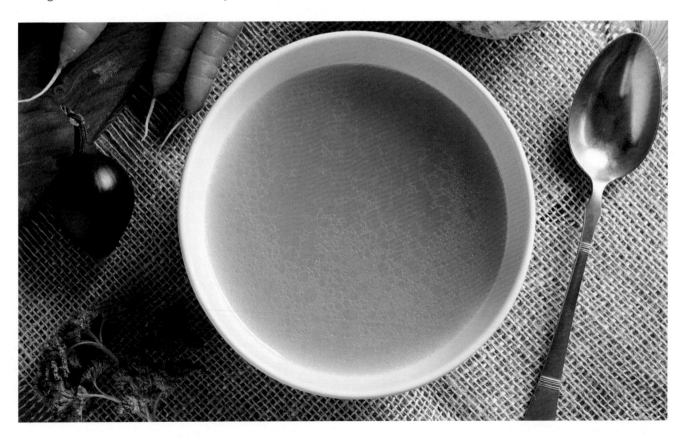

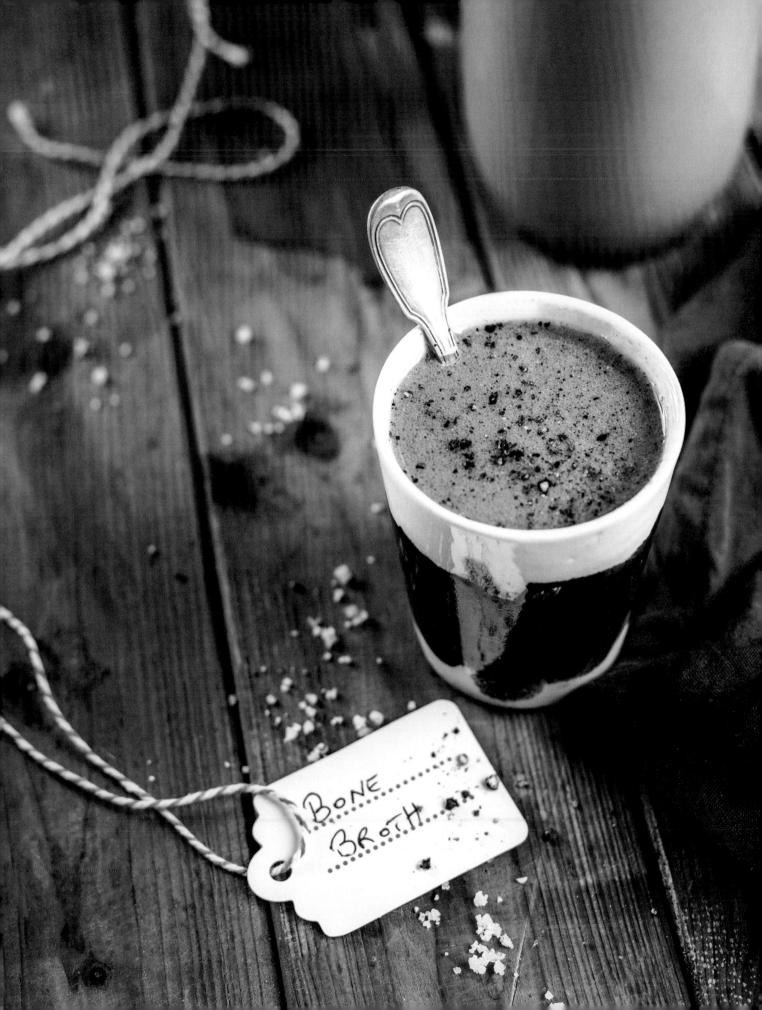

As a process of the immune system, inflammation also exercises adaptive immunity. This is when the body is encroached upon by an illness or other pathogens like bacteria, fungi, and other viruses, and the immune system learns what it is, destroys it, and then remembers it the next time it happens. This is why when individuals experience certain illnesses, they can build up immunities and either suffer fewer symptoms the next time, or none at all.

A pitfall of these bodily responses is that sometimes they can become chronic. Oftentimes this has to do with external stressors, like diet and environmental contaminants that are persistently causing inflammation in the body. This is severely detrimental to overall health, not just the affected areas, because it puts the body under constant stress and in perpetual defense mode. Foods that are filled with preservatives, made from processed vegetable oils, sourced from nonorganic farms, or otherwise exposed to toxins like chemicals and pesticides can all contribute to chronic inflammation. Considering these triggers, chronic inflammation is often a key symptom of serious illnesses like diabetes, heart disease, stroke, obesity, arthritis and osteoporosis, cystic fibrosis, fibromyalgia, and depression and anxiety.

Symptoms of chronic inflammation can be controlled with medicine, but not cured. The best way to prevent inflammation is to start with a healthy diet comprised of anti-inflammatory foods. By disrupting the causes of inflammation and removing them from the surrounding environment or regular diet, individuals susceptible to inflammation can prevent it from occurring at all. For those who have lived with chronic inflammation due to poor diet, illness, or environmental contaminants, making healthy lifestyle changes can drastically alter and even repair the damage that has been done to the body.

As a soothing home treatment that has been trusted for generations, bone broth has been proven to reduce, repair, and prevent inflammation and its underlying causes. Paired with healthy eating, activity, and awareness of the potential triggers of inflammation, individuals can reduce if not completely rid their lives of these ailments. With daily cups of bone broth or by adding gelled broth to recipes, the positive anti-inflammatory benefits can be an easy, unobtrusive way to regularly prevent these disruptive inflammatory disorders.

## Higher Energy

The extra boost in energy is just a few daily cups of bone broth away. Not only is the elixir packed with nutrients, minerals, protein, and vitamins that can replenish your system, but also in practice, drinking bone broth can replace some of the drinks that make us lethargic, unmotivated, and less likely to be active. Sugary energy drinks, sodas, and too much caffeine can stimulate momentary rushes of energy, but more often than not, they are followed by intense, regrettable energy crashes and adrenal fatigue. Not only this, but these kinds of beverages are filled with preservatives, chemicals, and coloring agents that can have severe health consequences, from weight gain and illnesses, all the way to cancer.

Drinking bone broth is a warm pick-me-up, but its nutrient and protein base sparks energy and jump-starts metabolism. Pair this with supercharged stews and soups made from bone broth, and the medley of vitamins, rich minerals, and nutrition yields a healthy, balanced diet that keeps your system from experiencing inflammation, digestive problems, and other stressors related to diet that can prevent us from getting up and moving. Studies show that individuals who take an active role in food preparation and health-conscious eating are more likely to exercise and relish activity. Some may chalk this up to be a personality trait, but the reality is that if your body feels good from the nutritious foods you put into it, you are more likely to want to get on your feet and use that body.

## Better Sleep

Most Americans suffer from sleep deprivation in some form or another. According to the National Center on Sleep Disorder Research at the NIH, 30–40 percent of adults in the United States report symptoms of insomnia, and 10–15 percent of those people suffer from chronic insomnia. What's more, the National Sleep Foundation has found that 38 percent of Americans awake from sleep feeling unrested, with others in that group experiencing tossing, turning, and an inability to return to sleep if woken. This is a very real problem because the stress on the body associated with lack of sleep can creep into the day, causing fatigue, low energy, and headaches, and can lead to more arduous health problems down the line. Sleep disorders are often associated with obesity, hypertension, diabetes, stroke, depression, cardiovascular disease, poor work performance, memory lapses, impaired cognitive function, gastrointestinal ailments, irritability, and anxiety. Excess weight and inactivity can cause disruptions in breathing during sleep, causing sleep apnea and other sleep disorders.

The benefits of bone broth to sleep are multifaceted. The first is that with healthy nutrition and bone broth as a part of an active lifestyle, individuals can reduce obesity and gastrointestinal-related sleep deprivation and have more restful nights. Additionally, the amino acid glycine has been found to facilitate the sleep cycle. Its interaction with brain receptors may be responsible for limiting muscle movement during REM sleep (rapid eye movement), increasing serotonin levels, and lowering core body temperature. Bone broth is rich with amino acids, including glycine, which can help transition the body into healthier and more restorative sleep cycles.

## Battling a Cold

Chicken soup has been the trusted home remedy for cold and flu season for generations. While the reasons behind this have long been anecdotal, recent studies have indicated that chicken soup can inhibit neutrophil migration, which typically leads to inflammation. The combination of fats and antioxidants in soup made from a whole chicken work together to achieve other health benefits, but the anti-inflammation qualities of chicken soup can deter a number of nutritional deficiencies and sicknesses. Additionally, sipping the warm broth stimulates nasal clearance. Drinking the broth throughout the duration of a cold can help improve painful symptoms of the upper respiratory tract.

## Fitness and Recovery from Injury

Sports and fitness have long been closely linked with high-protein diets, and for good reason. Protein provides energy and helps build muscle, but as a society, we tend to rely on lean cuts of meat and protein powders. While this can have many short-term benefits in the way of muscle building and strength, neglecting the other parts of the meat that include joint pieces, cartilage, and marrow is a missed opportunity for many other reasons. These lesser-chosen parts of the animal provide the vitamins, amino acids, minerals, and fatty acids that lean cuts do not. This can lead to vitamin deficiency and cause harm over the long term.

This is where bone broth comes in. The gelatin in bone broth contains many important, conditionally essential amino acids that can help athletes train, compete, and repair the wear and tear on their bodies that can result from intense physical exertion. Gelatin supplements have even been associated with over 200 percent higher performance output in athletes. Studies have shown that 15 grams of glycine paired with exhaustive exercise can increase dexterity, rebuild muscle tissue, bolster muscle strength, and fend off exhaustion.

Glutamine, another conditionally essential amino acid present in bone broth, can support the immune system, reduce muscle atrophy, and help the body recover from fatigue faster. When the body is overworked, particularly through athletics and intense training, muscles release glutamine to help make up for this exhaustion. When this happens, the muscles weaken. Drinking bone broth as an exercise supplement can replenish this glutamine so that this kind of negative result is never a problem.

When faced with injury, athletes can do astonishing damage. Constant training and strain on the body can break down cartilage and joints, tear ligaments, and add intense strain on the skeletal frame. With daily cups of bone broth, these joints, connective tissues, and bones receive constant nourishment and protection of amino acids and anti-inflammatory agents that can make injury less likely. In the case of injury, however, the typical response is for the athlete to take NSAIDs like ibuprofen to suppress inflammation and decrease pain. Dependency on these kinds of medicines can lead to a worn stomach lining. Instead, a holistic approach with bone broth can reduce injury-associated inflammation and speed up the healing process. The LA Lakers' nutrition consultant—a physician—has been prescribing bone broth to the players for years with phenomenal results. When the prognosis for a severely sprained ankle seemed to mean that Kobe Bryant would not play for the foreseeable future, bone broth brought him back in two games. Bone broth can offer athletes and people who live active lifestyles a healthy buffer, aiding in muscle strength, safeguarding bones and muscle tissue, and soothing recovery in the face of injury.

A couple of preparation notes before you get started:

1. As we are making a large quantity of hot liquid, take care not to put it immediately into your refrigerator or freezer. It must cool down to less than room temperature first. To expedite the process, simply put some water and ice into your kitchen sink. Once you pour the cooked broth through a strainer into a bowl, put the bowl into the ice water to bring down the temperature of the broth more swiftly. It should not take long before the broth is lukewarm and then safe to put into your refrigerator. Or, if you have some broth left over in the freezer, then you can put that frozen broth directly into the bowl with the just-prepared broth to lower the temperature without the ice bath.

2. I use three different preparation methods for the recipes, and each method can be used to make any type of broth. The only thing that will vary is the cooking time; bone broths require a longer cooking time to fully break down the collagen, which is the substance that gives the broth its nice "jelly" consistency when cooled.

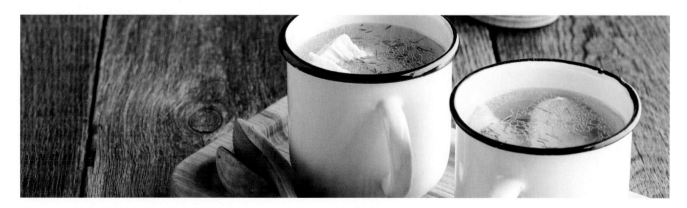

## Beef Bone Broth in the Instant Pot

Roasting meat bones in the oven before boiling them gives a little more depth of flavor to your broth. Also, I use relatively little salt, as I like to add some additional seasoning when I consume the broth. This may be a shake of soy sauce, a squeeze of lemon, and/or a dash or two of cayenne pepper. For this recipe I am using an Instant Pot, which is essentially a smart pressure cooker. This helps make the broth much faster than cooking on the stove or in a Crock-Pot.

If you don't have an Instant Pot, do not worry; if you have a slow cooker, follow the cooking instructions in the chicken bone broth recipe that follows. For stove top preparation, bring all ingredients to a boil and then simmer partially covered for at least 12 hours. The longer it goes, the better it will be!

*Yields 6–7 cups*

### Ingredients:

2 pounds beef bones, thawed
1 large onion, chopped
2 ribs celery, diced
4 cloves garlic, peeled and crushed
1 teaspoon sea salt
8 cups water
Optional and recommended: a handful of herbs, such as parsley, thyme, or rosemary

### Directions:

1. Place the beef bones on a roasting tray and place in an oven preheated to 400°F. Roast for 30 minutes.
2. After 30 minutes, places the bones into the Instant Pot.
3. Place the onion, celery, garlic, and salt into the pot on top of the bones.
4. Slowly add 8 cups of water (be sure not to fill the Instant Pot past the "max fill" line) then lock in the lid.
5. Set the Instant Pot for "Pressure cook, high" for 2 hours.
6. After 2 hours, let the pressure in the Instant Pot release naturally, about 20 minutes.
7. Vent any remaining pressure and then remove the lid.
8. Strain the contents of the Instant Pot through a sieve into a container for cooling and eventual storage.

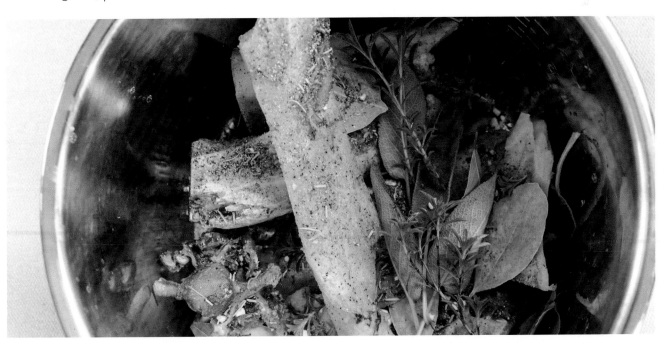

## Chicken Bone Broth in the Slow Cooker

We eat chicken a couple of times a week, and whenever I have leftover chicken scraps or a rotisserie carcass, I toss them into a ziplock bag in the freezer. When I have about 2 pounds' worth, it is time to make some chicken broth.

### Ingredients:
2 pounds chicken bones
1 large onion, peeled and chopped
2 ribs celery, diced
1 cup carrot pulp (or 2 medium carrots, diced)
2 bay leaves
1 teaspoon sea salt
8 cups water
Optional and recommended: a handful of herbs, such as parsley, thyme, or rosemary

### Directions:
1. Place all ingredients except for the water in the slow cooker.
2. Slowly add the water to the slow cooker and put on the lid.
3. Set the slow cooker for 12 hours on LOW setting.
4. Strain the contents of the slow cooker through a sieve into a container for cooling and eventual storage.

## Vegetable Broth on the Stove

If you do not consume meat, then you can still get the benefits of broth by going with a completely vegetarian version. This recipe is even vegan and, as a bonus, it takes much less time to make this broth than the meat broths!

### Ingredients:
1 cup mushrooms, cleaned and halved
2 large onions, peeled and chopped
2 cups celery pulp (or 4 ribs celery, diced)
2 cups carrot pulp (or 4 medium carrots, diced)
1 cup parsley, loosely chopped
6 cloves garlic, peeled and crushed
2 bay leaves
1 teaspoon sea salt
10 cups water

### Directions:
1. Place all ingredients except for the water into a large pot on your stove top.
2. Slowly add the water to pot and put on the lid.
3. Turn the stove burner to medium-high to bring the pot to boil.
4. Once a boil has been reached, turn the heat down to low and simmer for 1 hour.
5. Strain the contents of the pot through a sieve into a container for cooling and eventual storage.

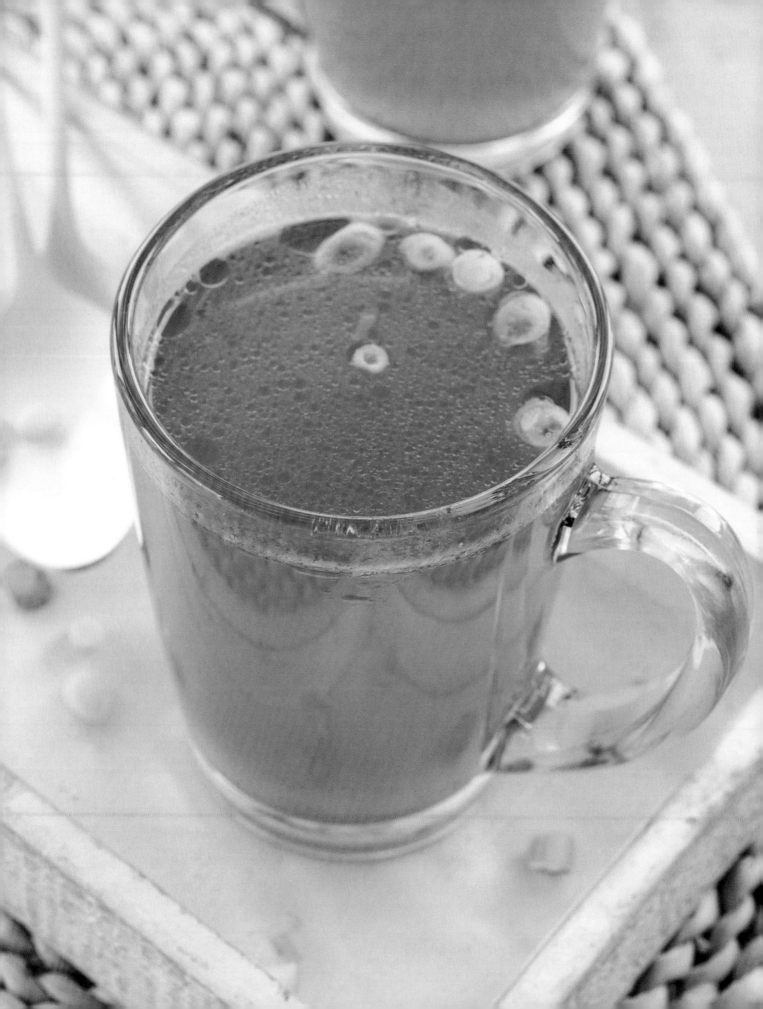

## Basic Lamb Bone Broth

Lamb: it may be adorable, but it's also chock-full of B vitamins, zinc, and even more CLA than beef. Though the taste is mild, the scent is strong and has what some might consider an off-putting level of "game" meat smell. Despite that, people love its gentle flavor, and it makes a great vehicle for all sorts of spice combinations.

Serves 8–10

### Ingredients:
5 lbs. lamb marrow bones, raw or cooked
    leftovers
5 quarts water
2 tbsps apple cider vinegar
1 tbsp salt
Optional: four sprigs of mint or two whole cloves

*If you would rather make a different quantity, use the ratio of 1 pound of bones to 1 quart water, with 1 teaspoon salt and ½ tablespoon vinegar per pound of bones.

### Directions:
1. In a stockpot, pressure cooker, or slow cooker, add bones.
2. If raw, brown if desired to increase flavor.
3. Add water, salt, and vinegar, cover, and bring to boil.
4. Reduce heat to a simmer, and cook, covered, 1–3 hours in a pressure cooker, 24–48 hours in a slow cooker, or 12–24 hours on a stove top. Add water as needed to stove top or slow cooker, and skim fat and film as it cooks.
5. Strain out bones and add salt to taste.

## Basic Fish Bone Broth

Though most people never notice, the gelatin from fish bones is used in commercial products from marshmallows to gummy candies. While this is one of the less good-looking types of broth to make, mostly according to those who don't like to be stared at by their food, fish has such a different nutrient profile from poultry or red meat that it is an excellent way to change things up.

Serves 8–10

### Ingredients:
5 lbs. fish heads and carcasses, raw or cooked
    leftovers
5 quarts water
2 tbsps apple cider vinegar
½ tbsp salt
Optional: several sprigs of dill

*If you would rather make a different quantity, use the ratio of 1 pound of bones to 1 quart water, with 1 teaspoon salt and ½ tablespoon vinegar per pound of bones.

### Directions:
1. In a stockpot, pressure cooker, or slow cooker, add bones.
2. If raw, brown if desired to increase flavor.
3. Add water, salt, and vinegar, cover, and bring to boil.
4. Reduce heat to a simmer, and cook, covered, 1–3 hours in a pressure cooker, 24–48 hours in a slow cooker, or 12–24 hours on a stove top. Add water as needed to stove top or slow cooker, and skim fat and film as it cooks.
5. Strain out bones and add salt to taste.

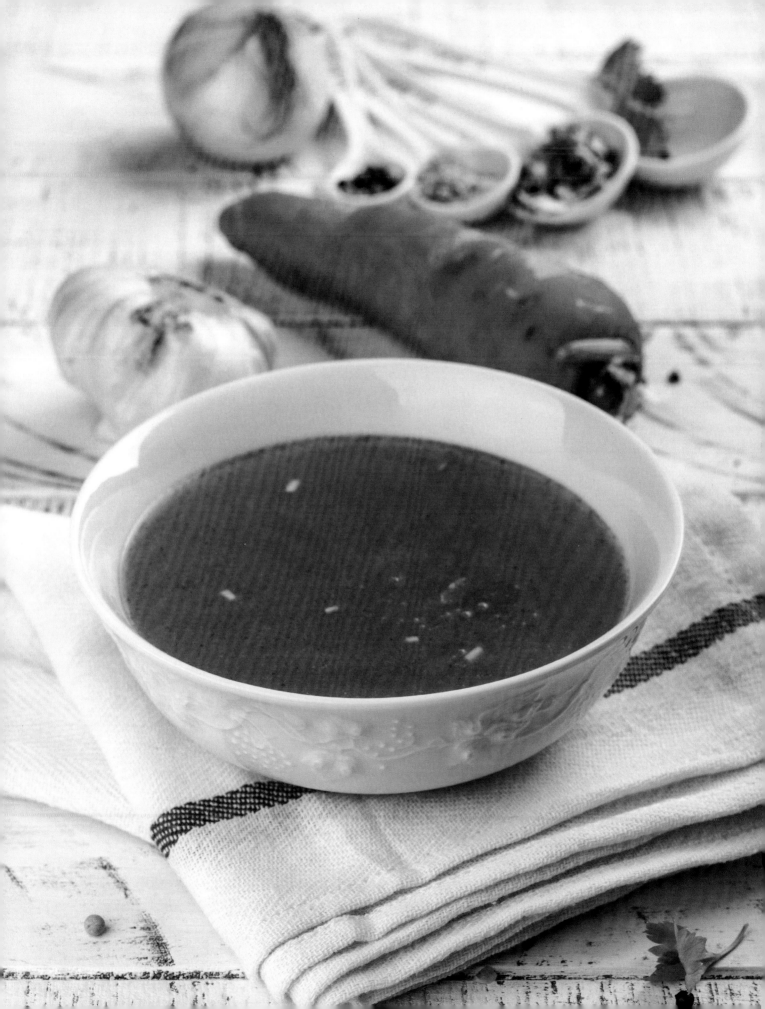

# Beautifier

While all bone broths contain collagen and help contribute to your body's own collagen production, this broth is the fast track there. Chicken and pig feet are dense with it, and lycopene-rich red foods such as tomatoes and hot peppers help your body create more. The flavor of these bones is surprisingly mild, so the tomatoes actually play a larger part here in taste than one would anticipate.

Serves 8–10

## Ingredients:
3 lbs. chicken feet
3 pig feet
1 lb. tomatoes, halved
5 quarts water
2 tbsps apple cider vinegar
1 tbsp salt
Optional: one hot red pepper, with or without
  seeds, halved

*If you would rather make a different quantity, use the ratio of 1 pound of bones to 1 quart water with 1 teaspoon salt, and ½ tablespoon vinegar per pound of bones.

## Directions:
1. In a stockpot, pressure cooker, or slow cooker, add chicken and pig feet.
2. If raw, brown if desired to increase flavor.
3. Add water, salt, and vinegar, cover, and bring to boil.
4. Reduce heat to a simmer, and cook, covered, 1–3 hours in a pressure cooker, 24–48 hours in a slow cooker, or 12–24 hours on a stove top. Add water as needed to stove top or slow cooker, and skim fat and film as it cooks.
5. Add tomatoes, and hot pepper if using, with one hour left on a stove top, two hours left in the slow cooker, or at the end of depressurizing if using a pressure cooker.
6. Strain out bones and tomatoes and add salt to taste.

# Inflammation Reducer

All broth made from grass-fed meat and wild fish will help lower inflammation, but if it's currently a problem you are dealing with, you may wish to amp up your defenses and tackle it as fiercely as possible. Packed with ginger, turmeric, and sweet potatoes, this recipe is like a chill pill for your system.

Serves 8–10

## Ingredients:
5 lbs. beef or lamb marrow bones, raw or cooked
  leftovers
5 quarts water
6 inches ginger root, sliced into ½-inch rounds
1 medium sweet potato, cut into quarters
4 fresh turmeric roots, sliced lengthwise
2 tbsps apple cider vinegar
1 tbsp salt

*If you would rather make a different quantity, use the ratio of 1 pound of bones to 1 quart water, with 1-inch ginger, 1 turmeric root, ¼ sweet potato, 1 teaspoon salt, and ½ tablespoon vinegar per pound of bones.

## Directions:
1. In a stockpot, pressure cooker, or slow cooker, add bones.
2. If raw, brown if desired to increase flavor.
3. Add water, salt, and vinegar, cover, and bring to boil.
4. Reduce heat to a simmer, and cook, covered, 1–3 hours in a pressure cooker, 24–48 hours in a slow cooker, or 12–24 hours on a stove top. Add water as needed to stove top or slow cooker, and skim fat and film as it cooks.
5. Add sweet potato, ginger, and turmeric with one hour left on a stove top, two hours left in a slow cooker, or at the end of depressurizing if using a pressure cooker.
6. Strain out all solids and add salt to taste.

## CBD Infusion for Beverage and Broth Recipe

Beverage infusion using tinctured CBD or CBDA and acacia gum powder is a convenient way to infuse CBD and CBDA into beverages—especially clear beverages and broth. High grades of acacia gum powder are best for all beverages, hot or cold. One serving of beverage or broth, for these purposes, is approximately 6 to 8 ounces (177ml–240ml).

### Ingredients:

CBD or CBDA tincture, 1 dropperful or up to 1 tsp (1ml–5ml), per beverage or broth serving

½ tsp–1 tsp (1g–2.5g) acacia gum powder, per beverage or broth serving 1 tbsp (15ml) room temperature water, per beverage or broth serving

### Directions:

1. Add the tincture and the acacia gum powder to each serving cup or bowl. Add the water.
2. Whisk vigorously until fully combined and emulsified.
3. Your serving cup or bowl is now ready for the beverage or broth you would like to add. Slowly add the beverage or broth while stirring. Serve immediately.

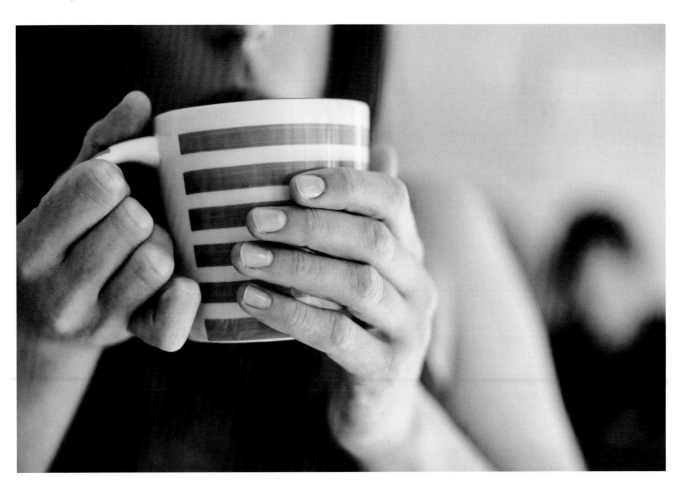

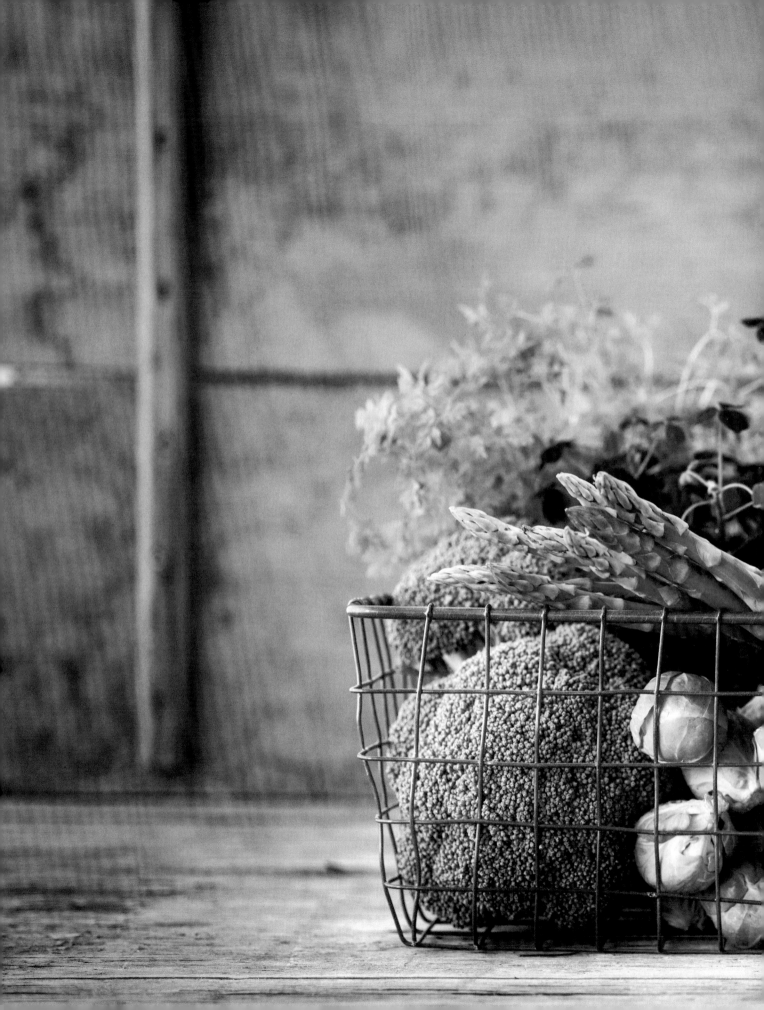

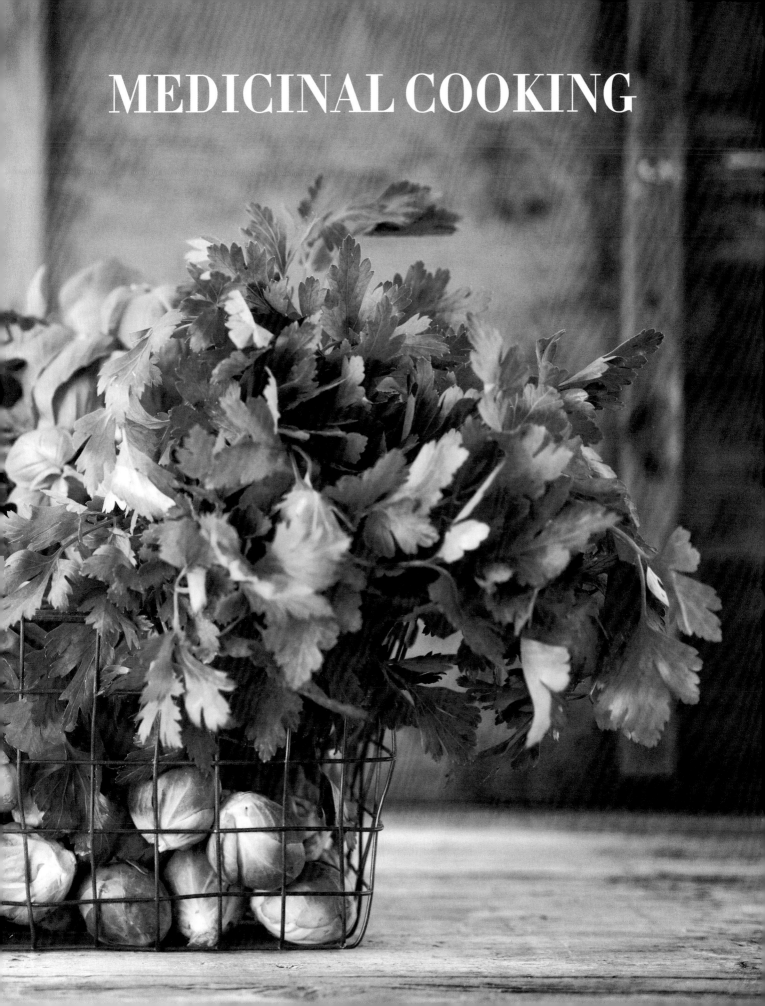

# MEDICINAL COOKING

## Healing Herbs and Spices

**Basil** has powerful antibacterial and antiviral properties. It's also an anti-inflammatory and a good source of vitamin A. It's sometimes used to treat constipation and indigestion. Try to have a tablespoon of fresh basil leaves or ½ teaspoon dried basil three times a week.

**Cinnamon** has a number of antioxidant properties. It also helps to regulate insulin, which regulates blood sugar. It may also inhibit the formation of amyloid plaques in the brain, reducing the risk of Alzheimer's. Aim to have ¼ to ½ teaspoon ground cinnamon daily.

**Cumin** helps to stimulate the production of pancreatic enzymes, which aid digestion. It's also a powerful antioxidant and anti-inflammatory, helps regulate insulin, and has anti-asthmatic properties.

**Garlic** has powerful antibacterial, antifungal, and antimicrobial properties—it's often used to fight infections, especially ear infections. It also helps to lower LDL cholesterol, protecting against heart disease, and is a pain reducer. Use fresh garlic rather than dried or powdered.

**Ginger** helps soothe nausea and stomach upset. It's also an anti-inflammatory and a pain reducer. Fresh ginger root is more effective than ground ginger.

**Rosemary** contains carnosol and rosemarinic acid, powerful antioxidants that counteract the cancer-causing effects of carcinogens. Use rosemary when frying, grilling, or broiling meats.

**Turmeric** is a spice that's used regularly in Ayurvedic medicine. It's a strong antioxidant that wards off cancer growth and Alzheimer's, among other things. It has anti-inflammatory properties, strengthens the immune system, and helps regulate insulin. Aim to have a teaspoon of ground turmeric at least three times a week. Fresh turmeric root is more effective than ground turmeric, but may be difficult to find.

## Almond Flour Waffles

Almond flour adds protein to these waffles, so you'll be energized rather than sluggish after consuming them. Almonds also contain a lot of antioxidants and vitamin E.

Makes 4 large squares.

### Ingredients:
3 eggs, separated
¼ cup milk (coconut, dairy, almond, or soy)
1 teaspoon vanilla
1 tablespoon maple syrup or honey
¼ cup butter or coconut oil, melted
1 cup almond flour
¼ teaspoon baking soda
¼ teaspoon salt

### Directions:
1. Turn on the waffle iron to heat.
2. Beat together the egg yolks and milk and add the vanilla, maple syrup, and melted butter or coconut oil. In a separate bowl, whisk or beat the egg whites until light and fluffy.
3. Whisk together the dry ingredients. Add the egg mixture and stir just until combined. Fold in the egg whites.
4. Grease waffle iron and cook according to the waffle iron instructions. For a standard waffle iron, pour about ¼ cup batter into the center of the iron, close the lid, and cook until lightly browned. Serve with maple syrup, apple compote (page 235) or fresh fruit and yogurt.

# Apple Compote

## Ingredients:

3 cups peeled and sliced apples

2 tablespoons butter

2 tablespoons brown sugar or maple syrup

½ teaspoon cinnamon

## Directions:

1. In a frying pan or cast-iron skillet, melt butter over medium heat.
2. Add all ingredients and sauté for about 5 minutes or until apples are tender.

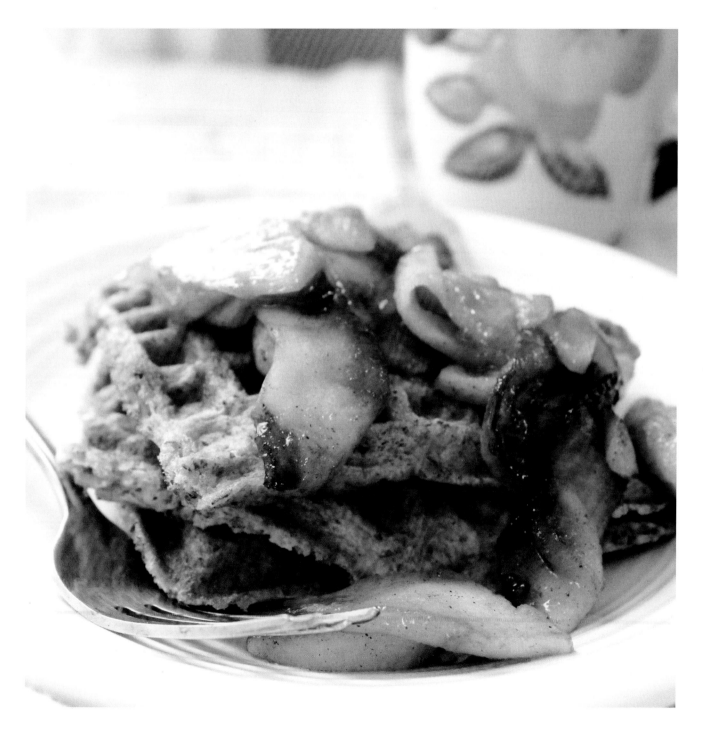

## Sweet Potato Pancakes

Sweet potatoes are full of the antioxidant beta carotene and may help reduce the risk of cancer. The coconut oil and cinnamon add more nutritional value to these tasty pancakes.

Makes about 12 medium pancakes.

### Ingredients:
Butter, coconut oil, or vegetable oil for the pan
1½ cups all-purpose gluten-free flour
3 teaspoons baking powder
½ teaspoon salt
½ teaspoon cinnamon
¼ cup butter or coconut oil, melted
2 eggs, beaten
1½ cups milk (dairy, almond, soy, or coconut)
1¼ cups peeled, cooked, and mashed sweet
   potatoes

### Directions:
1. Whisk together the dry ingredients and then pour the melted butter or oil over top and mix. Mix together the egg, milk, and mashed sweet potatoes and add to the dry ingredients. Stir just until incorporated—don't overmix.
2. Heat a griddle or frying pan and add enough butter or oil to lightly coat the surface. Have a plate nearby on which to place the pancakes when they're done (or you can put the oven on its lowest setting and place an oven-safe plate or pan inside to keep the pancakes warm until it's time to serve).
3. Ladle about ¼ cup of batter onto hot pan. If pan is big enough, you can do more than one pancake at once, as long as the edges don't touch. If they do run together, just use your spatula to cut them apart after they begin to firm up. Cook 2–3 minutes on the first side, or until bubbles begin to show on the top of the

pancakes and they're firm enough to flip. Cook another 1–2 minutes on the other side until pancakes are lightly browned.
4. Continue until all batter is used, adding oil to the pan as necessary. Serve with butter and real maple syrup.

## Hot Amaranth Cereal

Amaranth is high in protein and calcium and contains antioxidants and minerals.

Makes 2 servings.

### Ingredients:
½ cup amaranth
1 cup water
¼ teaspoon salt
1 cup milk (coconut, dairy, almond, or soy)
2 tablespoons honey or maple syrup
½ teaspoon vanilla
½ teaspoon cinnamon
Fresh berries or other fruit and/or nuts

### Directions:
1. Combine the amaranth, water, and salt in a medium saucepan and bring to a boil. Reduce heat to low and simmer for about 20 minutes or until the water is mostly absorbed. The amaranth grains should still look distinct—not like a pile of mush.
2. Stir in the remaining ingredients and serve warm.

Amaranth is very high in fiber, protein, calcium, iron, and magnesium. The first step of this recipe can be done the day before—in the morning, simply reheat and stir in the milk, sweetener and spices, and other desired toppings.

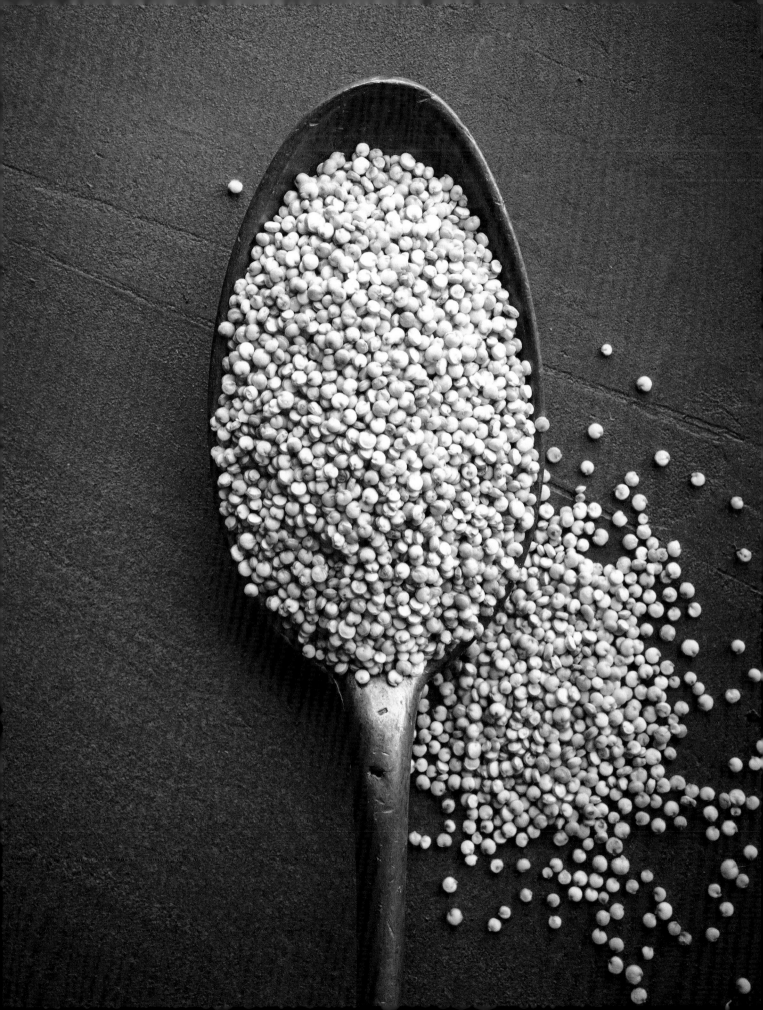

# Oatmeal Pumpkin Muffins

Pumpkin contains healing antioxidants, and oats are a great source of fiber. The cinnamon and ginger add nutritional benefits as well.

Makes 14 muffins.

## Ingredients:

1½ cups all-purpose gluten-free flour
1½ cups gluten-free old-fashioned oats
½ cup brown sugar or ⅓ cup maple syrup or honey
1 teaspoon baking powder
½ teaspoon baking soda
½ teaspoon salt
1 teaspoon cinnamon
1 teaspoon ground ginger
1½ cups pumpkin puree
3 tablespoon olive oil or melted coconut oil
¼ cup milk (dairy, almond, coconut, or soy)
2 teaspoons vanilla extract
2 eggs, lightly beaten
½ cup dark chocolate chips, raisins, cranberries, or peeled, chopped apple (optional)

## Directions:

1. Preheat oven to 375 degrees. Grease a muffin tin with at least 14 cups or line with cupcake liners.
2. Whisk together all the dry ingredients. In a separate bowl, whisk together the pumpkin, oil, milk, vanilla, and eggs and add to the dry ingredients, mixing until incorporated. Add the chocolate chips, raisins, or cranberries and stir just until evenly distributed.
3. Fill muffin tins nearly full and bake for about 20 minutes or until a toothpick inserted into the center of a muffin comes out fairly clean.

# Baked Frittata

Eggs, Greek yogurt, and fresh vegetables and herbs make this frittata a great way to start your day with a nutritional boost.

Makes 6 servings.

## Ingredients:

Olive oil for pan
1 small onion, finely chopped
½ cup finely chopped mushrooms (any variety)
1½ cups chopped fresh spinach
8 eggs
½ cup Greek-style yogurt
1 teaspoon salt
½ teaspoon black pepper
½ cup fresh chopped herbs, such as parsley, dill, cilantro, or tarragon (optional)
¾ cup freshly grated cheddar cheese (optional)

## Directions:

1. Preheat oven to 400 degrees. Heat a 10" cast-iron skillet on the stove top over medium heat. Coat bottom of pan with olive oil.
2. Sauté onions and mushrooms about five minutes or until onions are translucent. Add the spinach and herbs (if using) and sauté another few minutes to wilt the spinach. In a small bowl, beat together the eggs, yogurt, salt, and pepper. Reduce heat to low and pour the egg mixture over the top of the veggies. Cook uncovered, without stirring, for about five minutes. Sprinkle grated cheese over the top, if using.
3. Turn off stove top unit and transfer pan to the oven. Bake uncovered for another 3–5 minutes or until egg is set and cheese is slightly browned. Do not overcook. Slice and serve.

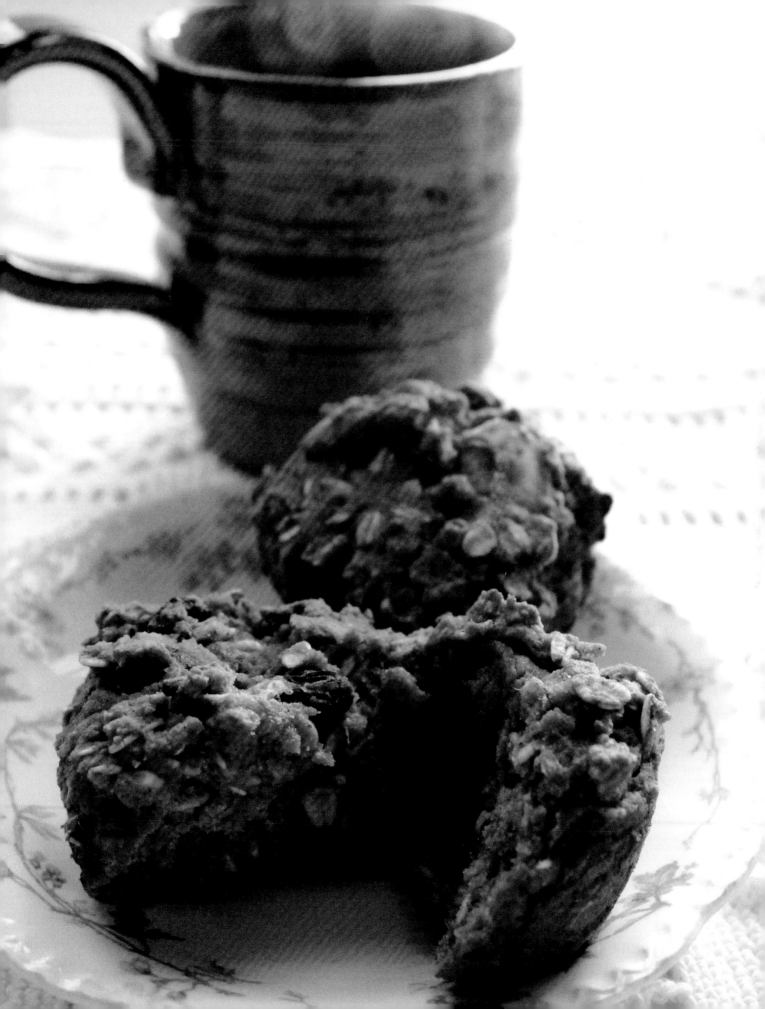

# Homemade Crock-Pot Yogurt

Homemade yogurt is surprisingly simple and is full of probiotics that contribute to a healthy gut. And a healthy digestive system is the foundation for healthy skin and a healthy mood and mind.

Makes about 4 cups of yogurt.

## Ingredients:

1 quart milk, preferably organic
1 tablespoon plain yogurt with live active cultures
1 tablespoon honey or maple syrup (optional)
2 teaspoons vanilla extract (optional)
Crock-Pot
Candy thermometer
Towels

## Directions:

1. Pour the milk into the Crock-Pot and turn heat on to medium-high. Add honey or maple syrup if using. Cover pot and allow milk to heat for about 30 minutes and then use the candy thermometer to take the temperature. The goal is to reach 180 degrees. If you're not there yet, return lid to pot and continue to heat. When milk reaches 180 degrees, turn off the slow cooker, remove lid, and allow milk to cool to 120 degrees (about 30 minutes).

2. While milk is cooling, place one tablespoon yogurt in a bowl and allow to warm to room temperature. When milk is at 120 degrees, add the yogurt to the milk, stir gently until yogurt dissolves, place the lid on the pot, and wrap thick towels around the outside of the pot to insulate it. Place in a safe place where it won't be moved or shaken for 6 to 8 hours or overnight. Then move to refrigerator to continue setting for about 4 hours or until desired thickness is reached. Add vanilla or other flavoring if desired and stir. Store covered in the refrigerator for 10–20 days.

# Almond Flour Banana Bread

The almond flour in this recipe adds protein, which helps to balance blood sugar and adds antioxidants and vitamin E. Bananas contribute potassium, magnesium, and a variety of other vitamins and minerals.

Makes 1 loaf.

## Ingredients:

1½ cups all-purpose gluten-free flour
1½ cups almond flour
1 teaspoon baking soda
½ teaspoon baking powder
½ teaspoon salt
3 eggs
2–3 very ripe bananas, mashed
⅓ cup brown sugar, honey, or maple syrup
¼ cup butter or coconut oil, softened
1 teaspoon vanilla extract
1 cup chocolate chips, raisins, or walnuts (optional)

## Directions:

1. Preheat oven to 350 degrees and grease a loaf pan. In a large mixing bowl, whisk together all dry ingredients.

2. In a separate bowl, mix together the wet ingredients. Fold the wet ingredients into the dry and mix to incorporate. Mix in chocolate chips, raisins, or walnuts if using.

3. Pour into the bread pan and bake 35–40 minutes or until a toothpick inserted into the center comes out fairly clean. Allow to cool until pan can be handled and then remove from pan and continue cooling on a wire rack.

You can use all almond flour in this recipe instead of the 1½ cups of all-purpose gluten-free flour. Using all almond flour will yield a somewhat denser (and more expensive) loaf.

## Maple Citrus-Glazed Salmon

Salmon is a great source of brain-boosting omega-3 fatty acids. Salmon contains lower amounts of mercury than larger fish, such as swordfish, shark, marlin, or king mackerel.

Makes 4 servings.

### Ingredients:
1 salmon fillet (about 1½ lbs), preferably wild Alaskan
3 tablespoons maple syrup
3 tablespoons balsamic vinegar
1 tablespoon orange juice
⅛ teaspoon kosher salt
⅛ teaspoon freshly ground black pepper

### Directions:
1. Heat oven to 450 degrees. Line a baking sheet with parchment paper and place salmon, skin-side down, on top.
2. In a small bowl, whisk together the maple syrup, balsamic vinegar, orange juice, and salt and pepper. Brush half of the glaze over the salmon.
3. Bake for 10 minutes, brush with remaining glaze, and bake about 5 minutes more or until fish flakes easily with fork.

Risotto is typically made with arborio rice, which is gluten-free and delicious, but it's also very starchy and doesn't have a lot of nutritional value. Quinoa is high in protein and fiber and other nutrients and is similar to arborio rice in its ability to absorb flavors.

## Quinoa Risotto with Shiitake Mushrooms and Arugula

Nearly all the ingredients in this recipe have super-food powers. Most notably, quinoa is gluten-free, high in protein, and full of healthy amino acids, and shiitake mushrooms boost the immune system and have a number of other health benefits. Garlic is a powerful anti-inflammatory and immune booster, as are onions.

Makes 4 servings.

### Ingredients:
1 tablespoons olive oil
½ yellow onion, peeled and chopped
1 glove garlic, peeled and minced
½ cup shiitake mushrooms, thinly sliced
1 cup quinoa, uncooked
¼ cup white wine
2¼ cups chicken or vegetable broth
2 cups arugula
½ cup grated Parmesan cheese (optional)
Salt and pepper to taste
Fresh thyme, minced (for garnish)

### Directions:
1. Rinse the quinoa in a fine-mesh strainer.
2. Place a large saucepan over medium heat and add the olive oil. Add the onion and sauté until soft, about 5 minutes. Add the garlic and mushrooms and sauté another three minutes.
3. Add the quinoa and cook, stirring, for two minutes. Pour in the white wine and simmer until the liquid is absorbed. Add ½ cup of the chicken or vegetable broth and allow to boil. Reduce heat to low and simmer, stirring occasionally, until the liquid is absorbed. Continue adding ½ cup at a time, stirring and allowing the liquid to be absorbed between each addition. Once all the liquid is absorbed and the quinoa is tender, toss in the arugula and cook until wilted.
4. Fold in the Parmesan, if using. Add salt and pepper to taste and garnish with fresh thyme, if desired.

# Vegetarian Chili

Garlic and onions are great immune system boosters, and beans are great sources of protein and may improve heart health.

Makes 6 servings.

## Ingredients:
1 tablespoon olive oil
1 medium onion, peeled and chopped
2 cloves garlic, peeled and minced
1 bell pepper (any color), chopped
1 jalapeno, seeds removed, diced (optional)
3 (15 oz) cans diced tomatoes, with liquid
2 (15 oz) cans red kidney beans, with liquid
2 (15 oz) cans black beans, with liquid
1 (15 oz) can corn, with liquid
2 tablespoons cumin
1 tablespoon chili powder
salt and pepper to taste

## Directions:
1. Heat oil in a large saucepan or Dutch oven over medium heat. Sauté the onion and garlic until onions are tender, about 5 minutes. Add the bell pepper and sauté another 5 minutes.
2. Add remaining ingredients, stir, and simmer for at least 20 minutes, stirring occasionally. Add salt and pepper to taste.
3. Serve with sour cream and shredded cheese, if desired. Great with cornbread.

# Quinoa-Stuffed Acorn Squash

Acorn squash is a great source of fiber, vitamin A, vitamin C, and a range of minerals. Kale is one of the most nutrient-dense vegetables you can find. Combined with the broth, olive oil, onions, and cinnamon, this recipe is a powerhouse of nutrition!

Makes 2 servings.

## Ingredients:
1 acorn squash, halved and seeded
2 tablespoons olive oil or coconut oil, divided
1 cup quinoa, uncooked
2 cups chicken or vegetable broth
¼ red onion, peeled diced (about ¼ cup)
3 cups kale, rinsed and broken into small pieces
1 tablespoon maple syrup
¼ teaspoon kosher salt
⅛ teaspoon black pepper
⅛ teaspoon cinnamon
¼ cup cranberries
3 tablespoons grated Parmesan

## Directions:
1. Heat the oven to 400 degrees. Brush the insides of the acorn with ½ tablespoon oil and place them facedown on the baking sheet. Bake for 20–25 minutes or until soft.
2. Place the quinoa and broth in a saucepan and simmer, covered, for about 12 minutes, or until all liquid is absorbed. Add the maple syrup, salt, pepper, and cinnamon, and mix. Add the cranberries.
3. Place a frying pan over medium heat and add remaining oil to coat the pan. Saute the onion until soft. Add the kale and sauté until wilted.
4. Mix together the quinoa mixture with the kale mixture and scoop into the squash hollows. Sprinkle with Parmesan and serve.

## Moroccan Chickpea Slow Cooker Stew

Sweet potatoes, butternut squash, and carrots are all good sources of vitamin A. The spices in this recipe contain anti-inflammatory properties. And chickpeas contain vitamin K, protein, and iron.

Makes 6 servings.

### For Slow Cooker:
2 medium sweet potatoes, washed and chopped (leave peels on)
1 pound butternut squash, peeled and chopped in bite-size pieces
2 carrots, washed and cut in ½ inch pieces
1 medium yellow onion, peeled and diced
1 can chickpeas, drained and rinsed, or 2 cups soaked dried chickpeas
1 (14.5 ounce) can diced tomatoes with juices
2 cups chicken or vegetable broth
2 teaspoons cumin
1 teaspoon turmeric
½ teaspoon ground ginger
½ teaspoon ground cinnamon
½ teaspoon salt
¼ teaspoon black pepper
2 cloves garlic, peeled and minced

### For Garnish:
Steamed basmati rice or quinoa for serving
1 cup pitted green brined olives
Toasted slivered almonds for garnish (optional)
Plain yogurt for serving (optional)

### Directions:
1. Place all ingredients (up until the olives) in a slow cooker, stir, and cook at low heat for about 6 hours or until vegetables are tender.
2. Stir in green olives, if using. Serve over steamed rice or quinoa. Garnish with sliced almonds and a dollop of yogurt if desired.

## Chai-Infused Coconut Milk Butternut Squash Soup

Coconuts contain lauric acid, which boosts the immune system. Butternut squash is a good source of vitamin A.

Makes 4 servings.

### Ingredients:
2 tablespoons butter or coconut oil
1 medium butternut squash
¼ cup minced yellow onion
1 tablespoon honey or maple syrup
½ teaspoon salt
½ teaspoon pepper
2 cups coconut milk
1 chai tea bag

### Directions:
1. Peel and seed the squash and cut into ½-inch chunks. In a stockpot or Dutch oven, melt the butter or coconut oil over medium heat. Add the squash and onion and sauté until squash is just barely tender, about 8 minutes. Add the honey or maple syrup, salt, and pepper, and sauté another couple of minutes.
2. Add the coconut milk, 3 cups of water, and the tea bag. Bring to a boil and then reduce heat and allow soup to simmer about 20 minutes.
3. Remove the tea bag and discard. Use an immersion blender to puree the soup. Alternately, you can use a blender or food processor, but you'll probably need to do a small portion at a time.
4. Taste and add additional salt and pepper as desired.

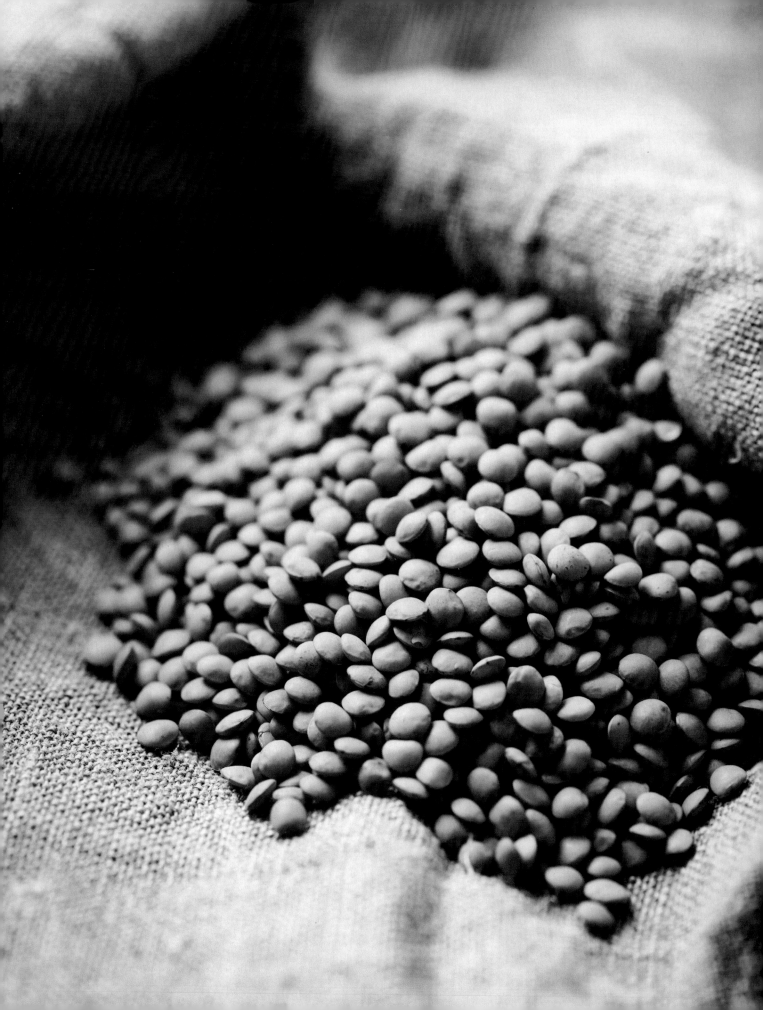

## Easy Lentil Stew

Makes 4 servings.

### Ingredients:

2 tablespoons olive oil or coconut oil
½ yellow onion, peeled and chopped
1 medium carrot, chopped
1½ cup dry lentils
4 cups chicken or vegetable broth
1 (14.5 ounce) can chopped tomatoes
1 medium potato, peeled and chopped into bite-size chunks
1 tablespoon dried parsley
1 teaspoon cumin
Salt and pepper to taste

### Directions:

1. Rinse the lentils in a fine-mesh strainer.
2. In a stockpot or saucepan, heat the oil. Add the onions and carrots sauté about 3 minutes, or until soft. Add all the remaining ingredients, cover, and simmer, stirring occasionally, for about 45 minutes, or until lentils and vegetables are tender. Taste and add more salt or pepper as desired.

## Roasted Vegetables

The combination of veggies, garlic, herbs, and spices packs a nutritional punch. Roasting the vegetables brings out their natural sugars, making them as yummy as they are good for you!

Makes 6 servings.

### Ingredients:

2 medium potatoes (yellow or red), washed and chopped into chunks
2 sweet potatoes, washed and chopped into chunks
1 red onion, quartered
1 medium carrot, washed and chopped into chunks
1 apple, washed, cored, and chopped into chunks
2 teaspoons fresh thyme
1 tablespoon fresh rosemary
3 tablespoons olive oil
2 tablespoons balsamic vinegar
1 tablespoon tamari
¼ teaspoon cinnamon
2 garlic cloves, peeled and minced
Pinch of sea salt and black pepper, to taste

### Directions:

1. Preheat oven to 475 degrees. Combine all the veggies and the apple in a large bowl. Add remaining ingredients and toss to coat.
2. Spread on a large roasting pan and roast for 35 to 40 minutes, or until veggies are soft, stirring every 10 minutes or so.

## Grilled Pear Salad with Green Tea Dressing

Green tea is good for your brain, metabolism, and skin! Pears are a low-glycemic fruit that is a good source of fiber and vitamin C.

Serves 4 as a side salad.

### Dressing
½ cup strong brewed green tea
2 tablespoons grape-seed oil
1 tablespoon unfiltered apple cider vinegar
2 tablespoons honey
1 tablespoon gluten-free tamari
½ teaspoon salt

### Pears
2 firm pears, halved and seeded
2 tablespoons honey

### Salad
4 cups arugula, rinsed and patted or spun dry
1 tablespoon coconut oil or butter
¾ cups shelled walnut halves

### Directions:
1. Preheat oven to 375 degrees.
2. Meanwhile, make the dressing. Combine all ingredients in a food processor or shake in a jar.
3. Place pear halves on a baking sheet, cut-side up, and brush the cut sides with honey. Bake for about 20 minutes, or until lightly browned. Cut into thin slices.
4. In a skillet, heat the coconut oil or butter and sauté the walnut halves until lightly toasted, just a few minutes.

Toss the arugula, pear slices, and toasted walnuts together with desired amount of dressing. If you don't use all the dressing, keep it in the refrigerator for another salad.

## Vegan Pumpkin Brownies

Pumpkin and applesauce make these brownies moist and delicious, while keeping them low in fat. You may find that you can use less than 1 cup of coconut sugar, given the natural sweetness of the fruit juice, applesauce, and oat flour.

Makes about 16 brownies.

### Ingredients:
1 cup all-purpose gluten-free flour
1 cup oat flour
1 cup coconut sugar
¾ cup unsweetened cocoa powder
1 teaspoon baking powder
1 teaspoon salt
1 cup fruit juice (apple is great, but any variety will do)
¼ cup coconut oil
1 cup pumpkin puree
½ cup applesauce
1 teaspoon vanilla extract
1 cup chocolate chips

### Directions:
1. Preheat the oven to 350 degrees F. Grease a 9 x 13-inch baking pan.
2. In a medium-sized mixing bowl, stir together the flours, sugar, cocoa powder, baking powder, and salt. Pour in juice, vegetable oil, pumpkin puree, applesauce, and vanilla. Mix until well blended.
3. Spread evenly in baking pan. Sprinkle chocolate chips evenly over the top.
4. Bake for 25 to 30 minutes or until the top is no longer shiny. Let cool for at least 10 minutes before cutting into squares.

## Amaranth Cracker Jacks

Amaranth gets its superfood status from its protein, lysine, calcium, and antioxidants.

Makes about 4 cups.

### Ingredients:
¾ cup amaranth
2 tablespoons honey or maple syrup
2 tablespoons coconut oil or butter
1 cup cashews
1 cup almonds
½ cup dried cranberries
¼ teaspoon coarse sea salt

### Directions:
1. To pop the amaranth, first heat a medium pot over high heat. To test that the pan is hot enough, add a drop of water. If it quickly forms a ball and evaporates, the pot is the right temperature.
2. Add 2 tablespoons of amaranth to the pot, cover with a lid, and gently shake the pot, sliding it back and forth in quick movements just above the burner. Within 10 to 15 seconds the amaranth should be fully popped. Be careful not to burn!
3. Empty popped amaranth into a bowl and repeat until all amaranth is popped.
4. Preheat oven to 275 degrees.
5. Combine popped amaranth with the nuts and dried cranberries. In a small saucepan, melt together the sweetener and coconut oil or butter. Pour over the amaranth mixture, add salt, and stir to coat. Place on a parchment paper-lined cookie sheet and bake for about half an hour, stirring with a spatula every 10 minutes or so.

Allow to cool completely before storing in an airtight container.

## Easy Coconut Mango Blender Sorbet

This recipe is so simple, so yummy, and really good for you, too!

Makes about 3 cups.

### Ingredients:
2 cups frozen mango chunks
½ cup unsweetened coconut milk
¼ cup honey or maple syrup
Dash cinnamon
Dash nutmeg

### Directions:
1. Combine all ingredients in a blender and blend until smooth. Enjoy immediately or store in a metal or glass dish in the freezer.

If your blender is not very powerful, you may need to combine ingredients in a bowl and then blend a little at a time, or add more liquid. Experiment with different frozen fruits to create your own sorbet recipe. Bananas, raspberries, and blueberries are great options. You can also use soy, almond, or cow's milk instead of coconut milk. For an elegant presentation, serve sorbet in hollowed-out citrus peels or coconut shells.

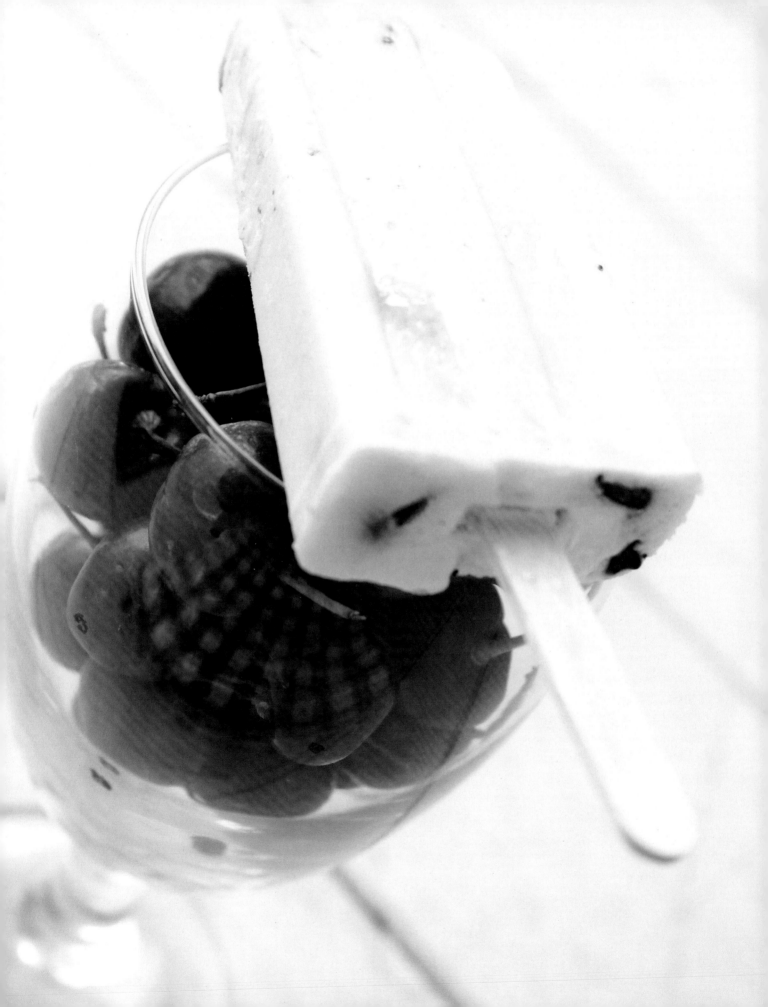

## Dairy-Free Chocolate Cherry Popsicles

Cherries have anti-inflammatory properties, helping with arthritis and a host of other conditions. Everything else in this recipe has healing properties, too!

Makes 8 Popsicles.

### Ingredients:
1 (13.5-ounce) can coconut milk
4 tablespoons honey
1 teaspoon vanilla or almond extract
2 tablespoons coconut oil
1 cup frozen cherries, thawed and chopped into small pieces
3 ounces dark chocolate, finely chopped (about ½ cup)

### Directions:
1. Combine coconut milk, honey, vanilla, and coconut oil in a blender and blend until smooth and creamy. Pour a little into the bottom of each of 10 Popsicle molds. Add a layer of cherry pieces, then chocolate chunks, then more of the liquid. Continue until all ingredients are used, finishing with the liquid. Freeze at least 3 hours.
2. To serve, run hot water over bottoms of molds to loosen the Popsicles. To display at a gathering, arrange Popsicles in a bucket of ice. Wrap leftover Popsicles individually in plastic wrap and store in a ziplock bag in the freezer.

## Energy Balls

Snack on one or two of these treats between meals or for dessert, or whenever you need a boost of energy and nutrients!

Makes about a dozen.

### Ingredients:
½ cup almonds, hazelnuts, or walnuts (or a mix)
¾ cup Medjool dates, prunes, dried cranberries, or raisins (or a mix)
1 tablespoon honey
3 tablespoons nut butter (almond, peanut, or cashew)
⅛ teaspoon almond extract
⅛ teaspoon vanilla
½ teaspoon cinnamon
⅛ teaspoon cloves

### Directions:
1. In a food processor, pulse together the dried fruit and nuts.
2. Add the remaining ingredients and pulse until mixture starts to clump together. Roll into balls.

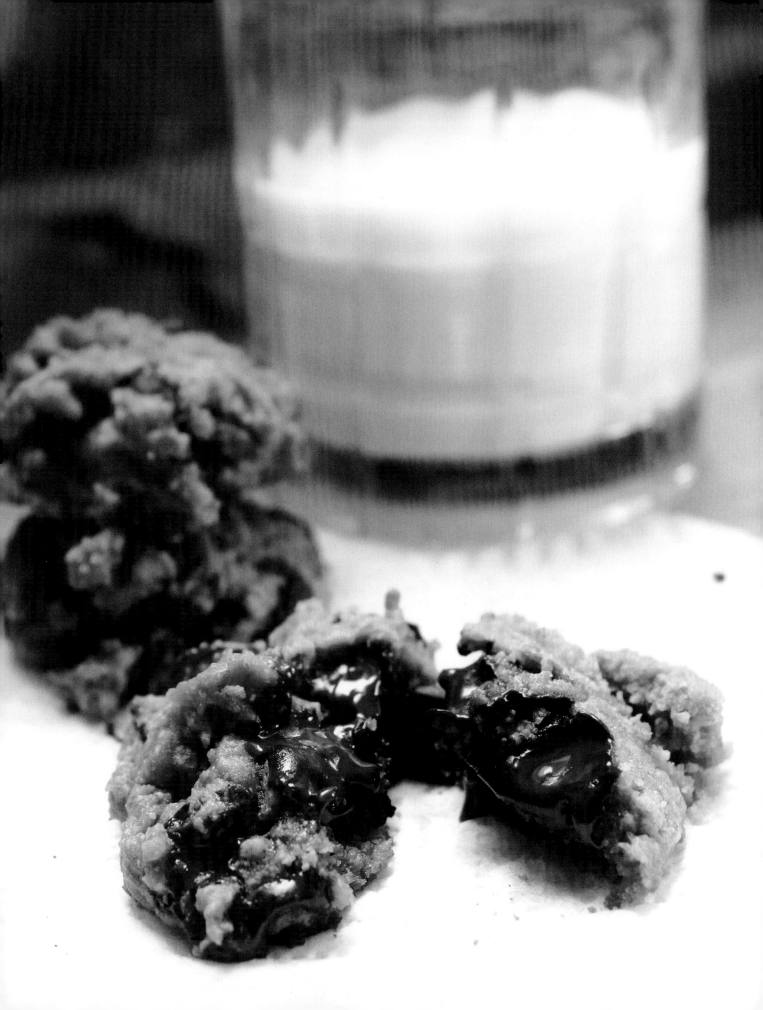

## Chickpea Chocolate Chip Cookies

You'll be surprised how addictive these cookies are, especially considering what a great source of protein and other nutrients they are!

### Ingredients:

1 (15–ounce) can chickpeas, rinsed and thoroughly drained
¾ cup peanut butter
1 teaspoon vanilla
2 tablespoons brewed coffee
¼ cup maple syrup
1 teaspoon baking powder
5 oz (½ bag) chocolate chips

### Directions:

1. Preheat oven to 350 degrees.
2. Combine all ingredients except chocolate chips in a food process and process until smooth. Add chocolate chips and stir.
3. Drop by teaspoonful onto a cookie sheet lined with parchment paper.
4. Bake for about ten minutes. Cookies will still be soft.

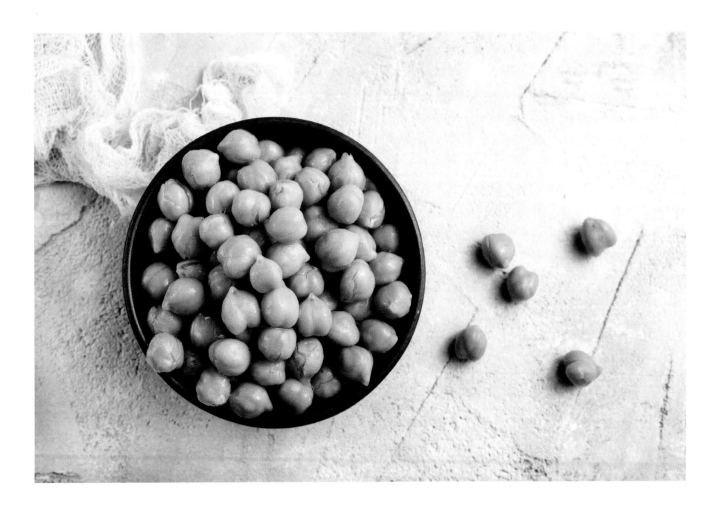

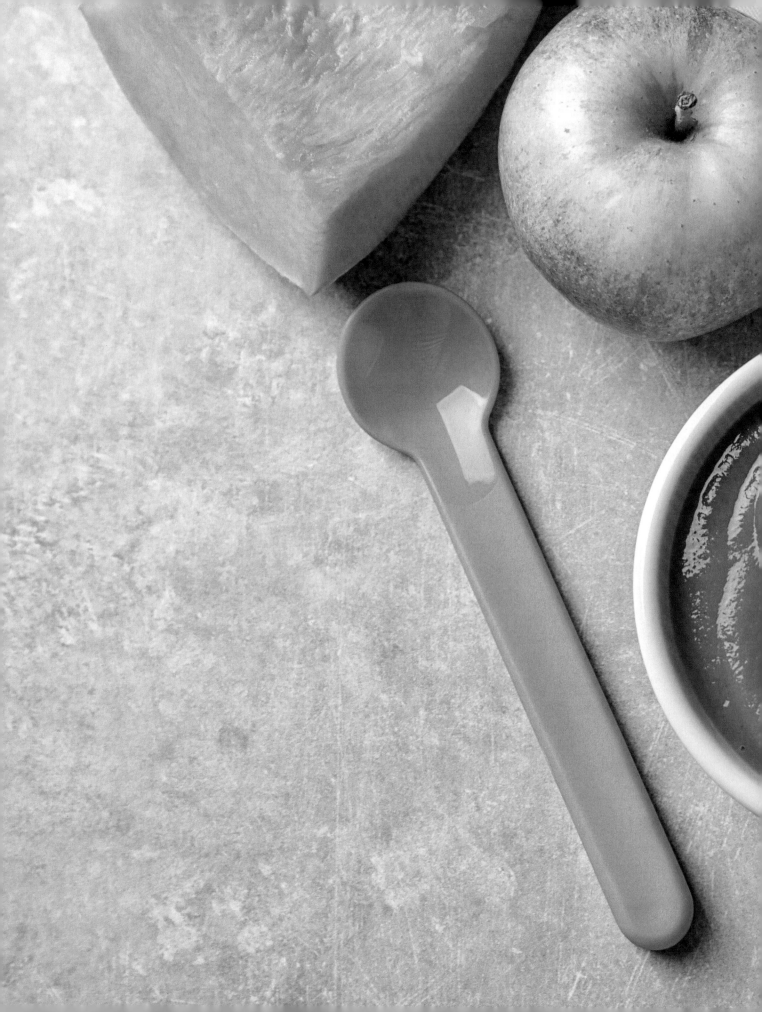

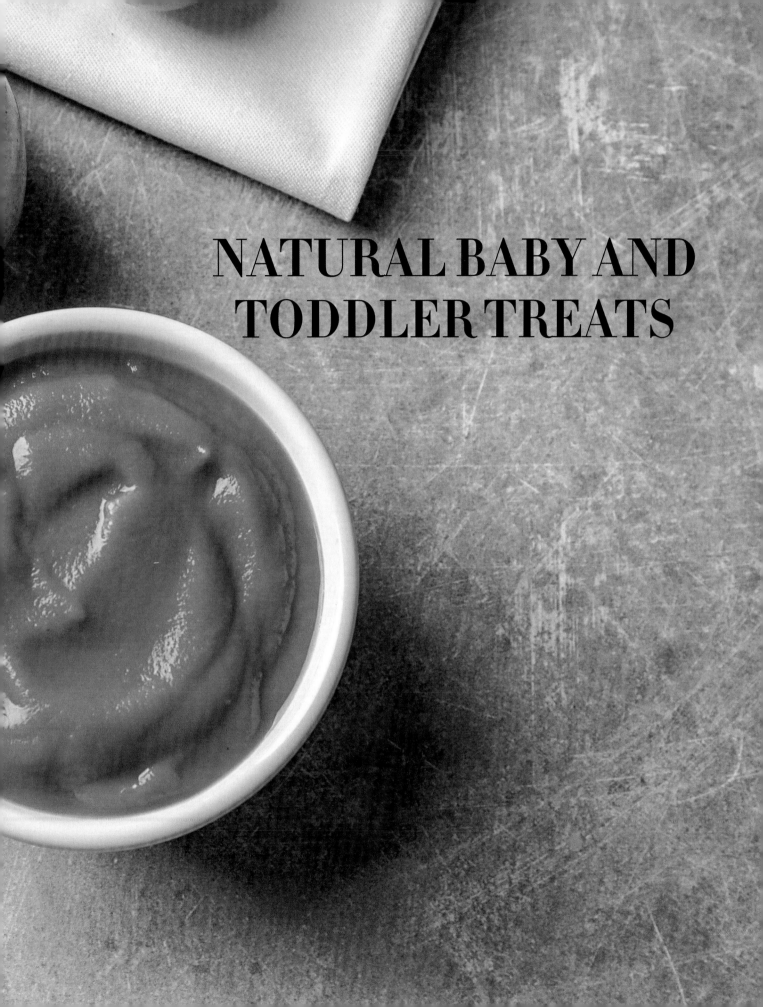

# NATURAL BABY AND TODDLER TREATS

# Baby Food

## Avocado Banana Smash

This creamy puree will be a sure favorite of your little one and is a great first combination for beginners to try out, with only two ingredients! What's even better than how much your baby will love this recipe is that you don't even need a food processor to get it to the perfect consistency!

### Ingredients:
½ avocado, peeled
1 ripe banana

### Directions:
1. Mash together avocado and banana with a fork until smooth.
2. Serve immediately.

### NOTE:
This recipe does not refrigerate or freeze well and should be eaten within the hour it is prepared.

## Persimmon Cantaloupe Puree

This puree requires no prep other than peeling the fruit and placing it into a blender! Cantaloupe is high in vitamins C and A and is so nutritious for your little one.

### Ingredients:
1 ripe persimmon, skin removed
1 cup ripe cantaloupe, peeled and seeded

### Directions:
1. Place ingredients into the blender and process until smooth.
2. Serve immediately or store in the refrigerator or freezer for a later date.

## Green Bean, Pear, and Tofu

Tofu is great for adding protein to your little one's diet. It's soft by nature, so it purees beautifully and is mild in flavor so it can pair with just about any other ingredient!

### Ingredients:
½ cup green beans
1 cup water
¼ cup soft tofu
½ cup very ripe pear

### Directions:
1. Boil green beans in water in a medium saucepan until they are tender, about 10 minutes.
2. Strain and add to a high-powered blender with the tofu and pear.
3. Blend until smooth. Add water for consistency if needed.
4. Serve immediately or store in the refrigerator or freezer for a later date.

## Turnip Leek Mash

Turnips are higher in nutritional value than white potatoes, and can make a yummy alternative to mashed potatoes!

### Ingredients:
1 tbsp. grass-fed butter
1 leek, washed thoroughly and sliced
⅛ tsp. black pepper
2 cups turnips (about 2–3 large turnips)

### Directions:
1. In a small saucepan, add the butter along with leek and black pepper.
2. Cook for 5 minutes until leek is tender.
3. Meanwhile, peel the turnips and steam for 15–20 minutes until tender.
4. Add all ingredients to a food processor and blend until smooth.
5. Add stock if needed for consistency.
6. Serve immediately or store for a later date.

## Roasted Carrots with Ginger and Pumpkin

Your baby is going to flip over this flavor-packed puree full of vitamins and healthy fats. Pumpkin and carrots are both great for developing eyesight, with their high content of beta-carotene, and taste even better with the addition of ginger, which is great for their tummies and immune systems!

### Ingredients:
4 carrots, peeled
1 tsp. coconut oil
½ cup pumpkin puree
1 tsp. fresh ginger, grated
Pinch of cinnamon

### Directions:
1. Preheat oven to 400 degrees.
2. Toss the whole carrots with coconut oil and roast for 30 minutes, or until tender.
3. In a high-powered blender or food processor, add roasted carrots, pumpkin puree, ginger, and cinnamon, and blend until smooth.
4. Serve immediately or store in the refrigerator or freezer for a later date.

## Cinnamon Stone Fruit Puree

### Ingredients:
2 ripe black plums
2 ripe apricots (can sub peaches)
¼ tsp. cinnamon

### Directions:
1. Peel and pit plums. Remove the pits from the apricots.
2. Add both the plums and the apricots to the blender along with the cinnamon.
3. Blend until smooth.
4. Serve immediately or store in the refrigerator or freezer for a later date.

### NOTE:
If fruit isn't soft and ripe, cook the fruit in water over the stove to soften before adding to the blender.

## Creamy Mango and Yogurt

Mango is full of vitamin C, potassium, and several other vitamins so good for your baby! I love mixing it with yogurt to give it some protein and creaminess for a truly yummy and nutritious puree.

### Ingredients:
1 ripe mango, diced and peeled
1 tbsp. water (if needed for consistency)
½ cup Greek or plain yogurt

### Directions:
1. Blend mango in a food processor or blender until smooth. Add water if needed at this time.
2. Stir in yogurt and serve.
3. Serve immediately or store in the refrigerator or freezer for a later date.

# Bigger Bites

## Baked Gluten-Free Chicken Nuggets with Homemade Ketchup

Makes 20–24 nuggets

There's no need to buy frozen nuggets filled with unknown ingredients when you can make your own taste this good, and are actually made healthy for your toddler with wholesome ingredients!

### For the Tenders
- 1 lb. chicken tenders (or use breasts and slice them yourself)
- 2 cups gluten-free crackers
- ½ cup gluten-free all-purpose flour
- 2 eggs, beaten
- 1 tsp. kosher or sea salt
- ½ tsp. black pepper
- Avocado oil spray or olive oil spray

### For the Ketchup
- 1 tsp. avocado oil
- ¼ cup onion, grated
- 1 clove garlic, minced
- 1 (15-oz.) can crushed tomatoes
- 1 tbsp. tomato paste
- 1 tbsp. Worcestershire sauce
- 1 tsp. molasses
- ½ tsp. kosher salt
- ¼ tsp. black pepper

### For the Tenders
1. Preheat oven to 375 degrees.
2. Cut chicken into 1-inch bite-size nuggets.
3. Place crackers in a food processor and pulse until the crackers are the consistency of bread crumbs.
4. Using wide bowls, place the flour, eggs, and ground crackers into 3 separate bowls.
5. Season the flour with salt and pepper.
6. For each nugget, lightly dust the chicken with flour to coat entirely. Dip the flour-coated chicken into the eggs and coat. Finally, dip the egg-coated chicken into the cracker crumbs and make sure it is coated.
7. Place nuggets on a wire rack on top of a baking sheet, and place into the oven.
8. Spray the nuggets with avocado oil spray and bake for 18–20 minutes.
9. Switch the oven to broil and broil for another 2 minutes to get a crispy crust.

### For the Ketchup
1. Heat oil in a saucepan over medium heat.
2. Add onion and garlic and sauté for 2–3 minutes.
3. Add in crushed tomatoes, tomato paste, Worcestershire sauce, molasses, salt, and pepper, and whisk to combine.
4. Bring to a boil, and then reduce heat and let simmer for 30 minutes, until ketchup has thickened slightly.
5. Serve immediately or store in an airtight container in the refrigerator.

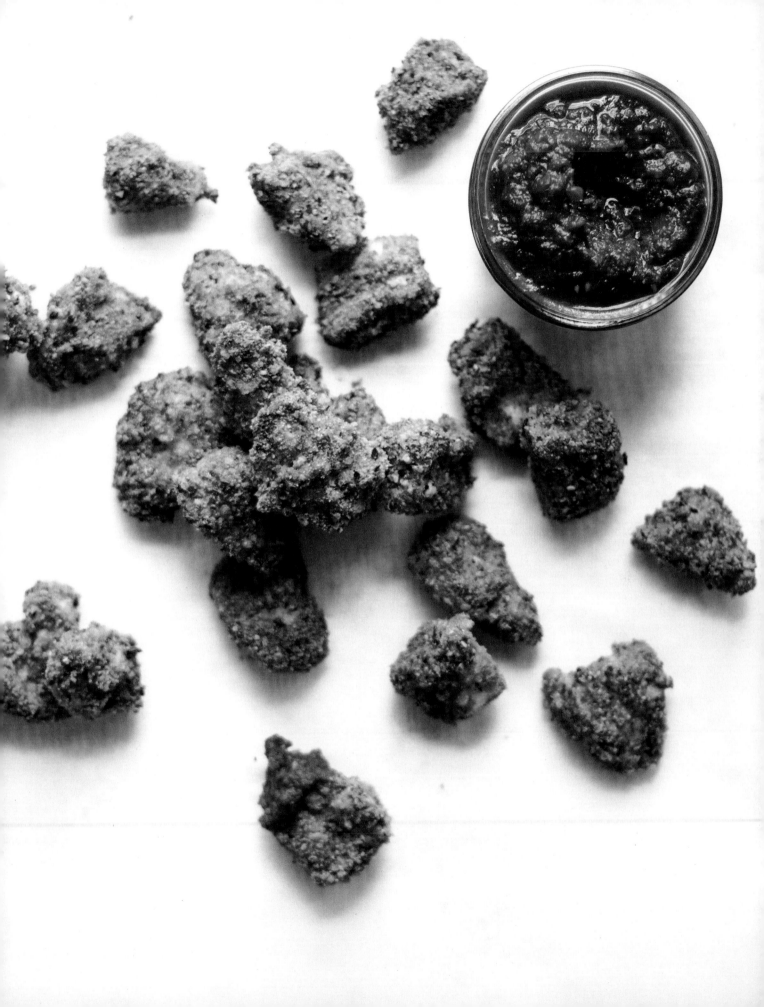

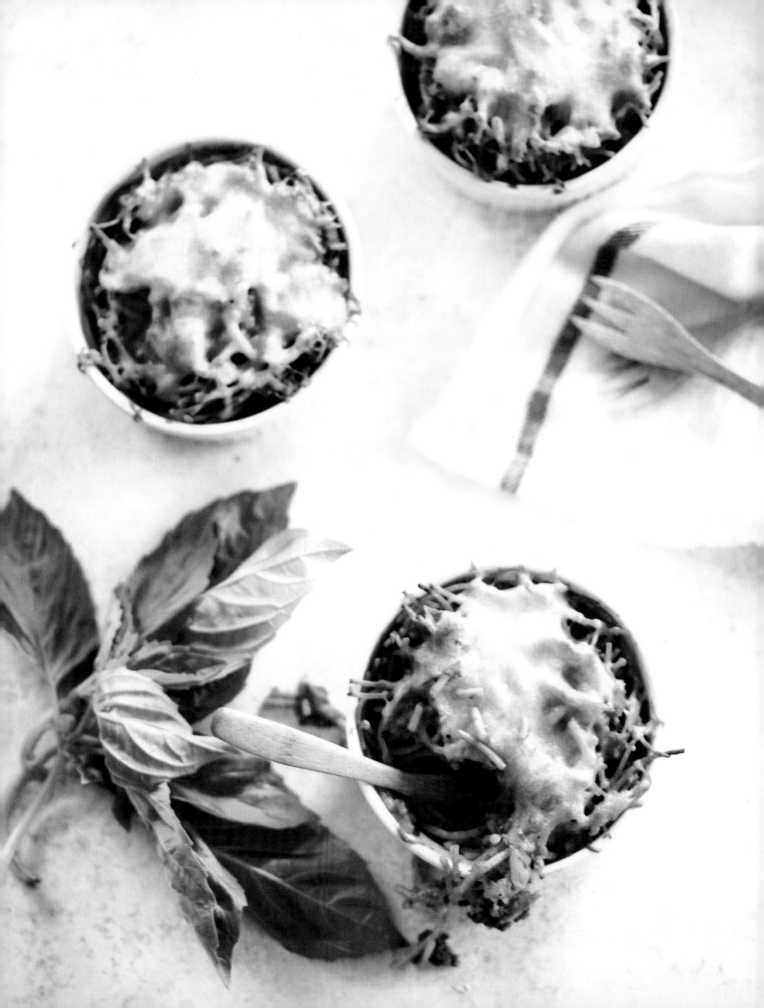

## Individual Whole Wheat Baked Skettis

Makes 8 individual servings

Spaghetti is always a kid favorite, and I love making individual baked versions for a fun take on a classic. Your toddler will love having their own dish all to themselves!

### Ingredients:

1 lb. whole wheat or gluten-free pasta
1 tbsp. olive oil
1 lb. ground bison or ground beef
½ cup onion, finely diced
2 garlic cloves, finely minced
2 (15-oz.) can crushed tomatoes
2 tbsp. Italian seasoning
1 tsp. brown sugar (optional)
2 tsp. salt
1 tsp. black pepper
2 tbsp. fresh basil
2 cups mozzarella cheese, shredded

### Directions:

1. Bring a large pot of water to a boil.
2. Add pasta and let cook until tender.
3. Heat a large skillet over medium heat.
4. Add olive oil and bison and brown the meat, about 10 minutes.
5. Add chopped onion and garlic to the meat, and continue to cook another 5 minutes.
6. Pour in both cans of tomatoes along with the Italian seasoning, brown sugar, salt, and pepper, and stir to combine all ingredients.
7. Let sauce simmer for about 15 minutes.
8. Taste and adjust seasonings if necessary.
9. Add fresh basil and stir in for the last minute of cooking. Turn off heat.
10. Drain pasta and snip noodles with kitchen shears to make it easier for little ones to eat, if desired.
11. Add both the pasta and the sauce to a large bowl and stir to combine.
12. Fill small oven-safe ramekins with the spaghetti filling and place on a baking sheet (in case of overflow while baking).
13. Sprinkle with cheese and bake for 20 minutes or until cheese is golden and bubbly.

## Spinach and Corn Quesadillas

Serves 1–2

Quesadillas are another great way to get your kiddos to eat their vegetables. They are easy to make and can be whipped up using whatever ingredients you have on hand. One of our favorite combinations is this recipe for my spinach and corn quesadillas!

### Ingredients:

1 tsp. olive oil
2 tbsp. red onion, finely diced
¼ cup corn kernels
¼ cup baby spinach, chopped
⅛ tsp. chili powder
⅛ tsp. black pepper
2 wheat tortillas
¼ cup cheddar cheese, shredded

### Directions:

1. Heat olive oil over medium heat, then add onion, corn, baby spinach, chili powder, and pepper, and sauté for 3–5 minutes until onion is translucent and spinach has wilted.
2. Remove from the pan and place one tortilla in the same pan.
3. Layer half the cheese onto the tortilla, then put the spinach and corn mixture on top of the first layer of cheese before layering the rest of the cheese.
4. Place the second tortilla on top and cook for about 3 minutes per side until the cheese has melted.
5. Cut into 4 pieces and serve immediately.

### NOTE:

You can make extra quesadillas to freeze for easy, make-ahead meals!

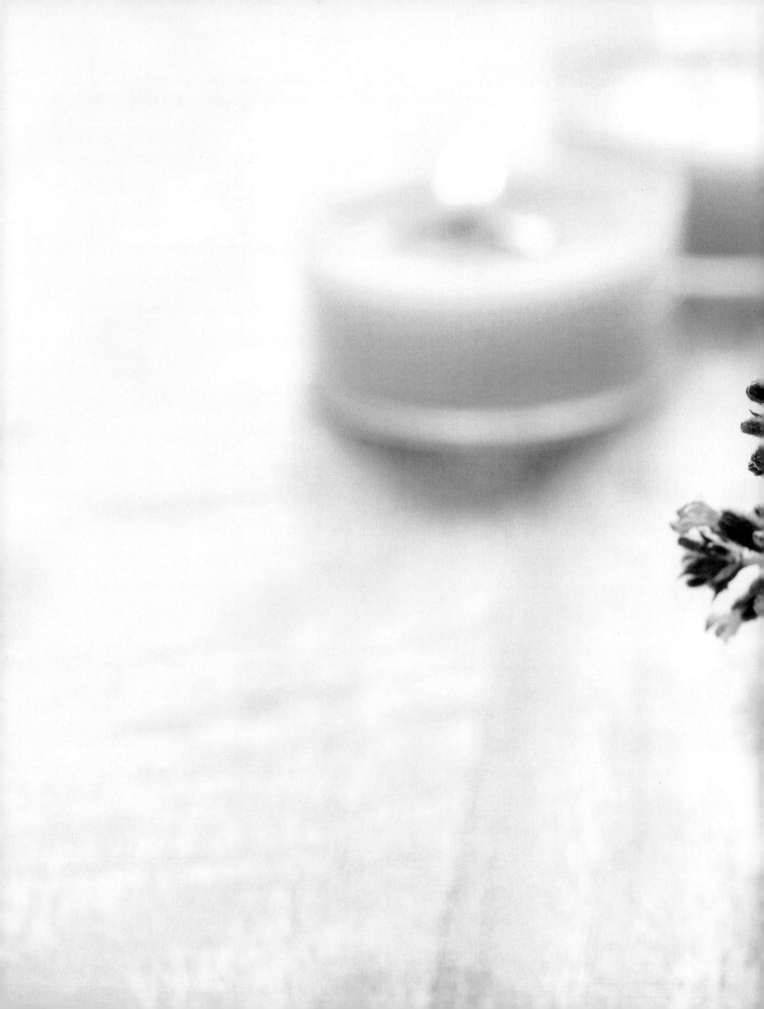

# PART THREE

# HOMEMADE COSMETICS AND NATURAL CLEANING PRODUCTS

Natural Cosmetics and Beauty Rituals      263
Natural Remedies for the Bedroom      295
Natural Cleansers for the Home      305

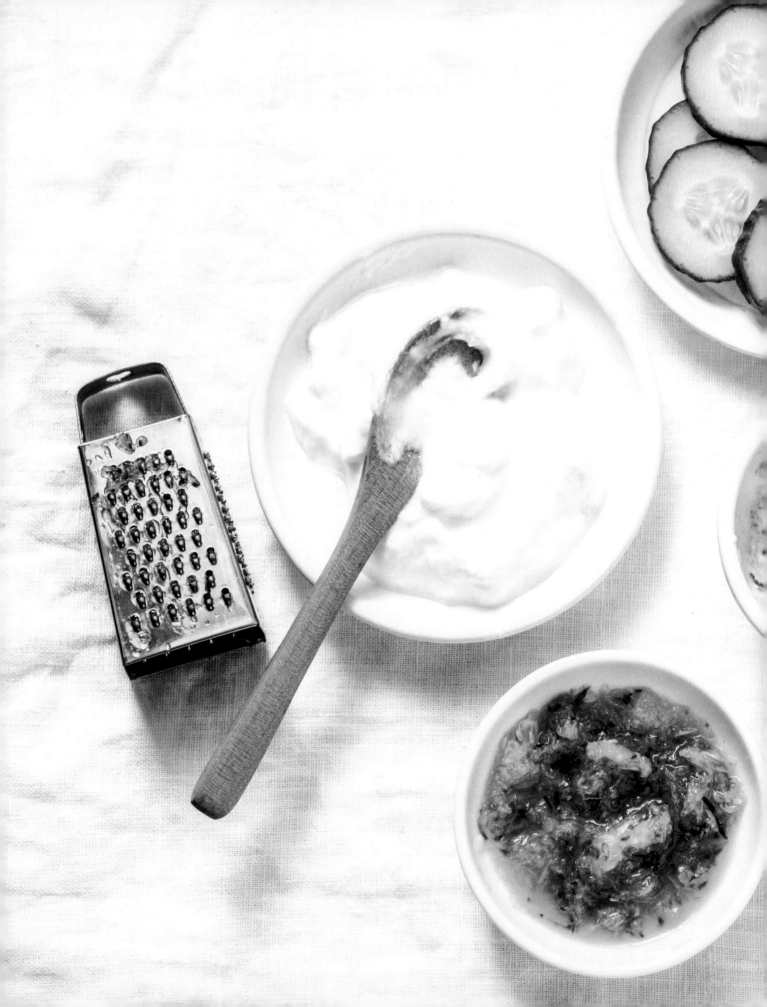

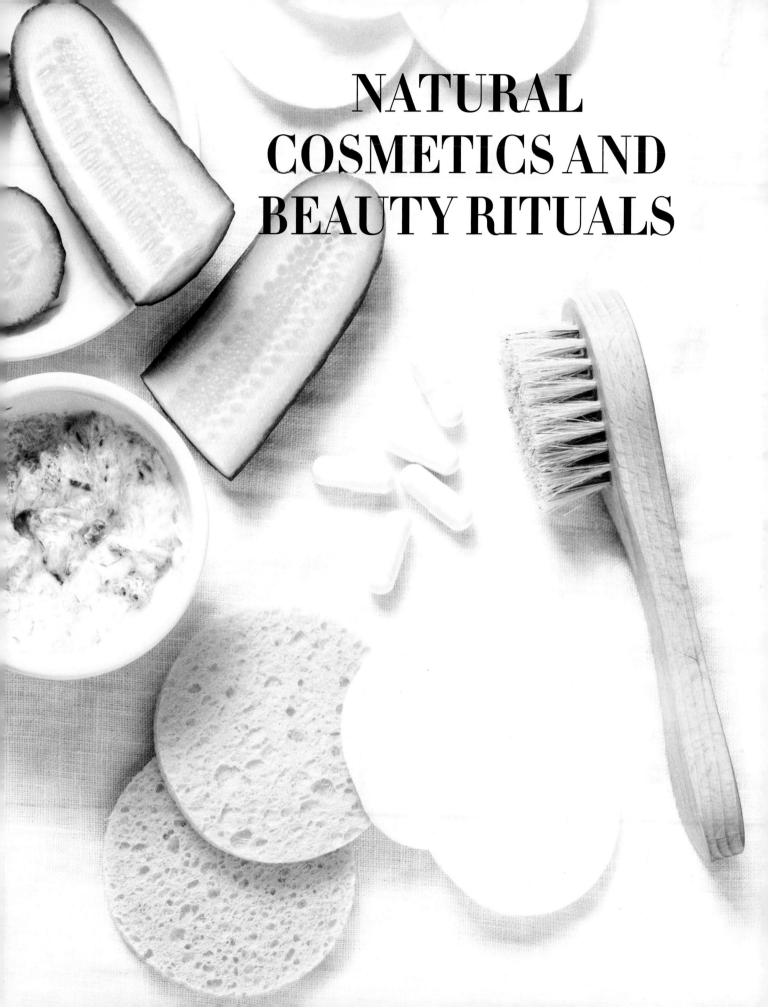

# NATURAL COSMETICS AND BEAUTY RITUALS

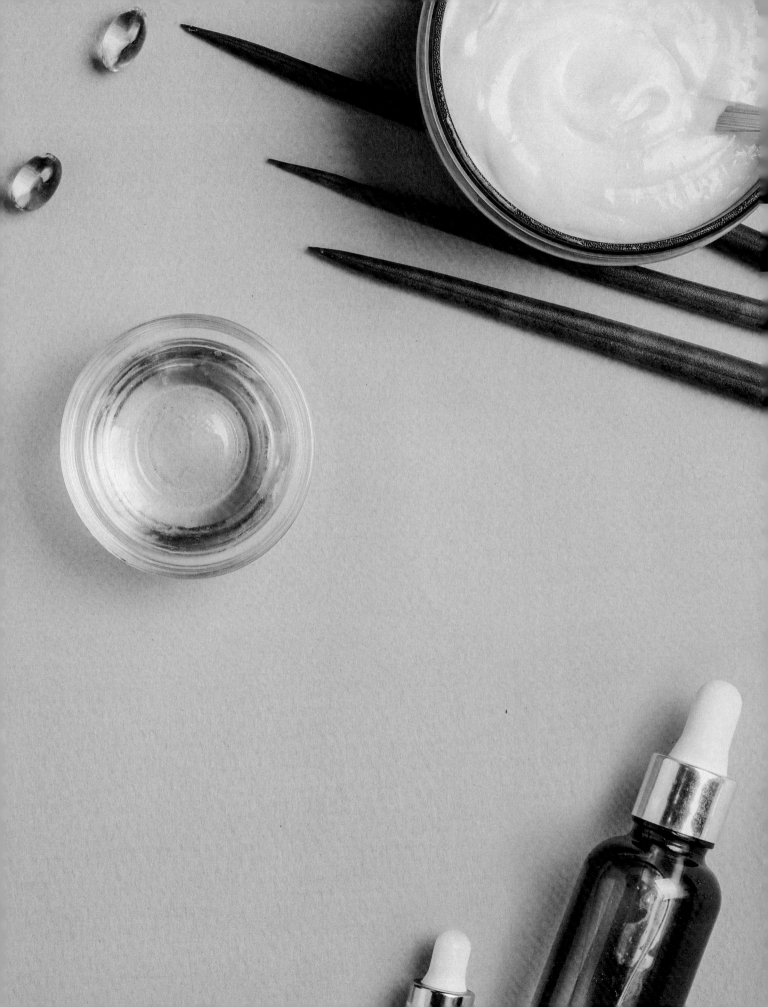

# Body Butters

## Whipped Coconut Oil Body Butter

Only a small amount of this luxurious all-over moisturizer will leave your skin glowing and replenished, soft, and smooth.

### Equipment:
- Electric hand mixer or stand mixer
- Mixing bowl
- Glass jar with sealed lid

### Ingredients:
1 cup solid coconut oil

1 teaspoon vitamin E oil

Approximately 6 drops of essential oils of your choice

### Directions:
1. Place coconut oil and vitamin E oil into the mixing bowl. Mix on high speed for about ten minutes, until light and fluffy.
2. Fold in the essential oils.
3. Spoon the body butter into a glass jar and secure the lid.
4. Store your body butter in a cool place and slather over your skin as required.

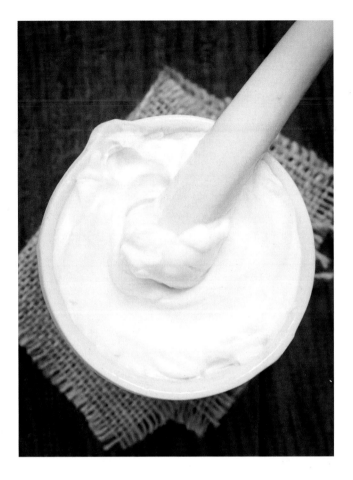

**Fruits and Vegetables for Your Skin**

**Beneficial for Oily Skin:** Lemons, grapes, limes, strawberries, grapefruits, apples

**Beneficial for Normal Skin:** Peaches, papayas, tomatoes, apricots, bananas, persimmons, bell peppers, cucumbers, kiwi, pumpkin, watermelwons

**Beneficial for Dry Skin:** Carrots, iceberg lettuce, honeydew melons, avocados, cantaloupes

# Body Oiling

Body oiling is an ancient technique used in Ayurvedic medicine—the oldest system of medicine on the planet. Our skin is aching to be cared for, yearning to be touched, and begging for natural medicines as opposed to the failed promises of synthetically perfumed potions and commercial creams. Nature always knows best.

According to Ayurvedic medicine, body oiling boosts the immune system, relaxes the mind and central nervous system, and makes muscles and tissues supple. Not surprisingly, body oiling feels really good on the skin. Pure essential oils combined with luxurious carrier oils deeply nourish skin and actively reduce wrinkles, bruises, burns, blemishes, age spots, and skin discolorations.

Body oiling is a totally luxurious process that yields tremendous results both for your skin and yourentire being. I like to body oil when I first get out of the shower and my skin is still warm and wet. Start by choosing your favorite carrier oil such as jojoba, cacao butter, rose hip oil, baobab oil, coco babacu, coco cream, and/or shea butter combined with an essential oil blend of your choice. Aim for a blend of ten drops in two tablespoons of carrier oil.

## Some effective essential oils to add to your body oil blend are:

- Juniper berry, basil, lavender—improves circulation and detoxification pathways
- Ylang-ylang, bergamot, cinnamon—heightens sexual desire and energy
- Cardamom, vanilla, immortelle—a stimulating euphoric blend
- Jasmine, hay, blood orange, black pepper—excellent blend for both men and women
- Lemongrass, lemon, lavender, rosemary—cleansing, energizing, purifying

Grace your body with a massage of long, firm, and loving strokes up the legs, over the stomach and buttocks, around the back and over the breasts, completing with arms always moving in the direction of the heart. Allow the oils to penetrate the skin. With high-quality natural oils, it doesn't take more than a couple of minutes to sink in. Smooth, touchable skin is just an added benefit to this time-honored technique.

In ancient Egypt, both men and women in all classes of society used body oiling. They saw that it was an effective way to maintain youth, vitality, and soft skin that would otherwise be dry and leathery in the hot desert sun.

## Beautiful Body Oil

### Ingredients:
Equal parts calendula, rose, and chamomile
2 parts olive oil
1 part sweet almond oil
½ part coconut oil
½ part jojoba oil
Essential oils of lavender, lemon grass, and sage (about 15 drops essential oil total per ounce of herbal oil)

### Directions:
1. Place herbs in a glass jar and add oils, being sure to cover the herbs by an inch or more of oil.
2. Screw the lid on tightly and shake the jar. Place jar in a sunny spot and allow to sit for 2–3 weeks, shaking once a day.
3. Strain out the herbs (cheesecloth works well), reserving the infused oil.
4. Store the oil in glass jar with a tight-fitting lid or cork. Label the jar and store away from direct sunlight.

## Skin Healing Oil

Ingredients:

2 parts comfrey leaf
1 part calendula
1 part elder flowers
1 part plantain
2 parts olive oil
½ part coconut oil

Directions:

1. Place herbs in a glass jar and add oils, being sure to cover the herbs by an inch or more of oil.
2. Screw the lid on tightly and shake the jar. Place jar in a sunny spot and allow to sit for 2–3 weeks, shaking once a day.
3. Strain out the herbs (cheesecloth works well), reserving the infused oil.
4. Store the oil in glass jar with a tight-fitting lid or cork. Label the jar and store away from direct sunlight.

## Simple Homemade Massage Oil

Ingredients:

1 cup jojoba, grape seed, or almond oil (olive oil can also be used, but can cause breakouts on sensitive skin)
12 to 15 drops essential oil of your choice (lavender, jasmine, myrrh, orange, or mint are all good choices)

Directions:

1. Combine the oils and store in a glass bottle with a tight-fitting lid or cork, away from direct sunlight.

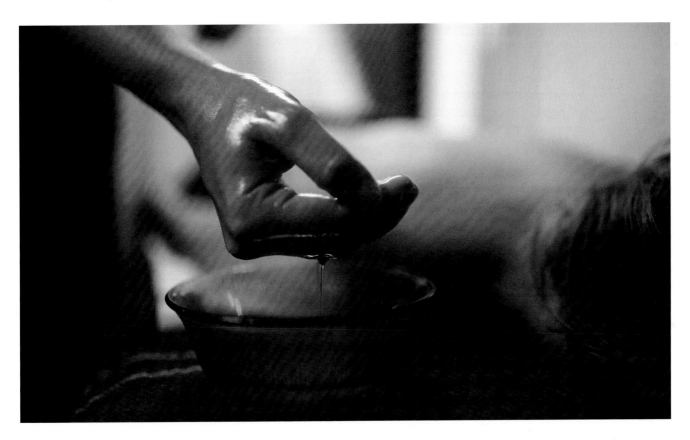

# Dry Brushing

Vibrant, glowing skin is the sign of a healthy body. As we age, our skin can thicken and take on a leathery, dry, dull appearance. Daily brushing is an ancient secret for retaining a vibrant, soft, glowing complexion.

The skin is the largest organ of elimination, known as the third kidney in holistic health. It is said that if the internal organs of elimination cannot keep up with the elimination of waste material, then the skin will take over the task. Skin brushing is a valuable addition to your morning routine and can be followed with a cool shower or Epsom salt bath. The invigorating brushing is invaluable to remove dead skin cells, allowing your skin to breathe while creating supersoft skin. More importantly, regular skin brushing will support detoxification and waste removal via the lymphatic system.

## Benefits of Dry Skin Brushing

1. Jump start the lymphatic system: Skin brushing assists the process of cleansing and detoxification by encouraging lymphatic drainage, speeding up removal of waste matter through the lymph vessels, improving venous circulation while encouraging the elimination of metabolic waste from our tissues. Unlike the heart, which is an automatic pumping machine, the lymphatic system relies upon the movement of surrounding muscles to keep fluid flowing and effective. Lymphatic congestion can contribute to swelling, fluid retention, inflammation, and chronic disease. In conditions of bed rest, chronic illness, or a sedentary lifestyle, the lymph can become congested and not drain as effectively. This is why movement is essential for our health.

2. Skin brushing stimulates circulation by getting the blood flow moving to the extremities, increasing blood flow through the veins and back to the heart while eliminating metabolic waste and cellular debris.

3. Ensures normal secretion of sweat and oil glands for the appearance of moisture-filled, soft and supple skin. In addition, gentle friction over the body's connective tissues and joints will help increase the production of collagen and elastin fibers, going a long way to slow the body's aging process.

4. Can improve digestion, assist with regular bowel function, and support the health of the kidneys through the repetitive and gentle stimulation of the underlying organs. Brush over the abdomen in a clockwise motion, mirroring the direction of the digestive tract (starting at the lower right quadrant, moving up to the belly button, and then over and down the left quadrant of the abdomen). Bloating and fluid retention may diminish as the body sheds excess fluid and toxins.

5. Skin Exfoliation: Dry skin brushing removes dead cells, leaving skin supersoft and allowing your skin to "breathe."

6. Can support breakdown of cellulite, remove agents which break down connective tissue, improve muscle tone, promote better distribution of fatty deposits, help remove congestion from local veins, and improve lymphatic stagnation.

## Skin Brushing as Part of a Daily Mindfulness Ritual

Each morning dry skin brushing is an invigorating way to start the day. Stay present, put your intention on gratitude, and focus on the optimal outcome for your day while invigorating the body; this practice has been said to stimulate the vital "chi" energy.

Brushing at night is a bit like a meditation; take a couple of minutes to brush down the skin before a nightly Epsom salt bath to unwind, release tension, and relax muscles.

For those who do not have regular massages, or for those who are less active, brushing is effective support for vibrant soft skin and to support the lymphatic system in doing its job.

Skin brushing is done on dry skin by using a dry bristle brush prior to showering or relaxing in a bath. Purchase a natural bristle brush (made from vegetable fibers—do not use a brush made from synthetic fibers or animal bristles). The brush will feel hard and a bit shocking for a new brusher. Persevere—your skin will thank you! Softer brushes can be used on the face. Periodically the bristle brush can be cleaned by using a mild cleanser or castile soap and left to air dry.

## How to Dry Brush Your Skin

Begin with the extremities first: starting from the arms and feet, brush in short circular motions and work towards the heart. Moving from the legs up to the abdomen, brush the abdomen in a clockwise manner, the buttocks and back, the fingers up the arms, and move in the direction of the heart. Avoid brushing areas of thin skin such as the breasts and neck and avoid open wounds, varicose veins, and areas of infection. Do not skin brush during cancer treatment if the tumor has metastasized.

A body at rest stays at rest. A body in motion stays in motion. No matter what state of health you are in, movement is your friend.

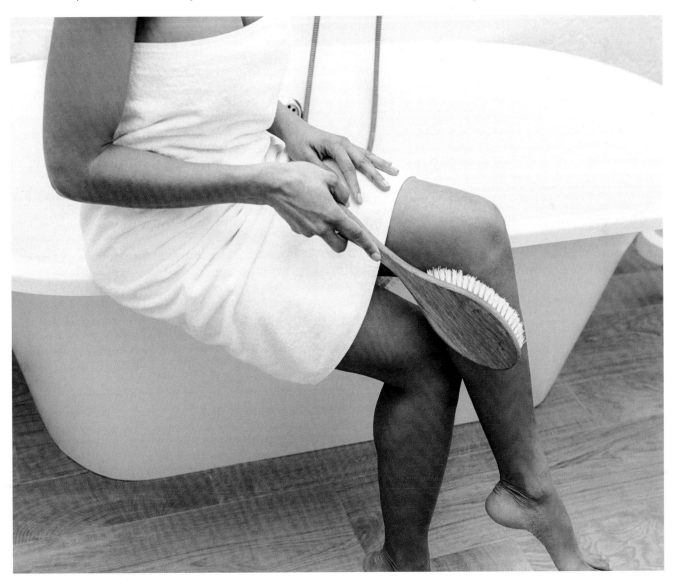

# Facial Oiling

We have a misguided understanding that applying oil to the face causes acne, blackheads, and breakouts. This simply isn't true.

Modern-day conventional soaps disrupt the endocrine, reproductive, digestion, and mental systems. They often contain cancer-causing sodium laurel sulphate, which creates bubbles or ethyl alcohol that strip the skin of valuable and necessary natural oils. In an effort to establish equanimity, our bodies need to recreate lost oils for normal skin balance once they have been removed. Cleansing the face with soap can lead to dry, excessively oily, or acne-prone skin, or premature wrinkles. Ditch the sudsy bar or liquid chemical "soap" and go Egyptian. Healing oils are where it's at.

Oils harmonize unbalanced skin, provide elasticity and tone, and even help remove the appearance of fine lines. I'm positively in love with jojoba for the face and body. Jojoba is an outstanding liquid wax that's one molecule away from skin sebum.

(Sebum is an oily or waxy matter, excreted from that skin than makes it dewy and youthful. It lubricates and waterproofs the skin and hair of mammals.) Jojoba is incredibly stable and is preferable to sesame oil or apricot seed oil, as it has a long shelf life that maintains its potency and medicinal qualities for years. Our bodies naturally and authentically understand jojoba.

To cleanse the face, simply moisten it with either water or, to pamper yourself more luxuriously, use rose hydrosol. Add a small amount of oil to the face. Massage it into the face and neck in circular motions. Use a clean towel or hemp cloth to remove the oil and exfoliate the face in circular motions. Another method is to moisten the edge of a towel. Apply the oil directly to the moistened towel and then cleanse and exfoliate the face in one easy step. To finish and moisturize, add a few more drops of jojoba or another carrier oil. You can also easily remove eye makeup by applying oil to a damp cotton swab and wiping it over the eye until it's clean. Beauty never felt so good.

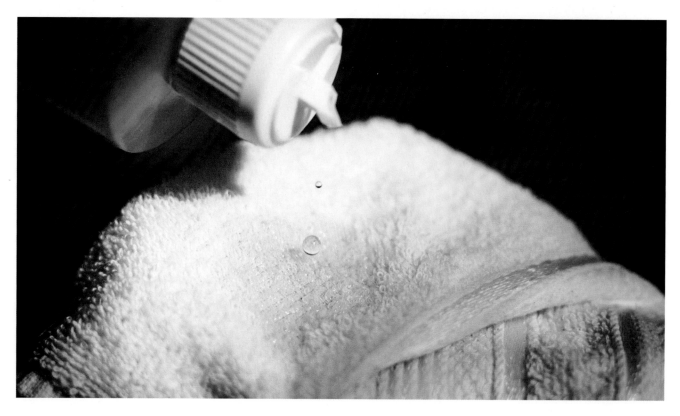

# Facial Steams

Facial steaming hydrates the skin during the long cold months of winter, removes blackheads and impurities, and adds a much-appreciated pinch of luxury. One of my favorite ways to facial steam is to use hydrosols as the base in place of plain water. Hydrosols are the aromatic waters left over after the steam distillation process and are prized for their medicinal, aromatic, and nutritive qualities. When you use them for facial steams, you're imparting the pure, homeopathic versions of rose otto, neroli, lavender, or ylang-ylang directly into the skin in a gentle yet highly effective way. Another benefit is that our lungs are treated to an aromatic steam bath, as hydrosols are powerful and prized liquid libations that promote health and vitality at the cellular level through the respiratory and circulatory systems.

If you don't have hydrosols available, you can easily replace them with pure essential oils and spring water or distilled water. Chemically treated, chlorine- and fluoride-laden tap water isn't suitable for the face or body. When we steam the face, the pores open to detoxify and draw in moisture, like the lungs. In using spring water, we shield the face from heavy metals, chlorine, fluoride, and nerve toxins found in many municipal water supplies.

Add two to three drops of geranium, rose otto, frankincense, cape chamomile, sandalwood, neroli, lavender, or fenugreek to a large bowl of freshly boiled water. These oils are high in monoterpenes (chemical properties that regenerate, soften the skin, and smell absolutely divine). They're so gentle that they will not cause irritation or an unpleasant reaction.

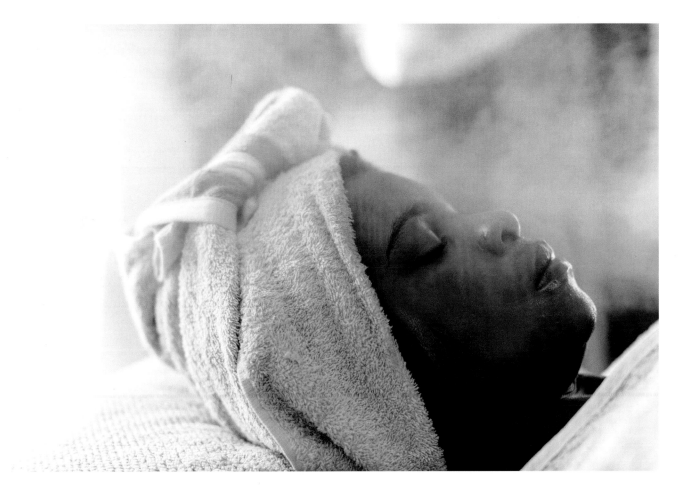

**Directions:**

1. Place your face close to the bowl of aromatic water and allow the steam to mist your face. For a more concentrated treatment, place a towel over your head. Come up for air quite often, because extreme heat over an extended period of time can cause burning and irritation to your delicate facial skin. Facial steaming should be a luxurious experience, not a torturous one. Use the steam treatment for ten to twenty minutes, followed with deep skin oiling. Feel free to gently exude blackheads and pimples after the facial steam because the pores will be open and pliable. Facial steams are a fabulous way to go from scaly lizard skin to perfect peach in a matter of minutes, and you'll smell glorious too. It's about the way we treat and honor ourselves every day that will reflect love and care back into our lives.

## Calming Aromatherapy Facial Steam

A few decades ago, facial steams were a regular part of many people's beauty routines, but they have since fallen out of popularity. Facial steams open the pores to allow all the good oils in the herb mixture you're steaming to get in. There's no real trick to it, except that you might get a few stares the first time you attempt the towel maneuver. Be careful not to do this when the steam is too hot; burning delicate facial skin is not beautifying by any means.

**Ingredients:**

½ cup dried rosebuds (pink or red)
½ cup dried lavender
½ cup dried chamomile
½ cup peppermint leaves

**Directions:**

1. Mix ingredients well in a 16-ounce jar with a tight-fitting lid.

**To Use:**

Fill a saucepan with a quart of water. Add ¼ cup of the above herbal mixture. Place a lid on the saucepan and let simmer for 15 minutes. Remove from heat and let cool for 5 minutes, not removing the lid. In the meantime, cleanse your face of any oil or makeup by wiping it with a cotton ball saturated in witch hazel or rose water. Tie back your hair and remove glasses if necessary. Take a hand towel and place it over your head like a hood, draped down at the sides, to create a barrier that will keep the steam in. Then remove the lid from the saucepan and gently lower your face to the warm steam. Start off high and lower your face as the steam gets cooler.

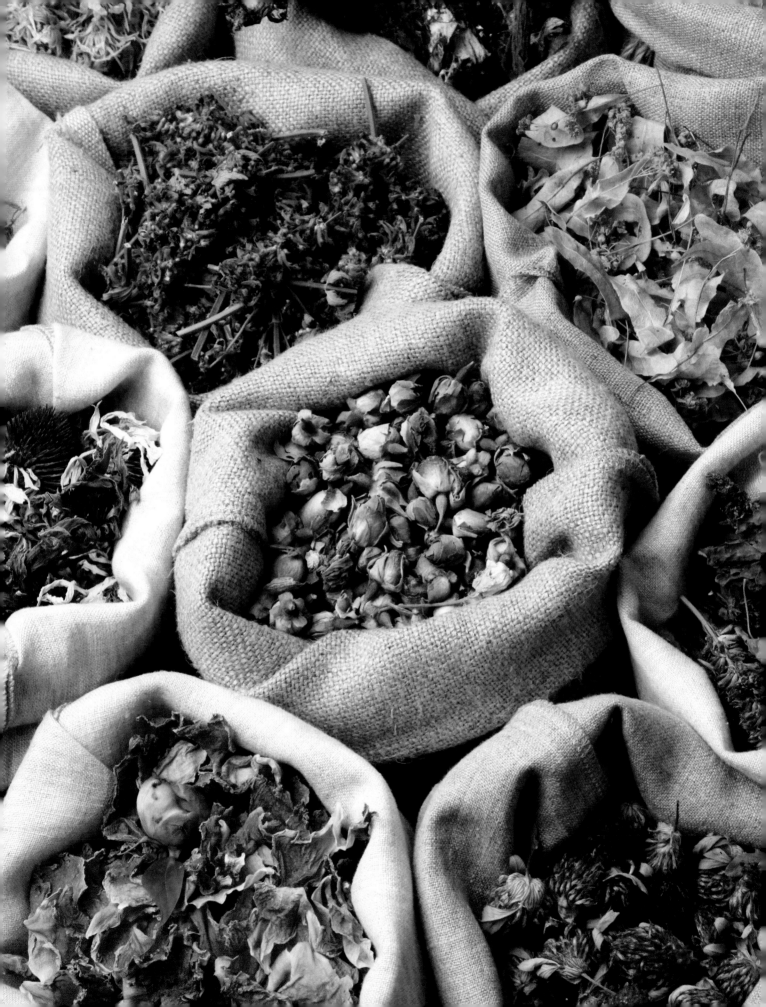

# Hair Treatments

## Replenishing Conditioner Treatment for Dry Hair

### Ingredients:
1 banana
1 avocado
3 tablespoons coconut oil
2 tablespoons mayonnaise

### Directions:
1. Mash the banana and avocado thoroughly until smooth and well combined.
2. Stir in the coconut oil and mayonnaise.
3. Apply treatment to dry hair, ensuring all strands are covered. Keep treatment on for thirty to forty-five minutes. For best results, wear a shower cap. Rinse treatment thoroughly in the shower. Shampooing your hair after the treatment is optional.

## Lavender Scalp Cream

If you suffer severely from eczema or dandruff, this scalp cream will remove the dead skin while soothing and healing irritated areas. This recipe also works well as a rejuvenating mask for dry hair.

### Ingredients:
3 tablespoons coconut oil
1 tablespoon olive oil
3 drops lavender essential oil (for dry hair mask, replace lavender with peppermint)

### Directions:
1. Melt coconut oil in a double boiler over low heat, and then add olive oil.
2. Once well combined, pour into bowl and add lavender.
3. Apply to dry hair, ensuring all hair is thoroughly covered. For best results, cover your hair with a shower cap. Keep the treatment on for a minimum of twenty-five minutes. If the scalp is severely inflamed, you can wear the mask all night. Rinse hair under the shower. Repeat the mask every few days until scalp is healed.

## Lemon Pepper Anti-Dandruff Mask

### Equipment:
- Double boiler
- Muslin straining cloth

### Ingredients:
2 tablespoons coconut oil
¼ teaspoon black pepper
3 drops lemon juice
3 drops lavender oil

### Directions:
1. Heat coconut oil in the top section of a double boiler over low heat until it melts. Remove from heat and add black pepper.
2. Strain the mixture by pouring it through a muslin cloth, then add lemon juice and lavender oil.
3. Stir until well combined. Set aside until the coconut oil is warm but still liquid.
4. Massage the oil deeply into your scalp. Apply any remaining oil onto your hair by stroking downward. Rub the tips so they are thoroughly covered with the oil. For best results, wear a shower cap over the mask and keep it on for a minimum of thirty minutes, or overnight if possible. Rinse off in cool water under the shower.

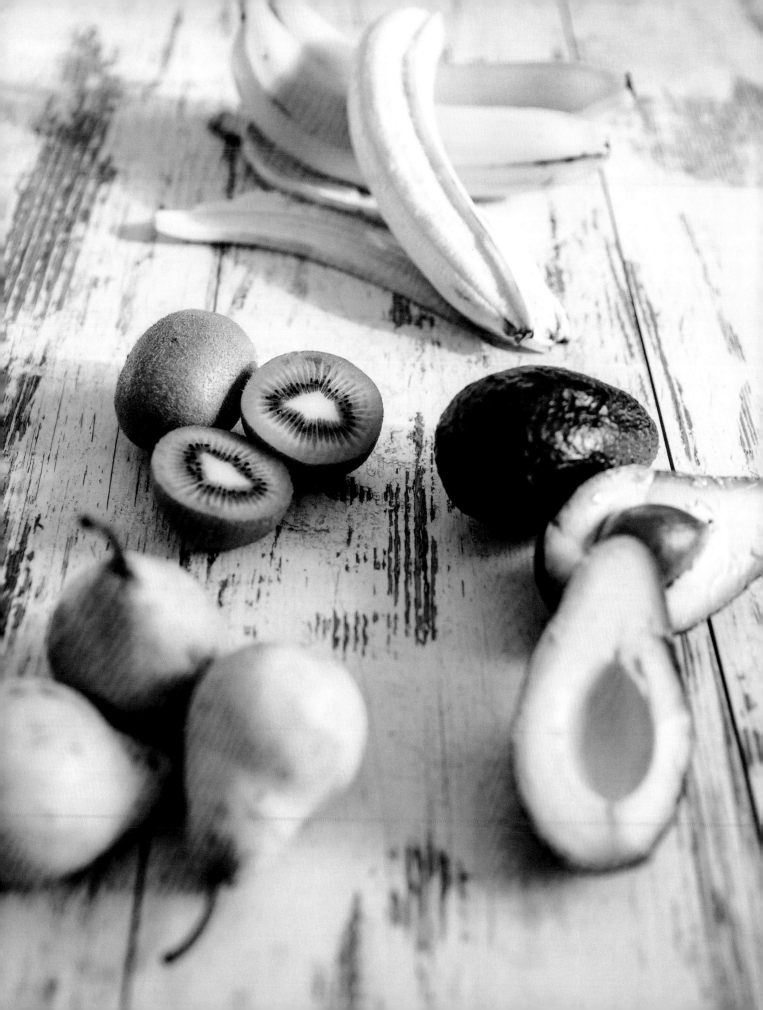

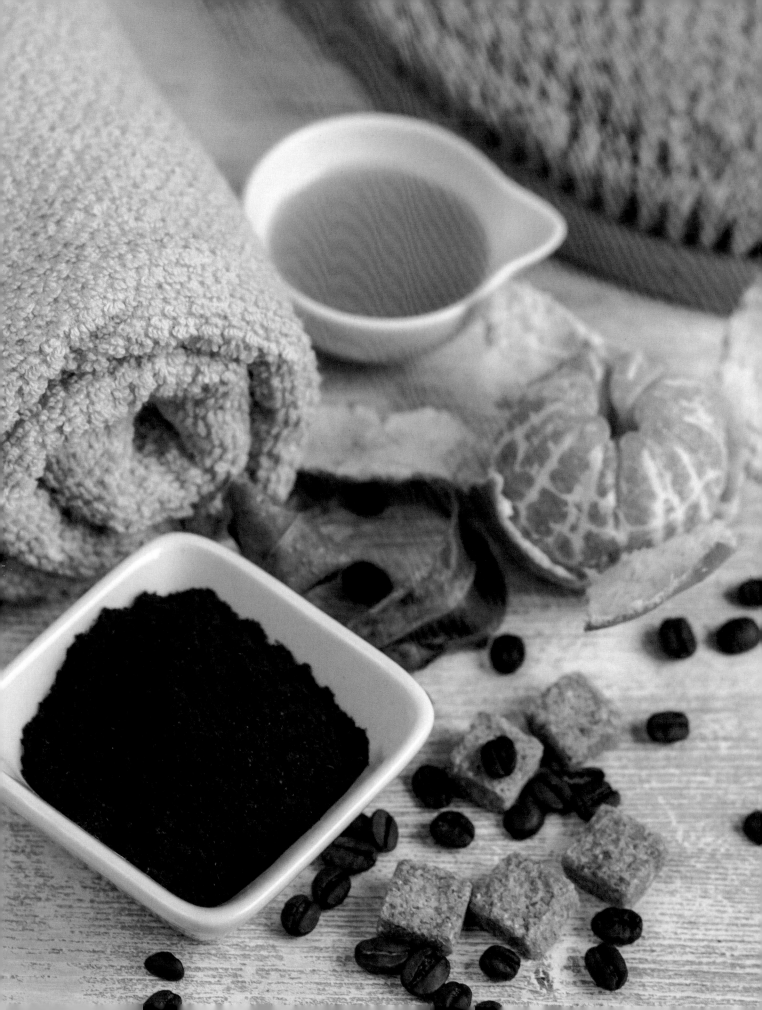

## Shampoo

Cleaning your hair can be as simple as making a baking-soda-and-water paste, scrubbing it into your hair, and rinsing well. However, if you enjoy the feel of a sudsy, soapy, scented shampoo, try this recipe.

### Ingredients:

4 ounces liquid castile soap
3 tablespoons fresh or dried herbs of your choice, boiled for 30 minutes in 2 cups water and strained

### Directions:

1. Pour the soap and herbal water into a jar, cover, and shake until well combined.
2. Wet hair, lather, and rinse.

## Hair Conditioner

This conditioner will add softness and volume to your hair. Avocado, bananas, and egg yolks are also great hair conditioners. Apply conditioner, allow to sit in hair a minimum of five minutes (longer for a deeper conditioning), and then rinse well. You may wish to shampoo a second time after using this conditioner.

### Ingredients:

1 cup olive oil
1 tsp lemon juice
1 tsp cider vinegar
2 tsp honey
6 to 10 drops essential oils, if desired

### Directions:

1. Whisk all ingredients together or blend in a food processor.
2. Store in an airtight container.

---

### Herbs for Your Hair

**Herbs for dry hair:** Burdock root, comfrey, elderflowers, lavender, marshmallow, parsley, sage, stinging nettle

**Herbs for oily hair:** Calendula, horsetail, lemon juice, lemon balm, mints, rosemary, witch hazel, yarrow

**Herbs to combat dandruff:** Burdock root, garlic, onion, parsley, rosemary, stinging nettle, thyme

**Herbs for body and luster:** Calendula, catnip, horsetail, licorice, lime flowers, nasturtium, parsley, rosemary, sage, stinging nettles, watercress

**Herbs for shine:** Horsetail, parsley, nettles, rosemary, sage, calendula

**Herbs for hair growth:** Aloe, arnica, birch, burdock, catmint, chamomile, horsetail, licorice, calendula, nettles, parsley, rosemary, sage, stinging nettle

**Herbs for coloring hair brown:** henna (reddish brown), walnut hulls, sage

**Herbs for coloring hair blonde:** calendula, chamomile, lemon, saffron, turmeric, rhubarb root

---

# Hand and Foot Treatments

## Stinky Foot Solution Soak

If you need a foot soak with some serious anti-stink properties, this is the one for you. The vinegar and tea tree oil bring antibacterial properties that will get the job done. I will admit this isn't the most lovely scented bath, and it probably won't inspire any vacation day dreams, but it will solve your stinky feet issues. Do this nightly or weekly to help detoxify.

### Ingredients:
1 cup vinegar
½ cup baking soda
½ cup Epsom salt
4–5 drops tea tree oil

### Preparation:
1. Mix the ingredients in the bottom of a basin and fill with the hottest water you can stand. Stir well to dissolve and mix the ingredients.
2. Put a folded towel right next to the basin before you put your feet in it so you can dry off when you're finished.
3. Submerge your feet in the bath for 20–30 minutes or until the water cools.

## Rosemary Peppermint Foot Scrub

Use this foot rub to remove calluses, soften skin, and leave your feet feeling and smelling wonderful.

### Ingredients:
1 cup coarse sea salt
¼ cup sweet almond or olive oil
2 to 3 drops peppermint essential oil
1 to 2 drops rosemary essential oil
2 sprigs fresh rosemary, crushed, or ½ teaspoon dried rosemary

### Directions:
1. Combine all ingredients and massage into feet and ankles.
2. Rinse with warm water and follow with a moisturizer.

## Beachside Break Foot Soak

There's little more relaxing at the end of a long day on your feet than plunging them into a warm bath that has tonics to ease pain and essential oils to bring you into a state of calmness. Epsom salt has been around for centuries and is well known to help detoxify, and magnesium keeps cramps at bay and relaxes muscles. Keep a basin handy, and a jar of this foot soak, and you can soak away your worries at the end of any hard day. I like to use a combination of vetiver, sandalwood, and lavender essential oils to invoke a calming, beachside scent. This will take you to that happy place of being in a beach chair with the sand under your toes and the salt air breezing by. If you prefer something more refreshing and uplifting, try peppermint or lime essential oils.

### Ingredients:
1 cup baking soda
1 cup sea salt
1 cup Epsom salt
15 drops of your favorite essential oil (I like 5 drops of vetiver, 5 drops of sandalwood, and 5 drops of lavender)

### Preparation:
1. Mix ingredients well in a bowl, being sure to evenly distribute the essential oils.
2. For each foot bath, use ¼ cup of the foot soak mixture and add it to a large basin that will fit both of your feet comfortably. Fill with warm or hot water, being careful not to make it too hot.
3. Put a folded towel right next to the basin before you put your feet in it so you can dry off when you're finished.
4. Keep your feet in the bath for 20–30 minutes or until the water cools.

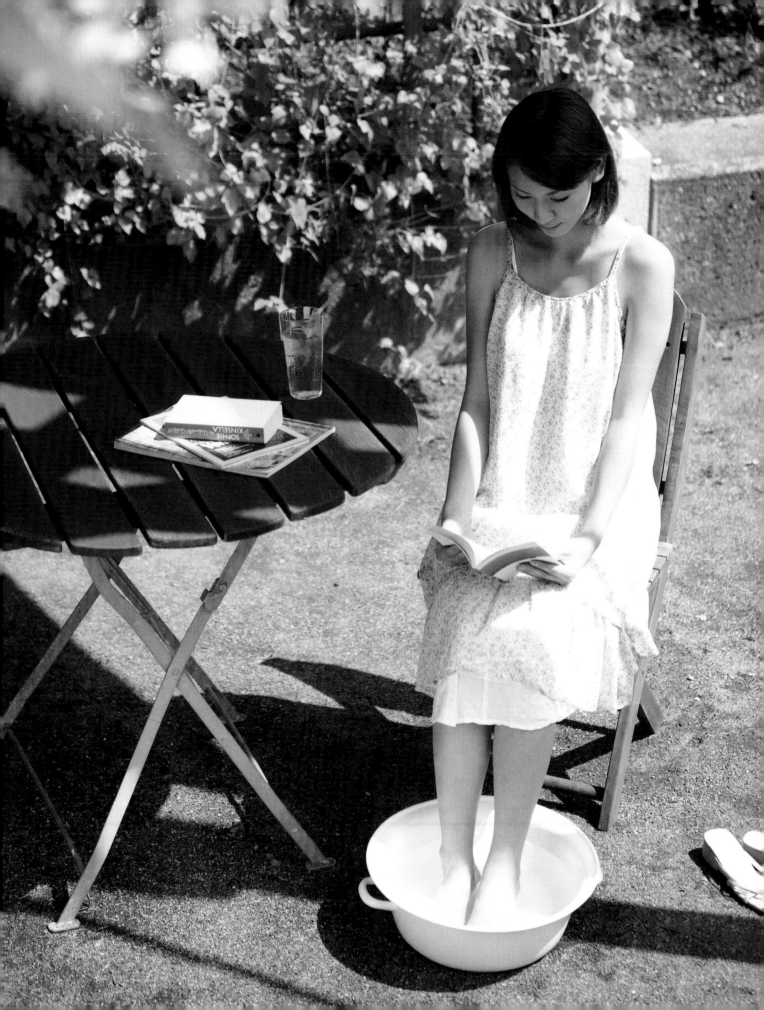

# Makeup Remover

## Eye'll Be Gentle Makeup Remover

This makeup remover is gentle on your skin but harsh on makeup, even waterproof makeup! Make sure you get a pure witch hazel free of alcohol, such as Dr. Thayer's. It's more expensive, but absolutely worth it, especially when you're putting it near your eyes! Making small batches of this is best; since you're using it near your eyes, you don't want to give bacteria a chance to grow. Since it's just two or three ingredients, though, it's no big chore; just add the witch hazel first and then add half as much jojoba oil.

### Ingredients:

4 tablespoons witch hazel
2 tablespoons jojoba or olive oil
The contents of 1 capsule of vitamin E oil, optional

### Preparation:

1. Mix well in a small pump bottle (travel-size works great).
2. To use, simply shake it up well, then pump a very small amount onto a cotton pad or small cloth and use to remove makeup. This may sting a bit around the eyes if you don't close them tightly!

## Tropical Face Cleanser

The vitamin C in kiwi has enzymatic and cleansing properties, and the apricot oil serves as a moisturizer. The ground almonds act as an exfoliant to remove dead skin cells. Yogurt has cleansing and moisturizing properties.

### Ingredients:

1 kiwi
¾ cup avocado, banana, apricot, peach, strawberries, or
papaya (or some of each)
2 tablespoons plain yogurt (whole milk is best)
1 tablespoon apricot oil (almond oil also works well)
1 tablespoon honey
1 teaspoon finely ground almonds

### Directions:

1. Puree all ingredients together. Massage into face and neck and rinse thoroughly with cool water.
2. Store excess in refrigerator for one to two days.

# Masks

## Lemon-Honey Facial Mask

Want a spa facial without the spa price tag? Too busy to leave the house, or have too many kids and/or animals to leave? Open the refrigerator! Chances are you have everything you need to whip up a facial mask. Unfortunately, you can't pull "time alone" out of the refrigerator, so you may have to retreat to a room with a locked door to enjoy your facial mask in peace.

### Ingredients:

3 tablespoons lemon or plain yogurt
1 teaspoon apple cider vinegar
1 teaspoon lemon juice
1 teaspoon olive oil
1 tablespoon honey

### Preparation:

1. Mix ingredients well in a small bowl.
2. Use your fingers to gently spread the mixture on your face. Yes, this might get a bit messy, so tip your head back and keep a towel handy.
3. Once you've smoothed this all over, avoiding your eyes, let it rest until it has dried out a bit and feels slightly tacky on your skin.
4. Gently wash off with warm water. Follow with a toner such as witch hazel or rose water to complete the experience.

## Avocado and Coconut Oil Hydrating Face Mask

This face mask will rejuvenate your skin, leaving you feeling fresh and invigorated. The antioxidant properties of honey will enhance coconut oil's natural healing properties. This recipe is for one instant face mask.

### Equipment:

- 1 bowl
- 1 fork
- Electric mixer

### Ingredients:

2 tablespoons virgin coconut oil
1 tablespoon honey
½ avocado
2 thin slices cucumber (optional)

### Directions:

1. Mash the avocado with a fork until it is a fairly smooth paste.
2. Add coconut oil and honey, and blend with mixer on a low setting until combined.
3. Spread the mask over your face and neck, avoiding the eyes.
4. Place cucumber slices over your eyes to rejuvenate the delicate skin.
5. Keep the mask on for fifteen to twenty minutes then wash off thoroughly with warm water.

## Honey and Coconut Oil Healing Mask

This mask combines the healing properties of coconut oil and honey with the antioxidant properties and smooth texture of Greek yogurt, making it ideal for anyone suffering from acne or dermatitis. It must be applied within a few hours of making it to ensure the ingredients remain fresh and potent.

### Equipment:
- Bowl
- Handheld mixer
- Ingredients:
- 1 tablespoon honey
- 1 tablespoon Greek yogurt
- 1 tablespoon virgin coconut oil
- 1 teaspoon arrowroot
- 5 drops of lemon juice or 3 drops tea tree oil

### Directions:
1. Place all ingredients in bowl and mix gently until well combined. If you don't plan to use the mask straight away, refrigerate it in a covered container.
2. To apply, smooth it over the T-zone, working down from the forehead. Then make a second application over the entire face and neck. Avoid the area around the eyes.
3. Leave on for approximately fifteen minutes then wash off thoroughly with warm water.

## Minty Cucumber Facial Mask

This is a revitalizing mask that reduces puffiness and refreshes the skin.

### Ingredients:
1 tablespoon powdered milk
1 teaspoon plain yogurt (whole milk yogurt is best)
1 teaspoon honey
1 teaspoon fresh mint leaves
½ cucumber, peeled

### Directions:
1. Blend ingredients thoroughly, using a food processor or blender if available.
2. Apply to face, avoiding eyes. Leave on for 10 to 15 minutes, then rinse.

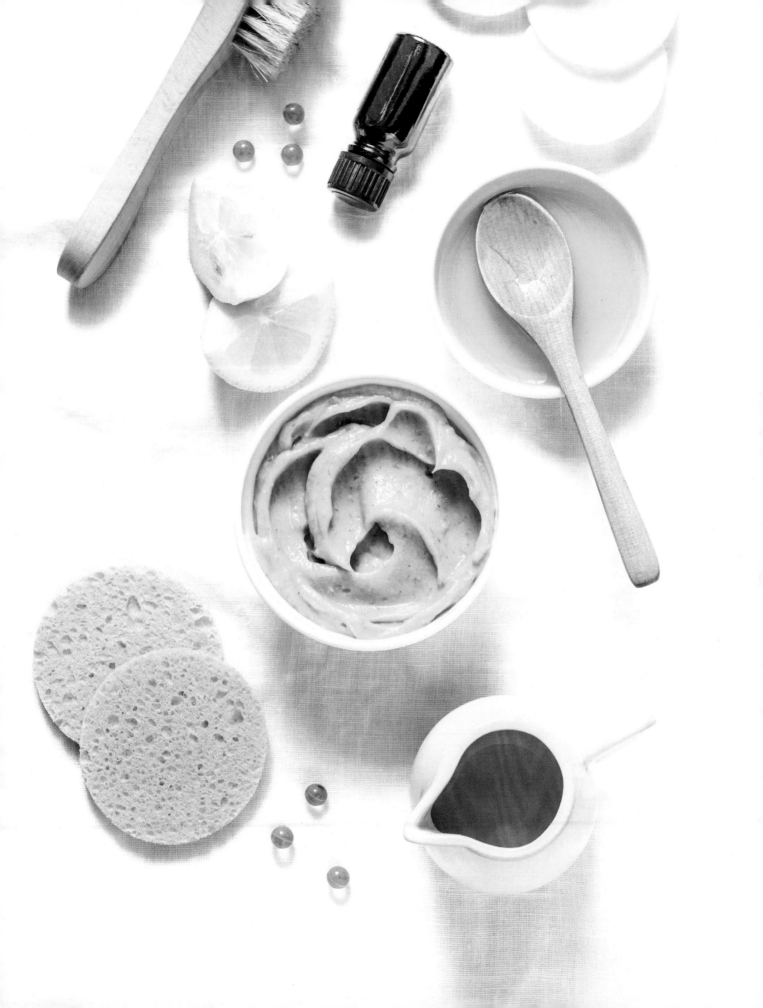

# Natural Deodorant

## Citrus Cream Deodorant

One of the best parts of aromatherapy—besides the health benefits—are the lovely smells of essential oils. Utilizing these aromas to keep ourselves smelling inviting is one of the benefits of incorporating essential oils into deodorant. Essential oils don't just mask unpleasant body odors, though—they deal with the cause of this odor. Our underarms are an excellent home for many different types of bacteria. While these bacteria may not be harmful, when they combine with sweat, they can be unpleasant to our senses. The essential oils in this recipe are antibacterial and mood lifting.

### Ingredients:
⅓ cup baking soda
2–4 tablespoons almond oil
2 drops bergamot essential oil
2 drops lemon essential oil
2 drops lime essential oil
2 drops orange essential oil
1 drop melaleuca essential oil
vanilla extract (optional)

### Preparation:
1. Pour ⅓ cup baking soda into a 4-ounce mason jar.
2. Start by adding 1 tablespoon almond oil and using a metal fork to stir in the oil.
3. Continue to mix in almond oil, a teaspoon at a time, until the baking soda is no longer powder. The consistency should be smooth without being oily. The amount of almond oil needed will depend on the where you live due to variations in the moisture content of the air.
4. Add 2 drops each of bergamot, lemon, lime, and orange essential oil, stirring between each oil.
5. Stir in 1 drop of melaleuca essential oil.
6. If desired, stir in vanilla extract, one drop at a time, until desired scent is achieved.
7. If needed, stir in more almond oil.
8. Use your index finger to pat mixture down into the mason jar.
9. Seal with mason jar lid.

### Administration:
1. Use your index finger to scoop out a dime-size amount of deodorant.
2. Rub the deodorant into one armpit, making sure to cover the entire armpit area.
3. Repeat on the other armpit.
4. Make sure to replace the lid tightly after using so the essential oils do not evaporate.

### Benefits:
- Sweating is an important part of the body's detoxification process, which is why this recipe does not call for ingredients that inhibit that process. While this is not specifically an antiperspirant, the baking soda in this recipe absorbs moisture.
- Melaleuca essential oil's antimicrobial properties have been valued by Aboriginal people for generation upon generation and are an important part of aboriginal bush medicine. The knowledge of the benefits of melaleuca—commonly known as tea tree oil—was passed on to settlers in New Zealand and Australia, who in turn shared the information with the Western world.
- Citrus essential oils are good for cleansing the skin due to their antimicrobial properties.
- Citrus essential oils are incredibly uplifting. Each citrus oil in this recipe has been researched for its mood-lifting properties. Using this deodorant in the morning gives you a mood boost to get your day going.
- Citrus essential oils have antioxidant properties giving this recipe additional health benefits.

## NOTES AND TIPS:

- Each person has a particular scent that blends best with their body chemistry. The amounts of the individual citrus essential oil can be adjusted—while maintaining the same overall number of drops—to create a recipe that works best with your body chemistry. Grapefruit oil may be substituted for any of the citrus oils to help achieve this balance.
- If you find skin sensitivity with this recipe, reduce the amount of citrus essential oils to one drop each and increase the amount of almond oil used. Discontinue use if sensitivity persists.
- Much of the skin sensitivity associated with citrus oils is due to their reaction with the sun. The underarm area is rarely exposed to the sun, which makes this less of an issue with this recipe. When going out in the sun for long periods or during peak sun times, make sure to apply sunscreen to your underarms.

## Basil Lavender Natural Deodorant

### Ingredients:

2 teaspoons coconut oil

8 drops rose geranium essential oil

8 drops basil essential oil

8 drops lavender essential oil

2 tablespoons cocoa butter

2 tablespoons shea butter

½ teaspoon grated beeswax for a more solid consistency

2 tablespoons arrowroot powder

1 tablespoon baking soda

5 drops vitamin E oil

### Directions:

1. In a double boiler, combine the oils, butters, and beeswax together; gently heat until melted.
2. Remove from heat and stir in arrowroot powder, baking soda, and vitamin E, adding in your essential oil blend last.
3. Pour into jars. Cover with a paper towel and let sit until cool and solid—about 5 hours or overnight.
4. Place the lids on securely and apply a small amount as needed in the morning to the underarms and on your feet as well, if needed. Options: Grapefruit and basil, orange, and lavender essential oils are other possible scents. Or choose your own favorite blend.

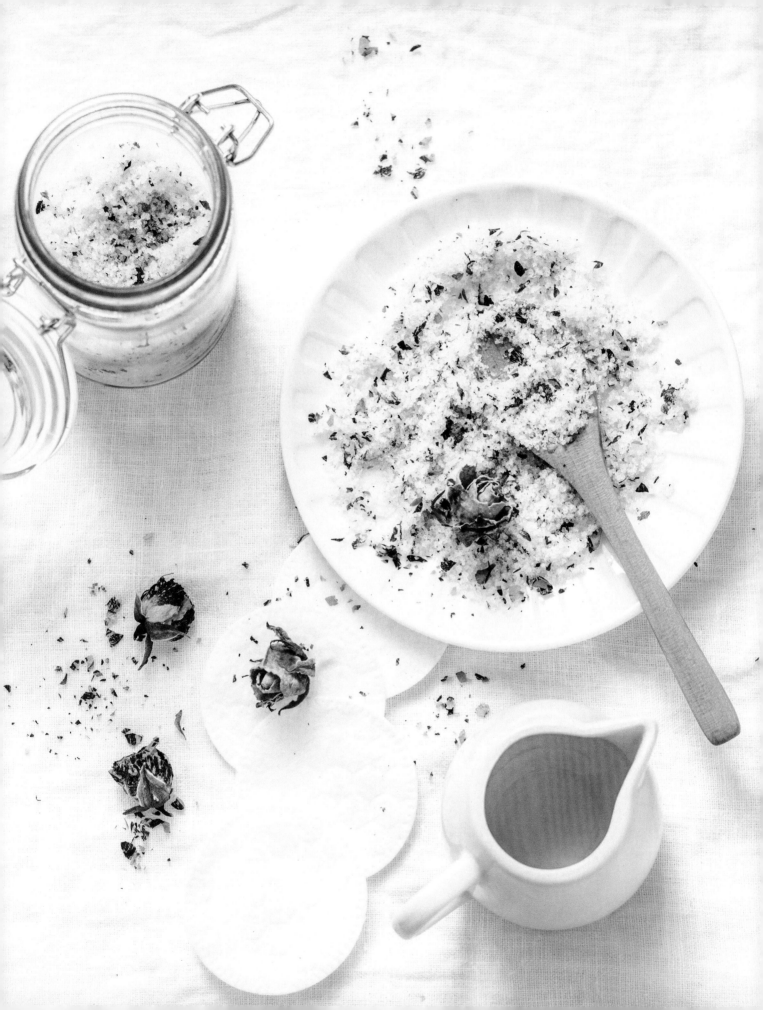

# Scrubs

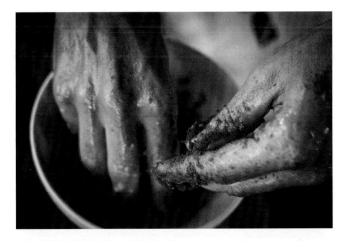

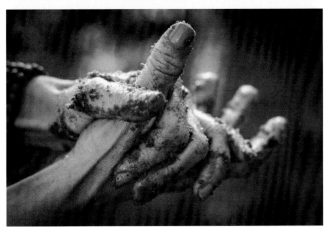

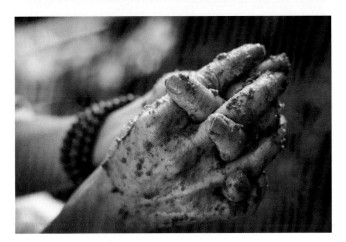

I recommend using scrubs on the body rather than the face. Facial skin is simply too delicate for the coarse grains of either sugar or salt. To exfoliate the face, use a soft towel and the facial oiling method.

Salt will draw impurities out of the skin and replace lost minerals back into it, whereas sugar is a humectant, meaning that it will help to retain moisture, unlike salt. Additionally, they work beautifully to soften the skin. Always use either fine-grain Himalayan pink sea salt or organic cane sugar for best results.

Table salt contains bleach, ammonia, and anti-clumping agents to make it presentable to the average consumer. Conventional sugar is genetically modified and toxic. It is saturated with pesticides, herbicides, fungicides, bleach, and other toxins that shouldn't be put in or on your body. It's very important to use the highest quality organic ingredients in your path to total beauty.

## Directions:

1. Slowly melt one cup of coconut oil in a pot over gentle heat. Allow it to totally liquefy.
2. Pour it into a glass bowl with four cups of salt or sugar in whatever combination that best suits you.
3. Mix well. Add more coconut oil to reach your desired level of creaminess. The blend should feel silky and cohesive rather than dry or overly oily. To amplify the pretty power, experiment by adding three tablespoons of aromatic herbs like rosemary, sage, mint, or thyme. You could also experiment with three tablespoons of dried violets, rosebuds, chamomile, jasmine, calendula, or lavender. Dried herbs and flowers give color and texture to your scrub creations.
4. Half-fill a five-milliliter bottle (approximately 50 drops) with your choice of pure essential oils.
5. Add your awesome essential oil blend to the salt or sugar mixture. Mix well.
6. Store in an airtight glass jar away from light, heat, and air.

7. Add one cup to a hot bath or use half a cup as an all-over body scrub.

Remember that herbs and flowers have aromatic and medicinal compounds. Consider the properties of the herbs when adding to your scrub blend.

An alternative base is pumice. It's a fine grain that's wonderful at sloughing off dead skin and can be used on the face. Always exfoliate with care. You can find pumice at health food stores, herbal apothecaries, or higher quality pharmacies.

Use scrubs on the hands, feet, elbows, knees, buttocks, thighs, or anywhere that needs a little scrubbing action. Scrubs are also very effective at breaking up the stagnation associated with cellulite. To treat stubborn cellulite, simply rub the scrub blend in circular and upward motions into dimpled points for five minutes every other day for at least three months. Try a fragrant combination of lemongrass, cypress, tangerine, lemon, and juniper berry. It's a powerful dimple-buster and smells oh so good.

## Some luscious salt or sugar blends are:

- Black pepper, ginger, clove, and lemon: This is an excellent winter warming scrub, especially on the feet, hands, and ears.
- Rose otto, vanilla, lavender, magnolia flower, and fenugreek: This is a "let's get groovy tonight" blend. It's sexy, sweet, and bursting with flower power.
- Peppermint, tansy, lavender, and hay: This is a heavenly azure blend that's slightly cooling in nature and helps to soothe frazzled nerves.
- Lemongrass, black spruce, and cypress: This is a "rise and shine" blend.
- Marjoram, lavender, cape chamomile, and vanilla: This is a "sweet dreams" blend. The combination of these oils is deeply relaxing and calming to the central nervous system.
- Vetiver, Douglas fir, white cedar, mitti attar, and spikenard: This is a "buffed body for men" blend.

In addition to scrubbing, cellulite can be diminished by avoiding greasy, fried, and rich foods; dairy products; and especially sugar (internally). Inappropriate dietary practices create and trap dampness in the body, which contributes to the appearance of unwanted cellulite.

# Coconut Lime Verbena Sugar Scrub

Sugar scrubs are wonderful way to exfoliate your skin, while at the same time allowing yourself a little bit of luxury. Store-bought sugar scrubs can be surprisingly expensive, but the ingredients for a homemade sugar scrub are simple and inexpensive. This coconut lime verbena sugar scrub brings a tropical spa feel into your bathtub or shower.

## Ingredients:

1 cup raw sugar
2 tablespoons raw coconut oil
10 drops lime essential oil
1 tablespoon dried lemon verbena leaves, crushed

## Preparation:

1. Soften your coconut oil either in the microwave (using a glass bowl) for 10 seconds at a time or on the stove at low heat.
2. Place 1 cup of sugar in a medium-size glass bowl.
3. Add 2 tablespoons coconut oil to the mixture slowly, stirring as you pour it into the sugar.
4. Add 10 drops of lime essential oil one drop at a time, stirring between each drop.
5. Sprinkle in the dried verbena and stir to evenly distribute it through the mixture.
6. Divide the sugar scrub between two 4-ounce mason jars and put the lids on tightly.

## Administration:

1. Before getting into the bath or shower, use a spoon to scoop out your desired amount of sugar scrub into a small dish.
2. After wetting your skin, use your hands to rub the sugar scrub over your arms, shoulders, stomach, back, hips, legs, and feet. Avoid your face and sensitive areas.
3. Rinse the sugar scrub off your body using warm water. As you rinse off the sugar and verbena, massage the coconut oil into your skin.

## Benefits:

- Raw sugar is larger and rougher than refined sugar and therefore is more exfoliating. The coconut oil protects your skin, while the raw sugar removes dead skin cells.
- Lime essential oil is uplifting to the mood.
- Lemon verbena leaves contain constituents with antispasmodic properties.

## NOTES AND TIPS:

- Additional raw coconut oil can be added to this recipe if you prefer a more oily consistency.
- Other citrus essential oils such as bergamot, lemon, or wild orange essential oils can be substituted for the lime essential oil as they have similar mood-lifting properties.
- Lime essential oil contains limonene, which causes sun sensitivity when used on the skin. So while this sugar scrub smells like a tropical beach vacation, it is not recommended that it be used directly before sun exposure. The raw coconut oil does provide protection from the sun, but the protective ability of coconut oil against limonene phototoxicity has not been studied.

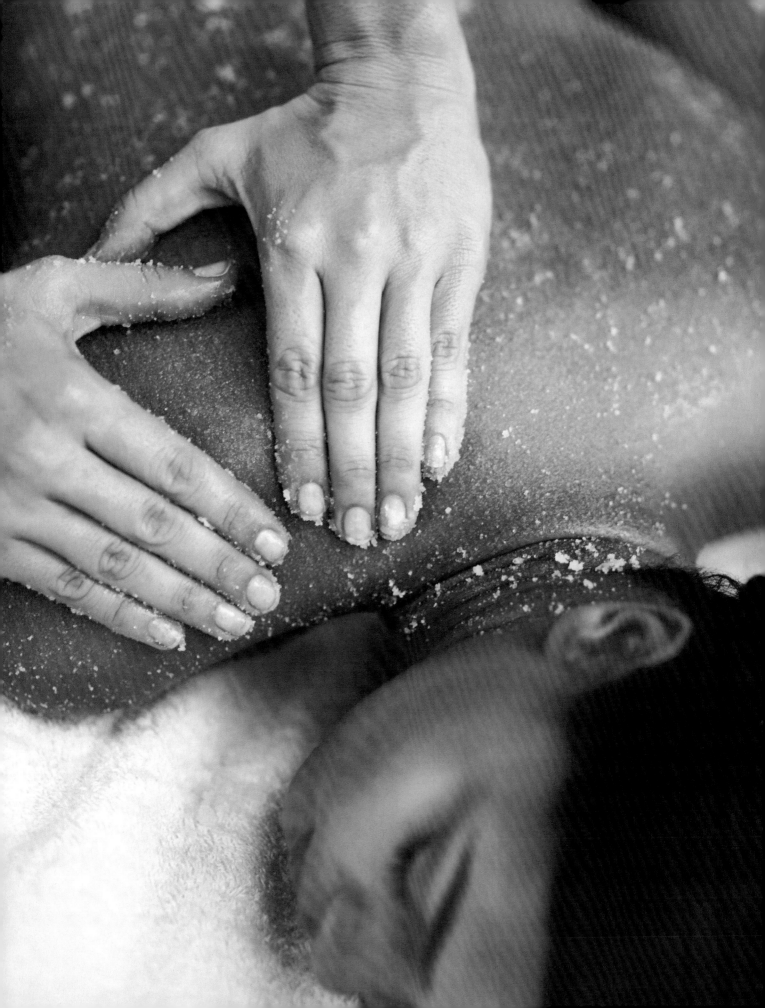

## Sweet and Subtle Sugar Scrub

Part of pampering yourself is giving yourself something sweet, but it doesn't always have to come in the form of food. Your skin deserves a sweet treat on those pampering days or even every day. This sugar scrub is that perfect gift to your body. It delights the senses, while being gentle on the skin.

### Ingredients:

1 cup refined sugar
2 tablespoons light olive oil
4 drops ylang-ylang essential oil
2 drops geranium essential oil
2 drops sandalwood essential oil

### Preparation:

1. Place 1 cup of sugar in a medium-size glass bowl.
2. Add 2 tablespoons sweet almond oil to the mixture slowly, stirring as you pour it into the sugar.
3. Add 4 drops ylang-ylang, 2 drops geranium, and 2 drops sandalwood essential oils, one drop at a time. Stir between each drop.
4. Divide the sugar scrub between two 4-ounce mason jars and put the lids on tightly.

### Administration:

1. Before getting into the bath or shower, use a spoon to scoop out your desired amount of sugar scrub into a small dish.
2. After wetting your skin, use your hands to rub the sugar scrub over your arms, shoulders, stomach, back, hips, legs, and feet. Avoid your face and sensitive areas.
3. Rinse the sugar scrub off your body using warm water.

### Benefits:

- Refined sugar is gentler on the skin than raw sugar and is ideal for softer or more sensitive skin.
- The germacrene in ylang-ylang, cintronellol in geranium, and α-santalol in sandalwood are all antioxidants. Olive oil is also an antioxidant due to its phenolic compounds.
- Antioxidants reduce skin roughness and scaling.

### Notes and Tips:

- Light olive oil is used in this recipe due to its subtle aroma. However, any olive oil can be used, and darker olive oils do have higher antioxidant benefits.
- Additional olive oil can be added to this recipe if you prefer a more oily consistency.
- Make sure to rinse your shower or tub thoroughly after using any scrub to keep the floor from becoming slippery.

## Invigorating Cellulite-Reducing Salt Scrub

Cellulite is a normal part of being a human. It affects women significantly more than men, but the presence of cellulite occurs in people of all sizes. Cellulite is not a medical condition, but it is a cosmetic one and many people would like to see a reduction in the appearance of dimpling on their thighs and buttocks. This salt scrub not only reduces the appearance of cellulite, it also helps you slim your thighs and hips.

You don't have to have cellulite to enjoy this scrub. The invigorating aspects of the scrub—coffee and grapefruit, orange, and rosemary essential oils—make this scrub a splendid way to start your morning. Plus, you still get to enjoy smoother, softer skin.

### Ingredients:

¼ cup Epsom salt
¼ cup ground coffee beans
3 tablespoons jojoba oil
8 drops grapefruit essential oil

5 drops orange essential oil
4 drops black pepper essential oil
3 drops rosemary essential oil
1 drop cinnamon essential oil
1 drop ginger essential oil

## Preparation:

1. In a glass bowl, combine 3 tablespoons jojoba oil with 8 drops grapefruit, 5 drops orange, 4 drops black pepper, 3 drops rosemary, 1 drop cinnamon, and 1 drop ginger essential oils. Stir oils together with a metal whisk.
2. Add ¼ cup Epsom salt to the oil mixture and stir until oils are evenly distributed throughout the Epsom salt.
3. Add ¼ cup coffee grounds to the mixture and stir until the salt scrub is evenly mixed.
4. Place two spoonfuls of the scrub in a small glass, metal, or ceramic bowl to use immediately.
5. Store the rest of the scrub in a 4-ounce mason jar for use later or to give as a gift.

## Administration:

1. Before getting into the bath or shower, use a spoon to scoop out your desired amount of Invigorating Salt Scrub into a small dish.
2. After wetting your skin, use your hands to rub the salt scrub over your arms, shoulders, stomach, back, hips, legs, and feet. Avoid your face and sensitive areas.
3. Rinse the salt scrub off your body, using warm water.

## Benefits:

- Caffeine is a common ingredient in cellulite creams. It reduces thigh and buttocks circumference and the dimpling appearance of cellulite. It does this by preventing the over accumulation of fat within cells.
- Jojoba oil increases the caffeine release from the coffee grounds and makes it more readily available for absorption by your skin.
- Used topically, orange, black pepper, cinnamon, and ginger reduce the appearance of cellulite.
- Use aromatically, grapefruit and black pepper essential oils affect the sympathetic nervous system. When combined with topical caffeine absorption, this has a slimming effect and reduces fat accumulation.
- Rosemary essential oil is invigorating and stimulating to the mind.

## NOTES AND TIPS:

- If kept in a cool, dark, and dry place, this scrub will last over two months and maintain its efficacy. How long it lasts will depend on the freshness of the ingredients, how infrequently it is opened and the moisture and heat levels in the air.
- Even though grapefruit is a citrus oil, it does not have the phototoxicity issues that other citrus oils can have. Therefore, it is safe to use on skin that will be exposed to the sun.
- The antioxidants in coffee protect skin from the effects of sun damage including early aging, skin cancer, and photosensitive erythema (a rash or redness due to oversensitivity to the sun).
- Using coffee from East Africa—such as Kenyan, Ethiopian, or Tanzanian coffees—for the coffee grounds will pair well with the grapefruit and orange essential oil in this recipe. Latin American coffees will also add a pleasant citrus aroma when used in this recipe. Asian Pacific coffees will emphasize the cinnamon essential oil.
- Lighter roasted coffees have a higher caffeine content than darker roasts.

## Orange Blossom Honey Salt Scrub

Smooth, nourished skin feels sensational. Pair that with the sweet smell of orange blossom honey, the bright aroma of orange essential oil, and fragrant geranium essential oil, and well, you've got yourself the recipe for a luxurious shower. Scrub your whole body with the Orange Blossom Honey Salt Scrub and feel the difference it makes to your skin.

### Ingredients:

½ cup Epsom salt
¼ cup ground Himalayan crystal salts
3 tablespoons orange blossom honey
2 tablespoons sweet almond oil
1 tablespoon evening primrose oil
10 drops orange essential oil
2 drops geranium essential oil

### Preparation:

1. In a large glass bowl, whisk together 2 tablespoons sweet almond oil, 1 tablespoon evening primrose oil, and 3 tablespoons orange blossom honey.
2. Whisk in 10 drops orange and 2 drops geranium essential oils.
3. Stir in ½ cup Epsom salt and ¼ cup Himalayan salts.
4. Stir until evenly mixed.
5. Divide between three 4-ounce mason jars and cap tightly.

### Administration:

1. Before getting into the bath or shower, use a spoon to scoop out your desired amount of Orange Blossom Honey Salt Scrub into a small dish.
2. After wetting your skin, use your hands to rub the salt scrub over your arms, shoulders, stomach, back, hips, legs, and feet. Avoid your face and sensitive areas.
3. Rinse the salt scrub off your body using warm water.

### Benefits:

- Evening primrose oil contains gamma-linolenic acid, an essential fatty acid for skin health, which improves skin elasticity and smoothness.
- Himalayan pink salts are nourishing to your skin, containing a variety of compounds not found in traditional table salts.
- The combination of orange blossom honey and orange essential oil cleanses your skin without drying it out.
- Geranium essential oil's anti-inflammatory properties are particularly effective against edema, swelling of the skin due to fluid build up.

### NOTES AND TIPS:

If you use the same tablespoon to measure the honey as you do the primrose oil, the honey will release from the tablespoon easily.

Getting water in your container of bath salts will decrease the longevity of the Orange Blossom Honey Salt Scrub due to the contamination of the almond oil putting it at risk for rancidity. Make sure to use dry hands or a spoon to scoop out the desired amount of scrub into a separate container before getting into the bath or shower.

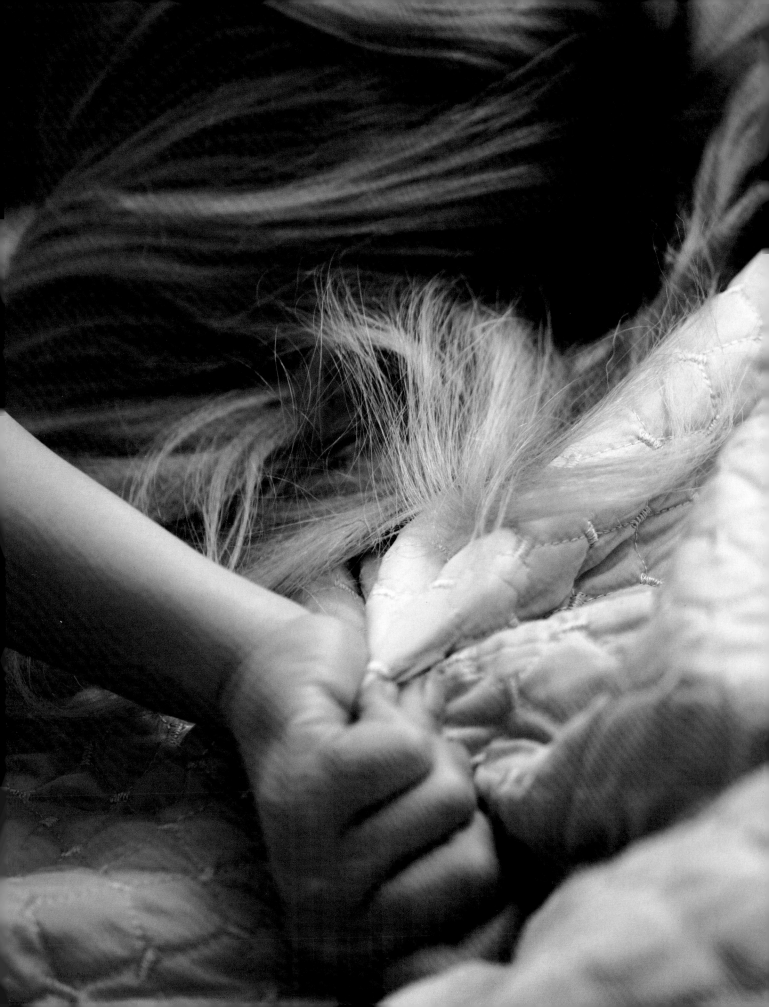

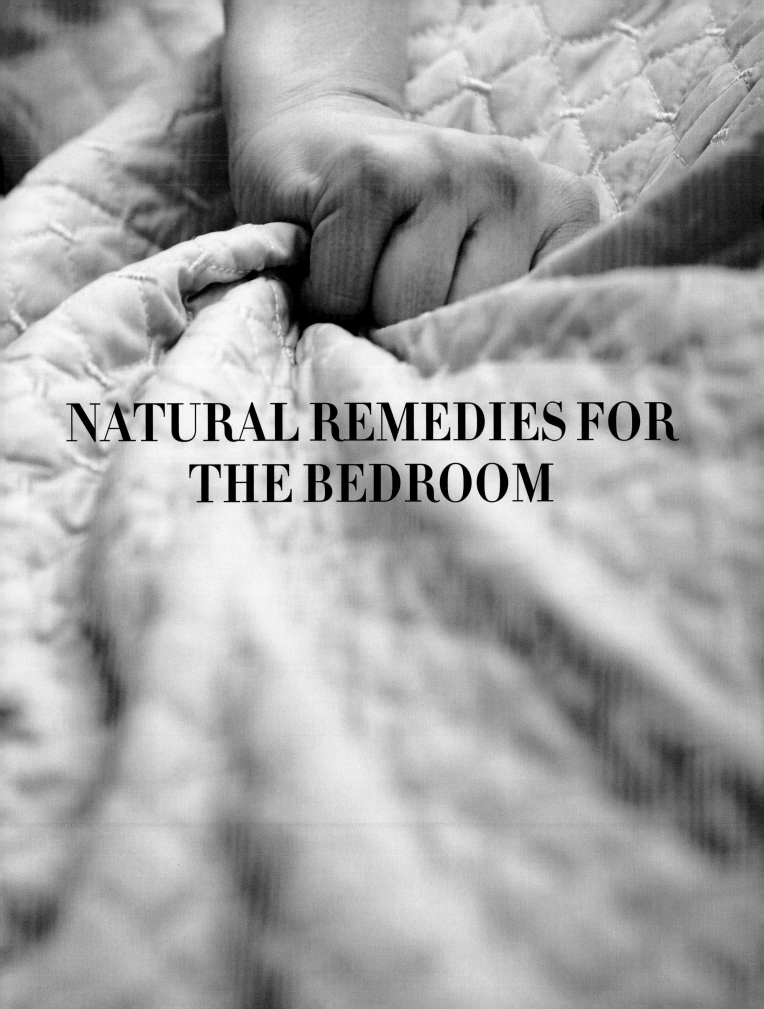

# NATURAL REMEDIES FOR THE BEDROOM

# Aphrodisiacs/ Stimulation

## An Introduction to Sex Drive and Libido

Sex drive, or libido, is more often than not the strongest urge in humans after food and sleep. But all too often, one partner ends up having a lower sex drive than another partner, who can end up feeling frustrated, neglected, or unloved.

Loss of sex drive is extremely common and is now the biggest single reason for consulting a sex therapist. A normal sex drive is needed, as your sexual health and general well-being are very closely linked. Just as the healthier you are, the more you are likely to want to have sex, increased sexual energy is also beneficial to the mind, body, and spirit.

Men are said to reach their sexual peak in their teens, while their psychological sex drive peaks after the age of fifty when testosterone levels fall. Women are said to reach their physical sexual peak in their thirties or forties, while their psychological sex drive reaches its maximum in their fifties, at the same time as that of males. But this is not to say that men and women cannot continue having and enjoying sex up to almost any age.

## Aphrodisiac Foods and Herbs

The following foods and herbs are considered to have libido-boosting properties. Not everyone will respond to these foods the same way, but preparing a romantic meal for your partner, perhaps with some of these ingredients, can be a wonderful way to get in the mood.

- Apples
- Asparagus
- Avocados
- Cherries
- Chilies
- Chilito cactus
- Chocolate
- Fenugreek
- Figs
- Ginkgo biloba
- Ginseng
- Horseradish
- Maca
- Mustard
- Myrrh
- Pine nuts
- Pomegranates
- Pumpkin
- Saffron
- Salmon
- Strawberries
- Valerian
- Vanilla
- Watermelons

## Cherry Chocolate Bars

What better way to make your partner feel loved than homemade chocolates? These happen to be full of aphrodisiacs, too. The toasted quinoa gives these a nice crunch, but feel free to substitute or add other treats, such as dried rose petals, hemp seeds, or sliced almonds.

Makes about ten 1-inch square pieces.

### Ingredients:
¼ cup quinoa, raw
5 tablespoons coconut oil
5 tablespoons unsweetened cocoa powder
1 tablespoon honey
½ cup dried cherries

### Directions:
1. Line a cookie sheet with parchment paper, spread quinoa on it, and bake at 350°F for 6 to 8 minutes. You're toasting the quinoa, so remove as soon as it's golden and well before it's blackened.
2. In a small saucepan, melt the coconut oil over low heat, add cocoa powder and honey, and stir. When fully combined, pour onto another cookie sheet lined with parchment paper.
3. Sprinkle toasted quinoa and dried cherries evenly over the surface. Place in the freezer for at least ten minutes, or until firm. Break into pieces and enjoy immediately or store in a sealed container in the freezer.

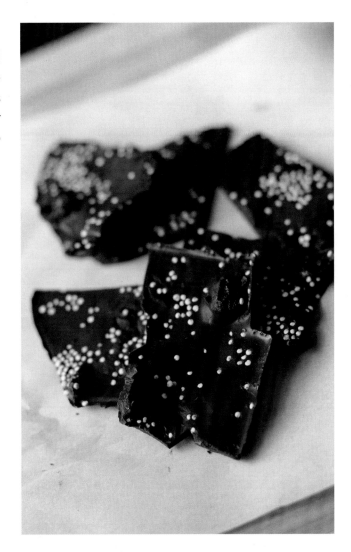

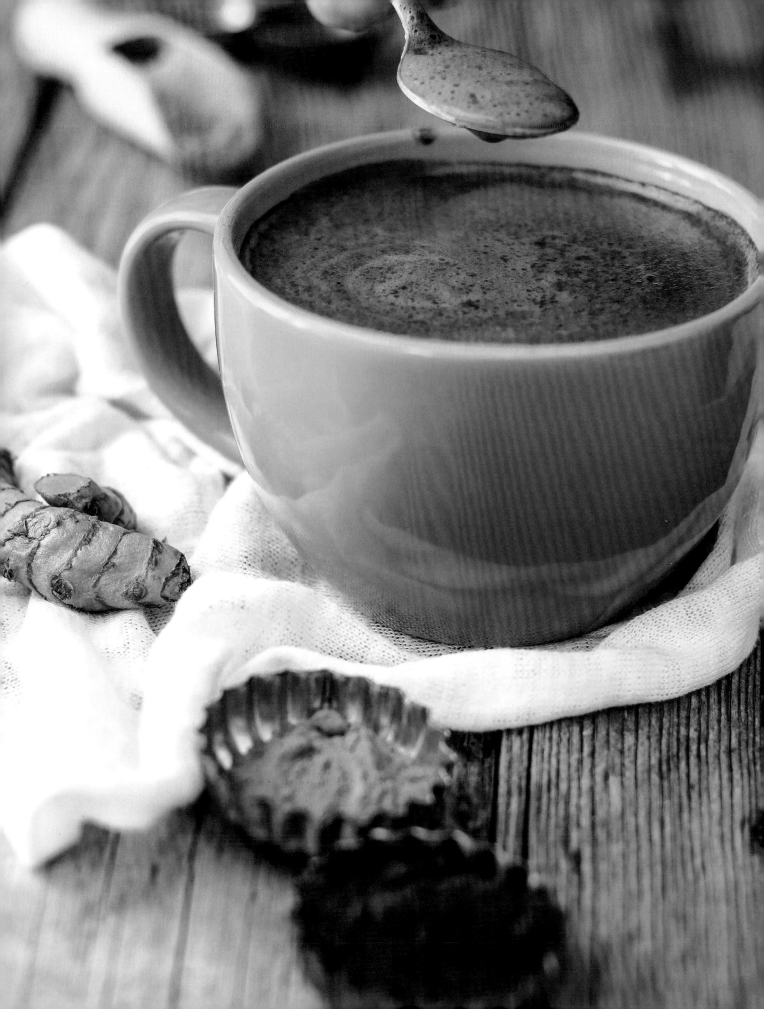

## Maca Hot Chocolate

Maca root powder is considered an adaptogen and is often used to increase sex drive, as well as to boost energy and to balance hormones. This drink is especially good for cold days, or enjoy it iced when the weather calls for it! Double the recipe if you're making a cup for your partner, too.

Makes 1 cup.

### Ingredients:

1 cup unsweetened almond or coconut milk
2 tablespoons unsweetened cocoa powder
2 teaspoons maca powder
⅛ teaspoon cinnamon
Pinch cayenne pepper
Tiny pinch black pepper
⅛ teaspoon turmeric powder
Honey or maple syrup to taste

### Directions:

1. Add all ingredients to a saucepan and heat over medium heat, whisking regularly.
2. Once hot and frothy, pour into a mug and enjoy!

---

### Mustard
*(Brassica nigra)*

Since ancient times, both mustard seeds and plant have been attributed with virility-promoting effects. For this reason monks were forbidden to use mustard. It is often documented that hot mustard baths are recommended to assist and enhance women's libido.

---

### Ginseng
*(Panax ginseng)*

Ginseng is a perennial plant native to northeastern China, eastern Russia, and North Korea; it is now rare in the wild. Ginseng is a true pro-sexual supplement and adaptogen, prized as a sexual enhancer and fertility aid. It can be grated and eaten in soups and salads or dried and powered for use in teas and tablets. The Chinese have revered this plant for thousands of years.

---

## Aphrodisiac Tea

A mildly euphoric tea, this blend gives an overall feel-good sensation and is wonderful for a date night, or just wanting to feel more loving and open.

### Ingredients:

1 part damiana
1 part rose petals
½ part shatavari
½ part orange peel

### Directions:

1. Steep herbs in boiling water for several minutes and then strain, or use a tea ball.

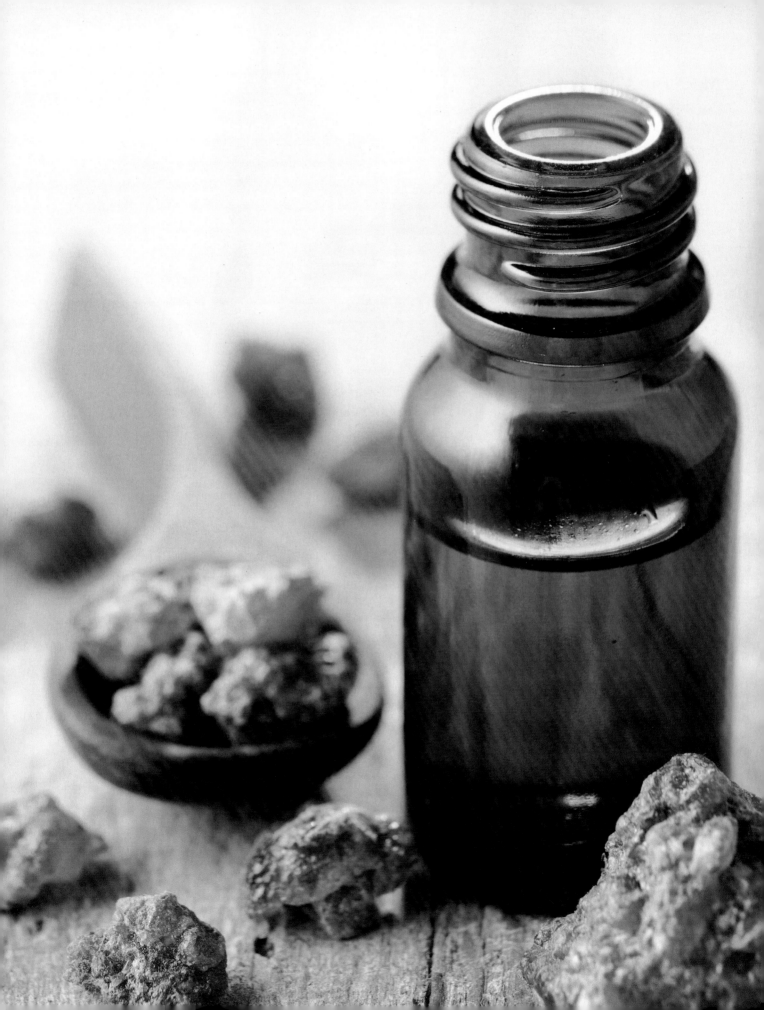

## Romantic Massage Blend

The thought of essential oils can conjure up images of a tent filled with colorful carpets, tapestries, scarves, and pillows; sensual music; and a romantic partner ready to give you a sensuous massage. Essential oils have long been prized as aphrodisiacs, and their ability to both relax and invigorate us make them ideal for use in the bedroom. A romantic massage brings intimacy to a relationship. This is especially important in long-term relationships, where the daily routine can interfere with the romantic bonds that are necessary to maintain a healthy partnership.

When using this romantic massage blend, don't forget to create a romantic mood with more than just essential oils. Light some unscented candles, create a visually appealing space, and get comfortable.

## Ingredients:

sweet almond oil
8 drops ylang-ylang essential oil
4 drops clary sage essential oil
2 drops bergamot essential oil
2 drops sandalwood essential oil

## Preparation:

1. Combine 8 drops ylang-ylang, 4 drops clary sage, 2 drops bergamot, and 2 drops sandalwood essential oils in a 1-ounce (15mL) blue or amber glass bottle.
2. Top with sweet almond oil.
3. Shake to combine ingredients.

## Administration:

A sensual massage is very personal, and individual preferences vary greatly. It is important to listen to your partner's desires and to express your own desires as well. Therefore, instead of step-by-step instructions on giving a massage using the romantic massage blend, this section will include some suggested massage techniques to use with your partner.

## Face massage:

Place a couple drops of the romantic massage blend onto the tips of your fingers. Lay your partner's head in your lap and gently stroke from the tip of the chin along the edge of the face to the forehead. Use the pads of your fingertips to stroke both cheeks. Run your fingers through your partner's hair. Use your thumb and pointer finger to gently rub the earlobe and outside edge of your partner's ears, going up and up and down several times. Use the tip of your ringer finger to gently touch the inner ridges of your partner's ears. Finish by stroking down on the earlobes.

## Back massage:

Straddle your partner's lower back (do not place your weight on your partner) and pour several drops of the massage oil down your partner's spine. Use your flat hands to spread the oil out along your partner's back from the shoulders down to the base of the spine. Draw your fingers up the spine and blow in a circular motion on the back of your partner's neck. Continue the massage by starting at the base of the spine and fanning upward toward the shoulders.

## Upper thighs and buttocks:

Drizzle a few drops of the romantic massage blend onto the back of your partner's thighs and buttocks. Use your pointer and middle fingers to rub the blend into the skin using circular motions. Then use your palms to knead the thighs and buttocks. Finish with a light brushing of the fingertips from the back of the knees up to the buttocks.

## Chest, stomach, and pelvis:

Put a dime-size amount of the romantic massage blend into your palm and rub your hands together. Use circular motions to massage the blend into your partner's chest and abdomen. Reduce the pressure and use a feathery touch to make circular motions on your partner's pelvis.

### Arms and inner thighs:

Place a couple of drops of the romantic massage blend on your fingertips and use a feathery touch to stroke the soft skin of the inner arms and thighs. Apply a little firmer pressure when stroking the tendons in the wrist or if your partner is ticklish. This part of a sensual massage is great for making eye contact.

### Benefits:

- The aromas in this massage stimulate the limbic system, which in turn plays a key role in sexuality.
- Ylang-ylang essential oil has pheromonal properties and has been used as an aphrodisiac by ancient Egyptians including Cleopatra.
- Clary sage is hormone balancing and an antidepressant. This improves your mood in the bedroom. It also has a gentle spasmodic effect on the uterus.
- Bergamot essential oil is a mood stimulator and relieves anxiety. Anxiety is often a barrier to romantic interaction and the addition of bergamot essential oil addresses that.
- Sandalwood essential oil acts as an aphrodisiac by increasing pulse rate, blood flow, and our perception of the attractiveness of others.

### NOTES AND TIPS:

- Due to the sensitive connection between aroma and sexuality, you can adjust the intensity of the aroma in the blend by adjusting the ratio of essential oils to sweet almond oil. For a lighter aroma, include half the number of drops of each essential oil.

### CAUTION:

Bergamot essential oil can cause sun sensitivity. If using this blend before going out, uncovered, into the sun, wash the blend off.

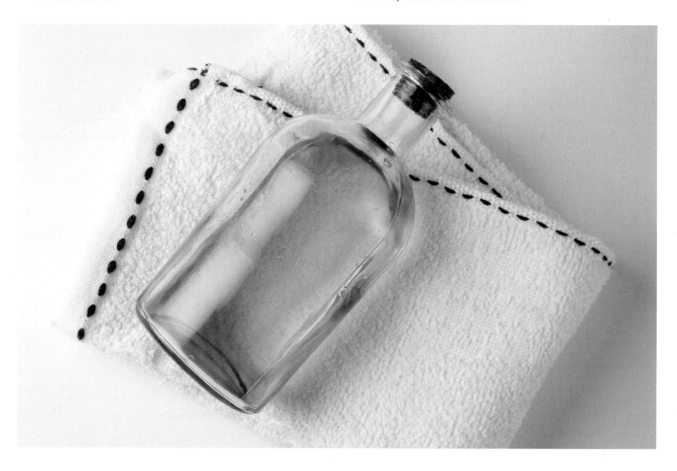

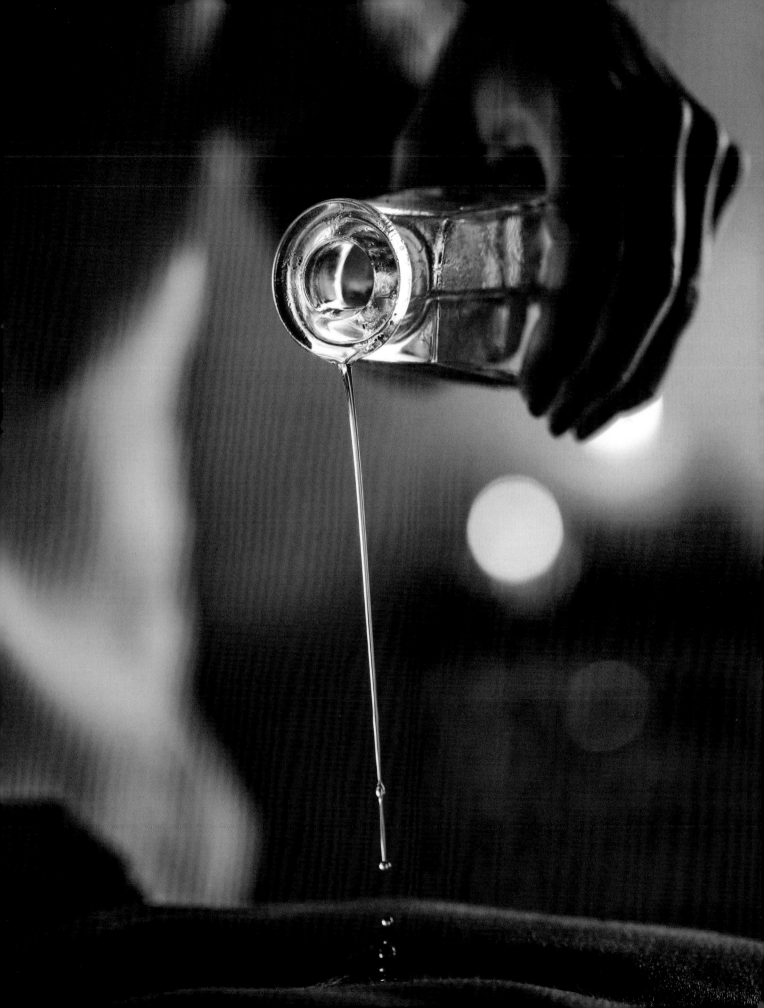

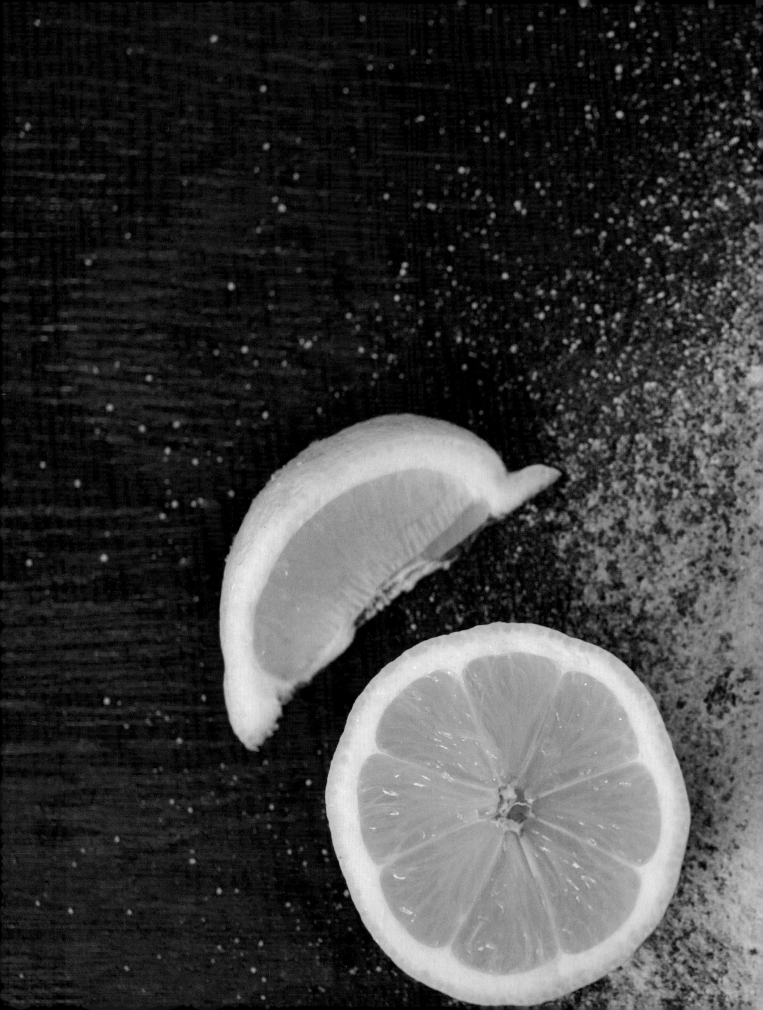

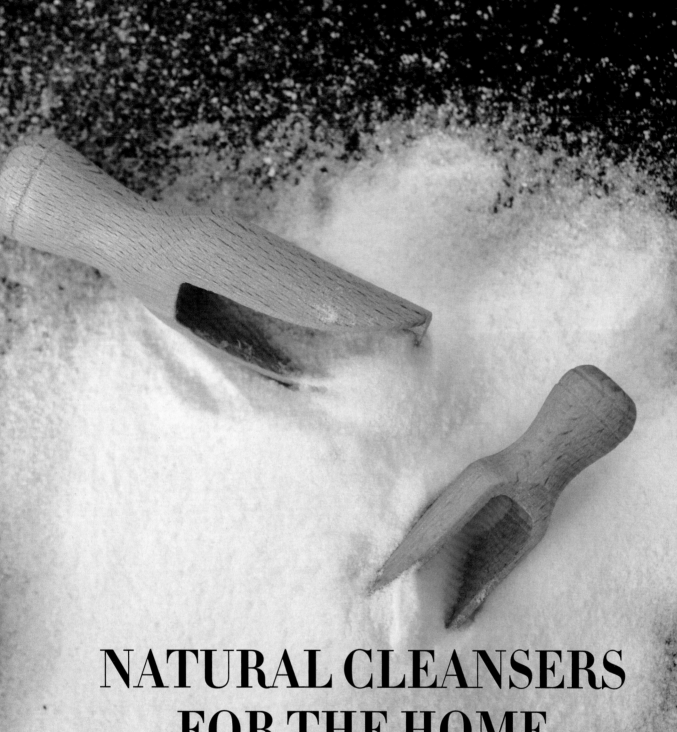

# NATURAL CLEANSERS
# FOR THE HOME

# Houseplants for Clean Air

Houseplants may conjure up thoughts of pleasant decor, added elements of design recommended by your favorite HGTV show, or background noise to an already busy home. The green and colorful flora aren't often thought of as much more than permanent fixtures on your grandmother's kitchen table, or some added kitsch to your neighbor's living room. But how often do you think of your jade plant as a health supplement? When was the last time you thanked your English ivy fern for filtering your air or reducing your stress? Or when did you last look at your philodendron and thank it for helping you concentrate and focus for an exam?

Plants are some of the healthiest additions you could add to your home, and you don't even have to ingest them. The simple act of having plants can help you heal more quickly, sleep better, focus more intently, reduce stress levels, boost the immune system, reduce depression levels, and more. And it's possible to reap these immense health benefits just by having these seemingly innocuous displays of nature sit in your house, doing absolutely nothing but look pretty.

Forget the dreaded agony of waking up at five in the morning to run three miles or the horror of meal planning based on a point system. Health is more than just following strict guidelines that are rare to achieve. Health is the accumulation of all your lifestyle choices, which include the addition of plants to your home.

Do you want to look younger, sleep better, reduce your stress, lower your depression, heal faster, and improve your focus? If you answered yes, there's good news. You can get all these amazing benefits without going to the doctor! In fact, plants are so good for you, if you could bottle

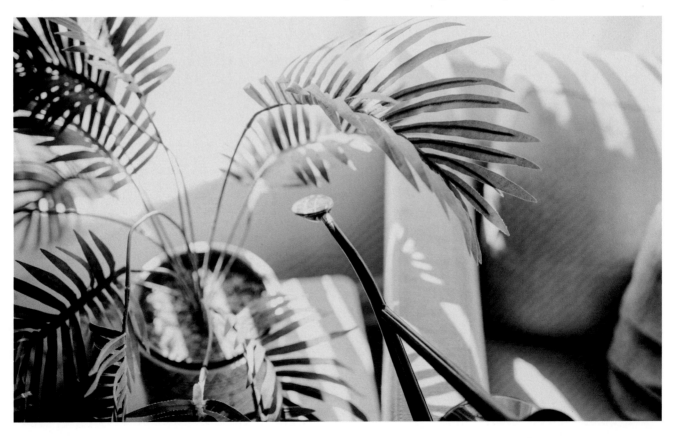

**306 The Illustrated Encyclopedia of Natural Remedies**

up all their amazing benefits into a pill, it would be a billion-dollar blockbuster. The first major benefit you receive from plants is better air. Yes, plants are able to filter contaminants and toxins out of our air, making us healthier and preventing costly long-term illnesses from appearing in the first place.

Humans spend a whopping 90 percent of their lives indoors, mostly in their homes, continually breathing in recycled air. Our cultural allergy to the outdoors is providing us with a unique experience of a myriad of physical reactions to our dirty interiors. The air you breathe inside your home could be a contributing factor to a variety of illnesses, and more damaging than the air in the most polluted cities. From frequent colds to dry skin, chronic cough, eye irritation, and memory lapse, the stagnant particles we call "air" are making us sick. There's even a term for this phenomenon called "sick building syndrome." Very original.

Virtually every home is overrun with a variety of toxic pollutants, including carbon monoxide, hydrocarbons, chemicals in pesticides, paints, cleaners, deodorants, hairsprays, laundry detergents, fireplaces, rugs, clothing, sheets, off-gases from furniture, carpets, glue, and even your air fresheners. **Newsflash: Your ocean breeze–scented air fresheners are in fact synthetic, toxic pollutants, and their smell resembles the interior of your last Uber ride rather than the actual ocean.**

Air quality is pertinent to good health, and if we are continually breathing in pollutants, we're putting ourselves at risk for serious long-term health complications such as asthma, cancer, and other chronic illnesses. While not often talked about, this public health issue is something that needs to be addressed. Luckily, going to your nearest garden center is an easy way to prevent the harms of our indoor lifestyle. A good rule of thumb is to have a clean-air plant for every one hundred square feet of your home.

## The NASA Clean Air Study

Even NASA understood the importance of our leafy friends, conducting a study in 1989 examining their ability to clean and filter the air for space stations, and what they found was impressive. The research demonstrated that common houseplants not only recycle our air, absorbing the carbon dioxide we breathe out while releasing precious oxygen back into our atmosphere, but they also have the ability to filter out carcinogenic chemicals, such as benzene, formaldehyde, trichloroethylene, ammonia, and xylene. But how?

Plants absorb carbon dioxide and also particulates in the air, which are then processed into the life-affirming oxygen we breathe in, but that's not the whole story. There are also microorganisms in the potting soil that are responsible for a big part of this cleaning effect. You heard it, the dirt that we so often avoid touching is the very dirt that is keeping us healthy and saving our lungs from toxic compounds. The leaves, roots, soil, and all the microorganisms of a plant have a part to play in their ability to clean our precious air, and every plant we place inside our airtight homes is another win for our air quality.

One Japanese researcher went as far as to identify how these microbes are affecting our health, and what he found will change the way you look at tree huggers. Forests are more than just trees and dirt; they are an ecosystem filled with airborne antifungal and antibacterial compounds called phytoncides. It seems as though when you inhale these compounds, they boost your white blood cells, especially a type which attacks tumors and viruses. Taking a hike reduces cancer, and not in the way you'd imagine. Forget cardio, bring me more phytoncides! For those of us who don't have regular access to a forest for a daily hike, we can still get the benefits of microbes from our indoor gardens. High five!

So while we're trying to inhale certain microbes and bacteria, what should we be avoiding and what are the top chemicals that our homegrown friends are able to filter away? The following is a list of the most common indoor air pollutants, ones that are easily filtered away by clean-air plants.

## The Most Common Indoor Air Pollutants

**Benzene**: A widely known carcinogen often found in gasoline fumes, cigarettes, and car exhausts, and used in industries related to plastic, oil, gasoline, rubber, and more. What's startling is that benzene is found at high levels in indoor air, which could be from car exhaust, paints, adhesives, and even in your new furniture. The more time you spend indoors could equal the more exposure you have to benzene. The World Health Organization states that exposure to benzene is a major public health concern, citing exposure can lead to cancer and aplastic anemia.

**Formaldehyde**: Another widely known chemical, this colorless, flammable, strong-smelling gas is found in a variety of household products and building materials. Often used in glues; adhesives; wood products such as particleboard, plywood, and fiberboard; and fungicides, germicides, and disinfectants. The Environmental Protection Agency states that formaldehyde can cause short-term irritations of the skin, eyes, nose, and throat, and high levels of exposure may cause some types of cancers.

**Trichloroethylene**: Another chemical commonly used as an industrial solvent. Chronic exposure has been linked to cancer and other chronic illnesses.

**Ammonia**: One of the most widely produced chemicals in the United States, ammonia is actually found in nature and is produced in the human body. Often found in fertilizer and the manufacturing of plastics, explosives, fabrics, pesticides, dyes, and other chemicals, you're most likely exposed to it via your household cleaning solutions. Overexposure to this chemical can cause irritation; burns; eye, nose, and throat irritation; and lung damage.

**Xylene**: Widely used as a chemical solvent, cleaning agent, and paint thinner, xylene has been shown to cause irritation to the mouth and throat, dizziness, headache, confusion, and liver and kidney damage.

Plants may appear docile, but their ability to filter out harmful substances and chemicals from your air proves that their strength is more than meets the eye. According to NASA, some houseplants are better than others at cleaning and filtering our air; below are the ten best plants to add to your polluted home (I'm not judging).

## My Top Ten Favorite Plants to Filter the Air

### Boston Fern

If you're looking for a dependable presence in your life, search no further. The Boston fern is the ultimate houseplant, a favorite of indoor gardeners since the Victorian age. The good old fern ranks number nine in NASA's top fifty air-purifying plants list, and is the most efficient at removing formaldehyde from the air, not to mention its ability to remove other contaminants.

### English Ivy

English ivy is a workhorse when it comes to cleaning your air, filtering out trichloroethylene, formaldehyde, benzene, and xylene. It also amazingly clears out fecal matter from the air, so you're in luck if you have any pets or children! This vine looks beautiful in a hanging pot or around your windowsill, and will make you look way more elegant. This is a great plant for beginners and is easy to take care of. However, be careful if you have pets, as it can cause problems for both dogs and cats.

### Golden Pothos

Also known as Devil's ivy, the golden pothos is one of my favorite houseplants due to its indestructible nature. This plant thrives on neglect, and if you

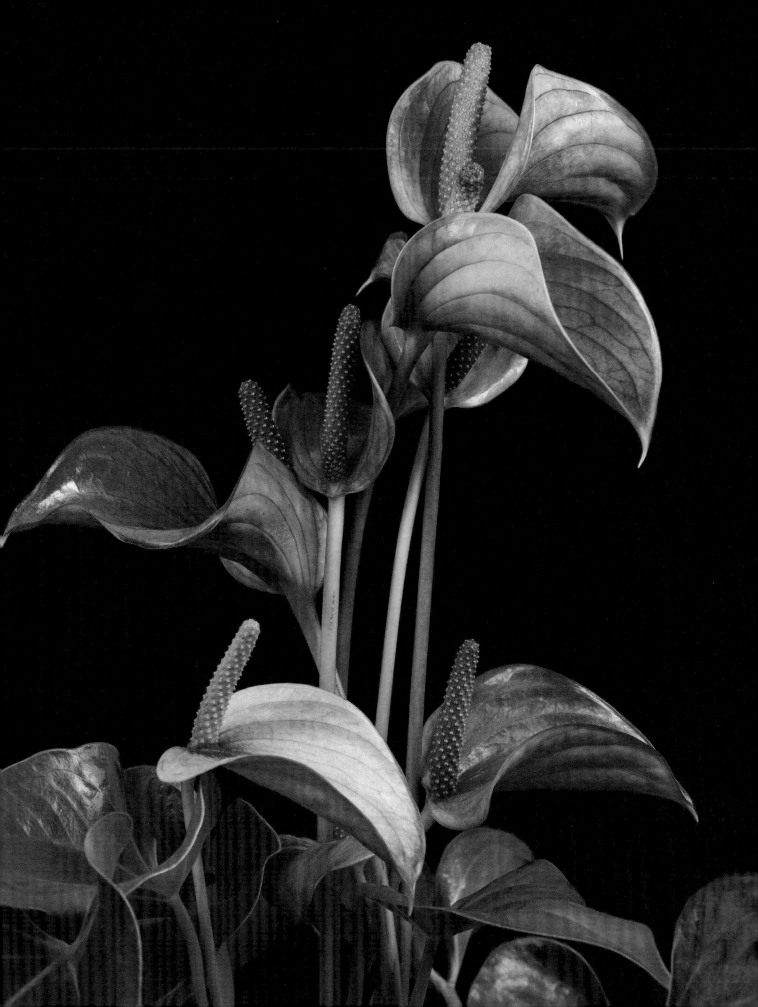

are new to indoor gardening, start with the classic pothos. The golden pothos also does an amazing job of filtering the air of formaldehyde, xylene, toluene, benzene, carbon monoxide, and more.

## Peace Lily

The name alone should make you want to grab one of these plants for your home. What's better is that NASA found the peace lily to be one of the top three plants for removing indoor air toxins, such as ammonia, formaldehyde, and benzene. However, the peace lily is toxic to animals and children. Keep it away from reach, as it can cause skin irritation, burning, and swelling.

## Spider Plant

The ever interesting spider plant will eliminate formaldehyde and xylene from your air and grows very quickly indoors. If you're lucky, it'll even produce beautiful white blossoms. This plant is nontoxic.

## Snake Plant

A classic houseplant often used in offices for its ability to survive in low light or artificial light environments, the snake plant has been found to clean out benzene, formaldehyde, trichloroethylene, and xylene.

## Chinese Evergreen

The Chinese evergreen is one of the most beautiful and unique-looking houseplants around. Native to tropical forests in Asia, these plants can filter out benzene, carbon monoxide, formaldehyde, trichloroethylene, and more! However, this is toxic to dogs, so make sure to keep it out of their reach.

## Flamingo Lily

One of the more unique and beautiful houseplants, the flamingo lily is easy to grow and will thrive for many years on your kitchen table if provided with ideal conditions. It should be kept away from pets, children, or any adult who acts like a child, as it contains calcium oxalate crystals, which can be harmful if chewed. Flamingo lilies been found to filter formaldehyde, ammonia, and xylene.

## Aloe Vera

Not just for your skin anymore! Aloe vera has been found to filter out formaldehyde from the air. Aloe is also very easy to maintain, only requiring watering when the soil is dry. The leaves hold a fluid that is known to be an anti-inflammatory and to possess wound-healing properties!

## Bamboo Palm

An overachiever when it comes to filtering formaldehyde out of the air, the bamboo palm can grow to be as tall as twelve feet high, making it one of the most efficient air filters around. The bamboo palm also removes benzene, as well as trichloroethylene, and is a pet-friendly plant.

With so many options, our air doesn't have to make us sick anymore. It's clear now that we can't live in the vacuum of our tidy, chemical-laden homes. It's not possible to thrive indoors without plants, and in order to live healthy lives, we must bring nature with us. Luckily for us, many plants can thrive indoors with us, helping us breathe cleaner air and making our homes beautiful representations of health and wellness.

# Plants Lower Stress and Depression

Stress is all too common in our contemporary lifestyles. From traffic jams, long and boring commutes, the twenty-four-hour news cycle, and the constant pings of emails and cell phones to the never ending break of social media and the Internet, it's no wonder we're all about to burst a communal blood vessel. Life may be getting more efficient, but it sure isn't getting any easier, or happier. Don't get me wrong, we are living in very exciting times, but *Dancing with the Stars* is not a cure for depression, it's just a distraction from our hectic lives.

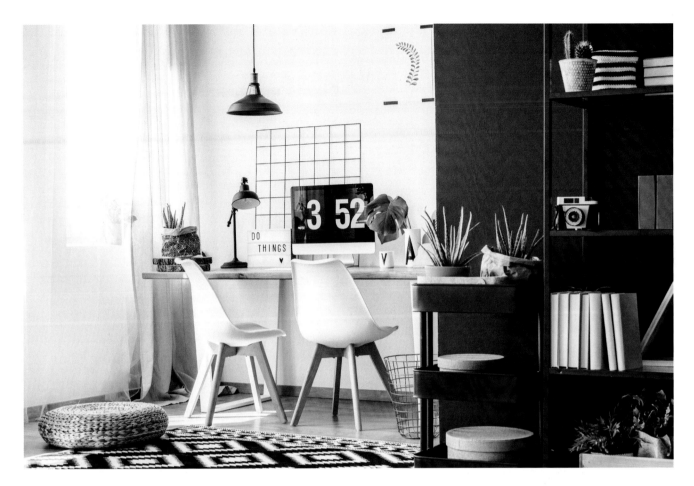

When asked about stress, many people reply with "I'm fine" or "I have no more stress than anyone else!" This is not a good sign. Our criterion of stress should not be how you compare to your next-door neighbor, Joe, who works seventy hours a week and drinks five gin and tonics to unwind. In fact, forget everyone you know because chances are they're all stress balls who don't know the definition of relaxation.

Let's get dramatic for a second: stress is killing you. It's one of the main causes of 60 percent of all human illnesses and disease, such as heart attack, stroke, and heart disease. How is this so? Well, the body can't distinguish between the stress of getting cut off by another BMW on your way to work, or the stress of being chased by a mountain lion. This means your body reacts just as strongly to a seeming annoyance as an actual life-threatening situation.

The problem with this scenario is that these stressful occurrences are happening on a daily basis, constantly pinging your nervous system and flooding your body with hormones meant to be used only in times of actual, dire need. Long-term and chronic exposure to stress disrupts nearly every system of your body, suppressing the immune system, increasing heart rate and blood pressure, contributing to infertility and irritable bowel syndrome (IBS), and even rewiring your brain to be more prone to anxiety and depression.

And stress isn't the only cause of depression. There are many variables that contribute to depression, including genetics, life circumstances, grief, changes in hormone levels, and newer research pointing towards the gut biome and nutrition. According to the National Institute of Mental Health, 16 million adults had at least one major depressive episode in 2012, or around 6.9 percent of the population. And that's reported cases. According to the World Health Organization, more than 350 million people suffer from depression worldwide.

Depression is a huge topic, with many causes and many types; however, it's generally known to suck. This is some stressful news, but there are some remedies to help. With that said, plants have been shown to increase levels of happiness, lower levels of stress, and lower the incidence of depression. The unseen mental benefits of plants is yet another reason to add some greenery to your home and start gardening.

Research from the Norwegian University of Life Sciences and Uppsala University in Sweden found that the mere presence of plants in an office or home increased levels of happiness, reduced stress and fatigue, and reduced the amount of sick leave workers took. Another study found that indoor plants may reduce psychological stress by suppressing the sympathetic nervous system (our fight-or-flight response), making us less stressed and our bodies more relaxed.

Even more research found that when plants are placed in already high-stress work environments, people reported feeling calmer and experienced an increased sense of happiness. Having contact with nature, whether it be indoor plants, increased visibility of nature, or even better access to parks or outdoor spaces, improved health promotion efforts and reduced perceived stress, and general health complaints decreased. Just thirty minutes of walking surrounded by the natural world reduced depression in 71 percent of participants!

In fact, the research keeps pointing back to nature leading to happiness in humans. A 2010 study found that hiking or walking through the forest for two hours per day over a two-day period lowered stress hormone levels, blood pressure, and pulse rate. And science is showing that just being able to see a natural setting with your own two eyes increases your brain's pleasure receptors.

Add a hot tub and some bubbly, and you'll be the happiest you've ever been in your life.

## Plants Increase Focus

While technology is increasing at lightning speeds, our focus is dwindling at the speed of sound. Yes, we carry minicomputers in our back pockets, travel the world via virtual reality, and drive high-performance electric vehicles. However, it seems as though we can't get through a conversation anymore without checking our Instagram, our ability to read a book dwindles in comparison to our Netflix bingeing abilities, and our listening skills only last for approximately 2.1 seconds.

According to a new study from Microsoft, humans now lose focus after eight seconds, one second less than our goldfish competition. Our increased dependence on Google, GPS systems, and everything in between has made us less focused, impatient, and perhaps a little dumber. Since the year 2000, our attention spans have dropped from an average of twelve seconds down to eight, and our minds are constantly waiting for the next bing, click, ping, beep from our phones, emails, and computers. Good luck getting through this book; if you make it to the end, make sure to congratulate yourself!

There's good news, however, for those of us who love plants. We're beginning to understand that the mere presence of plants in our workplace or home environment can drastically change how we think and how we focus. One study published in the *Journal of Environmental Psychology* found that having plants in your workspace can boost your ability to focus and maintain attention. The human mind can stare at boring spreadsheets and Google docs for only so long, and don't get started on expense reports and billing—we can only do so much. Our brains are complicated biocomputers, and we have only a limited capacity for what is known as "directed attention." Directed attention basically means anything we do at work:

controlled, focused, concentrated attention. And of course, it diminishes the more we use it in a day. No wonder Google has Ping-Pong tables and nap pods at its workplace!

With this in mind, when we engage with nature, walk in a park, or look at plants in our office, our mind is able to continually draw its attention to something new—a leaf, a blade of grass, a bird pooping on a stranger. Your senses are continually being engaged, capturing your attention over and over again. This second kind of attention is known as "undirected attention." Undirected attention allows us to rest our directed minds and rejuvenate for the next round of intense, directed thinking. Plants are some of the most effective ways to bring forward our undirected minds, thus leading us to a more focused work day.

Other studies have looked specifically at plants in the workplace, comparing sparse desks with those decorated with your average fern or snake plant. What they found was that people who sat at a desk with flowers and plants were better at paying attention to a task than those sitting at an empty, lonely desk. The restorative breaks that plants give us should not be underestimated. Imagine a world where every classroom was a mini jungle and every office resembled a beautiful forest. These oases would provide us with the ability to work more diligently, learn more intently, and happily focus on our next task.

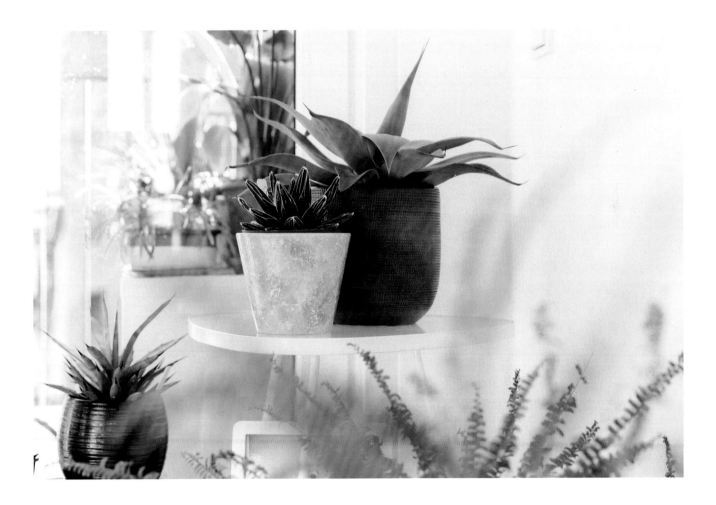

# Kitchen and Bathroom Cleaning

## All-Purpose Cleaner

Keeping your home clean is key in staying healthy, but most commercially available cleaning products are full of unhealthy ingredients. Natural cleaning solutions are generally safer for us and our families. When making your own cleaning products, you want ingredients that are simple and effective. This all-purpose cleaner is perfect for counter surfaces, floors, walls, and even toilets, sinks, and tubs. The best part about this cleaner, though, is that you can invite your children to clean with you. The essential oils contained in this recipe are safe for children ages two and older. You don't want them to drink it, of course, but spraying this while they help you clean won't irritate their little lungs like traditional cleaners will.

### Ingredients:

½ cup white vinegar

1½ cup water

1 teaspoon borax

10 drops lemon essential oil

5 drops melaleuca essential oil

5 drops lime essential oil

5 drops lemongrass essential oil

5 drops white fir essential oil

### Preparation:

1. Use a metal funnel to combine all ingredients in 16-ounce blue or amber glass bottle.
2. Screw on a spray nozzle top.
3. Shake to mix ingredients thoroughly.

### Administration:

1. Spray directly on the surface you wish to clean.
2. Use a cloth or natural sponge to scrub area and wipe clean.

### Benefits:

- Vinegar is often used alone as an effective natural disinfectant.
- Borax reduces mold growth in both hard and porous surfaces. This is especially important when cleaning in the bathroom and kitchen.
- Lemon, lemongrass, and melaleuca essential oils are all effective antimicrobials against multiple strains of staph, strep, and candida.
- Lemongrass is particularly effective against listeria strains.
- Citrus oils (including lemon and lime) contain limonene, which has a wide range of antimicrobial properties. These oils disinfect against food-related microorganisms, and have insecticidal properties as well. White fir essential oil also contains limonene.

### Notes and Tips:

- To increase the longevity of this cleaner, store it in a cool, dark place or even in the refrigerator.
- If this spray gets in your or your child's eyes and is irritating, rinse with a carrier oil such as olive oil, sweet almond oil, or coconut oil. Do not rinse with water.

## Sanitizing Counter Spray

Kitchen counters are one of the dirtiest places in our homes, even if they look clean. Foodborne pathogens are not visible to the naked eye, and small splatters from uncooked meats and eggs, dairy products, and even fruits and vegetables can harbor harmful bacteria, viruses, and fungi. A safe cooking surface is paramount to serving healthy foods. The problem with most commercial cleaners for the kitchen is that they aren't safe to be used around food and definitely are not safe for ingestion. Warning labels tell you to make sure to clean any surfaces that will come in contact with food again after cleaning with those products. This kitchen counter spray is safe for cleaning your counters and for keeping your counter microbe free after you use it. Lemongrass and oregano essential oils are highly antimicrobial without damaging your lungs or skin. This spray leaves your kitchen smelling fresh and ready to use.

### Ingredients:
½ cup white vinegar
1½ cup water
1 teaspoon borax (optional)
25 drops lemongrass essential oil
15 drop oregano essential oil

### Preparation:
1. Use a metal funnel to combine all ingredients in 16-ounce blue or amber glass bottle.
2. Screw on a spray nozzle top.
3. Shake to mix ingredients thoroughly.

### Administration:
1. Spray directly onto your kitchen counter, refrigerator, or stove surfaces.
2. Use a cloth or natural sponge to scrub area and wipe clean.

3. If you do not include the borax, use the misting setting on the spray bottle nozzle to spray a fine mist over your countertops to protect the surfaces from contamination before you use them.

### Benefits:
- Both lemongrass and oregano essentials are highly effective against bacteria, viruses, and fungi including—but definitely not limited to—multiple strains of listeria (a common foodborne bacteria), *Escherichia coli*, *Salmonella enterica*, *Klebsiella pneumoniae*, *Acinetobacter baumannii*, *Pseudomonas aeruginosa*, *Enterococcus faecalis*, *Serratia marcescens*, *Staphylococcus aureus*, and *Candida albicans*. Many of the microbes inhibited by lemongrass and oregano essential oils have become drug-resistant, but not resistant to essential oils.
- Lemongrass essential oil is one of the strongest antifungal essential oils.

### NOTES AND TIPS:
- CAUTION: Oregano essential oil is not recommended for topical use in children under the age of six. It is safe to use this spray in areas where children will be, but it is not safe to let young children use this spray to clean.
- If you do not have oregano essential oil, or want to add a festive touch to your counter spray, you can substitute cinnamon essential oil for the oregano.
- Borax is not safe for ingestion in large doses, but is not harmful in the amount included in this spray. However, do not use borax in this recipe if food will come in contact with this spray.

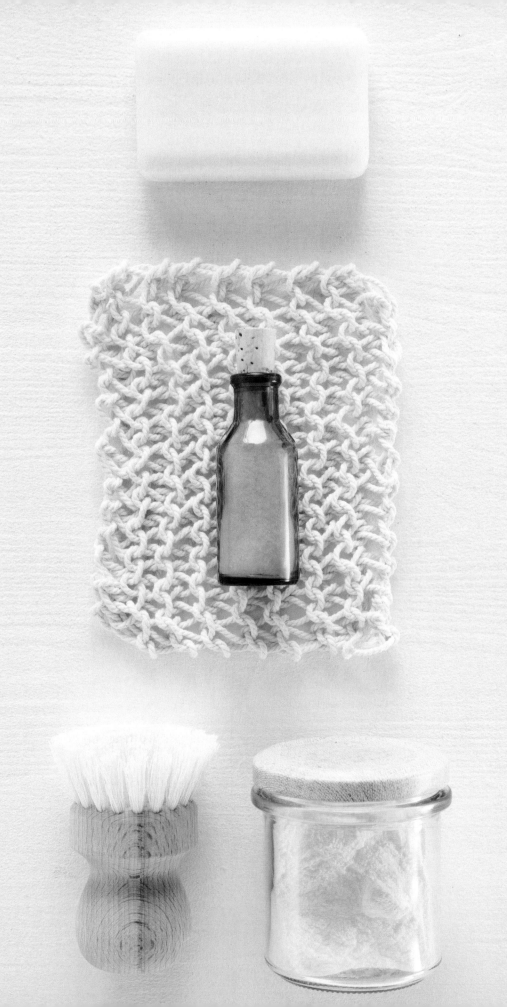

# Citrus-Fir Dish Soap

Properly washing dishes is an important part of preventing foodborne pathogens from contaminating our cooked food. This is especially true when washing cutting boards and other food prep materials. Essential oils are effective against many of the microbes that are carried in raw meats and unwashed fruits and vegetables. This dish soap cleans your dishes, kills microbes, and leaves your kitchen smelling pristine and uplifting.

## Ingredients:

1 cup boiling water
¼ cup grated bar soap
¼ cup unscented liquid castile soap
1 tablespoon washing soda (optional)
10 drops lemon essential oil
10 drops lemongrass essential oil
5 drops lime essential oil
5 drops white fir essential oil

## Preparation:

1. Bring 1 cup water to a boil.
2. Turn off heat and add ¼ cup grated bar soap.
3. Stir until bar soap is melted into the water.
4. Add ¼ cup unscented liquid castile soap.
5. Stir in 1 tablespoon washing soda (optional).
6. Use a funnel to pour the mixture into a 16-ounce blue or amber glass bottle
7. Allow to cool.
8. Add 10 drops lemon, 10 drops lemongrass, 5 drops lime, and 5 drops white fir essential oils.
9. Cap with a pump top.
10. Shake well.

## Administration:

1. Shake before using.
2. Wet dishes.
3. Pump out desired amount of Citrus-Fir Dish Soap onto a natural sponge.
4. Scrub dishes to remove food build up and grease.
5. Rinse dishes with hot water.
6. Air dry dishes in a dish rack or hand dry with a towel.

## Benefits:

- Lemongrass essential oil is highly effective against bacteria, viruses, and fungi including multiple strains of listeria (a common foodborne bacteria), *Escherichia coli, Salmonella enterica, Klebsiella pneumoniae, Acinetobacter baumannii, Pseudomonas aeruginosa, Enterococcus faecalis, Serratia marcescens, Staphylococcus aureus,* and *Candida albicans.*
- Lemon essential oil works both as a cleanser and a degreaser.
- Lemon, lime, and white fir essential oils contain limonene, which has a wide range of antimicrobial properties, especially against foodborne pathogens.

## NOTES AND TIPS:

- This dish soap is safe to use with children ages two and up who want to help out with washing the dishes. If you find that it irritates their skin, reduce the amount of lemon and lemongrass essential oils in the recipe to 5 drops each.
- In colder months, use less washing soda or replace the washing soda with baking soda to prevent clogging of the dish soap pump.

## Gunk- and Grease-Removing Spray

Oily gunk and grime can build up on kitchen surfaces quite quickly. Counter, stoves, ovens, stove hoods, refrigerators, floors, and even walls end up with splatter from cooking or mysterious sticky spots from who knows what. Soap and water, or even kitchen sprays, are hard pressed to remove all this residue. Surprisingly, the best solution is more oil! The slickness of olive oil, combined with the degreasing powers of lemon and eucalyptus essential oils, whisk away the gunk and grease that was so hard to get rid of before.

### Ingredients:
⅓ cup olive oil
8 drops lemon essential oil
6 drops eucalyptus essential oil

### Preparation:
1. Use a funnel to pour ⅓ cup olive oil into a 4-ounce blue or amber spray bottle.
2. Add 8 drops lemon and 6 drops eucalyptus essential oils.
3. Apply spray cap and shake well.

### Administration:
1. Shake before using.
2. Spray the Gunk- and Grease-Removing Spray directly on any sticky, greasy, or gunky surfaces that need to be cleaned.
3. Allow to set for a few minutes and then use a cloth or natural sponge to remove spray and gunk from the soiled surface.

### Benefits:
- Limonene, found in lemon and other citrus essential oils, works as a solvent and degreaser.
- The cineole in eucalyptus oil has industrial-strength grease solvent properties.

### NOTES AND TIPS:
- This spray can also be used to remove grease from hands.
- Store the Gunk- and Grease-Removing Spray in a cool, dry, and dark place to prevent the combination of oils from losing their efficacy or going rancid.
- This spray is not intended for wood, carpet, or fabric surfaces.

## Looking Good Enough to Eat Fruit and Veggie Cleaner

Even when we purchase organic fruits and vegetables, they are still coated with food wax, transported, handled by picky customers, and have most likely acquired mold spores and germs along the way. It makes good sense to rinse them clean in this mixture before storing and eating. All but the softest of berries (raspberries) can be cleaned using this method.

### Ingredients:
½ cup vinegar
2½ cups water
A few drops of grapefruit seed extract, optional

### Directions:
1. Mix together in a medium-size bowl. Place this mixture in a clean basin in your sink and add your fruit or vegetables. Do all of your soft fruits in one batch, your hard fruits in another, and your vegetables in a third. Dry fruits and vegetables thoroughly using soft cloth or paper towels before storing, and throw a small cloth rag or paper towel in the container with them to absorb the moisture that escapes from the fruit and makes them go soft.

**Extra Tip:** You can also place fruits and vegetables inside pillowcases or specially made small fabric bags to store them. Just be sure to wash the bags regularly, too.

# Bathroom Scrub

Cleaning ourselves leads to having to clean our bathrooms regularly. Toilets, sinks, showers, and tubs get dirty from dust, water stains, beauty products, and even just daily use. Getting to these areas clean takes some elbow grease and a great cleaning product. Many commercial products are harsh on our lungs and leave us needing to shower to get them off our skin. This bathroom scrub is tough on dirt and stains, but gentle on your lungs and skin. It's even safe for children over the age of two to use when helping out with household cleaning.

## Ingredients:
1 cup baking soda
1 cup witch hazel
8 drops lemon essential oil
6 drops geranium essential oil
6 drops melaleuca essential oil
4 drops orange essential oil
2 drops lemongrass essential oil

## Preparation:
1. Pour 1 cup witch hazel into a 16-ounce wide-mouthed blue or amber bottle.
2. Add 8 drops lemon, 6 drops geranium, 6 drops melaleuca, 4 drops orange, and 2 drops lemongrass essential oils.
3. Swirl to combine.
4. Use a funnel to add 1 cup baking soda.
5. Cap with a powder-releasing cap.
6. Shake well to combine ingredients.

## Administration:
1. Shake well before use.
2. Open the holes side of the powder-releasing cap.
3. Sprinkle the Bathroom Scrub over the area you desire to clean.
4. Use a scrub brush or sponge to clean the area.
5. Rinse with water.

## Benefits:
- Baking soda has long been used as a household cleaner. It gets rid of odors and acts as an abrasive to make scrubbing easier.
- Lemon essential oil cuts oily buildup that can occur from using bath and beauty products.
- Geranium, melaleuca, and lemongrass essential oils all deter fungal infections including athlete's foot. Making sure your shower/tub is free of this fungus is an important part of keeping your feet clean and healthy.

All the essential oils in this recipe are cleansing and antimicrobial.

# Lemongrass-Peppermint Toilet Drops

When we use the restroom at home or as a guest, we don't want to leave unpleasant odors. Wouldn't it be great if the bathroom smelled better after we used it than it did before? Well, it's quite simple to achieve, actually. Simply use the Lemongrass-Peppermint Toilet drops before and after using the bathroom and leave the room smelling lovely.

## Ingredients:

30 drops lemongrass essential oil
25 drops peppermint essential oil
10 drops geranium essential oil
5 drops basil essential oil

## Preparation:

1. In a 5mL blue or amber vial, combine 30 drops lemongrass, 25 drops peppermint, 10 drops geranium, and 5 drops basil essential oils.
2. Place an orifice reducer in the mouth of the vial.
3. Apply a tight-fitting cap.
4. Shake well.

## Administration:

1. Shake before use.
2. Before defecating in a toilet, add 3 drops of the Lemongrass-Peppermint Toilet Drops onto the surface of the toilet water.
3. Use the toilet.
4. Flush the toilet.
5. Add 3 more drops of the Lemongrass-Peppermint Toilet Drops to the surface of the toilet water and leave there until the toilet is used again.

## Benefits:

- Geranium essential oil is effective against airborne bacteria.
- Toilet smells can come from contagious gut bacteria, viruses, and parasites. Lemongrass and basil essential oils protect against the spread of these microbes.
- Lemongrass essential oil is particularly hearty at getting rid of stinky toilet smells.
- The combination of peppermint and lemongrass essential oils leaves behind a pleasant aroma.

## NOTES AND TIPS:

- Essential oils are hydrophobic so they stay on top of the toilet water's surface. This traps unpleasant odors underneath the essential oils.
- If stored in a cool, dark, and dry location, the Peppermint-Lemongrass Toilet drops can be stored for up to a year.

## Air-Freshening Diffuser Blend

There are a lot of reasons why your house—and especially your bathroom—might not smell so fresh. Funky smells can be caused by simply using the bathroom for its intended use, laundry that may be piling up, or even just having a teenager living in your house. Instead of just masking the odors with air sprays that aren't particularly good for your lungs, use the Air-Freshening Diffuser Blend to rid your bathroom—or other rooms!—of the sources of those odors.

### Ingredients:

½ cup water
5 drops lemon essential oil
5 drops lime essential oil
2 drops melaleuca essential oil
2 drops lemongrass essential oil

### Preparation:

1. Pour ½ cup water (or amount recommended for your particular diffuser) into your diffuser.
2. Add 5 drops each of lemon and lime essential oils.
3. Add 2 drops each of melaleuca and lemongrass essential oils.

### Administration:

1. Place your diffuser on a flat surface near a plug in your bathroom.
2. Turn on the diffuser.

### Benefits:

- Lemon and lime essential oils cleanse the air.
- Melaleuca and lemongrass essential oils get rid of mold and fungi that may be spreading through the air and causing unpleasant odors.
- Lemongrass essential oil stamps out toilet-related odors.

### NOTES AND TIPS:

- Note that some essential oils are not safe to diffuse around small children or pets. Melaleuca, for example, is harmful to dogs.
- This blend can be used anywhere in the house that needs some freshening up.
- If you don't have a diffuser, you can add this blend (minus the water) to ½ a cup of baking soda in a 4-ounce mason jar. Just cover with a circle of fabric to create a simple jar air freshener.

# Sparkling Glass Cleaner

Mirrors and glass surface can get just as gunky as countertops, but cleaning them can be a little bit harder. With glass, you have to be careful not to use regular oils that might leave streaking, which water can leave, too. Vinegar and essential oils are the perfect alternative solution due to quick evaporation, leaving your glass surfaces sparkling.

## Ingredients:

1½ cups white vinegar
½ cup water
6 drops bergamot essential oil
6 drops lemon essential oil
6 drops orange essential oil

## Preparation:

1. Use a funnel to pour 1½ cups white vinegar and ½ cup water into a 16-ounce blue of amber spray bottle.
2. Add 6 drops each of bergamot, lemon, and orange essential oils.
3. Cap with a spray nozzle.
4. Shake well to combine.

## Administration:

1. Shake before use.
2. Spray the Sparkling Glass Cleaner onto any glass surface or mirror.
3. Wipe the area you want to clean with a lint-free towel.
4. Allow to air dry.

## Benefits:

- Citrus essential oils—including lemon, bergamot, and orange—are excellent degreasers and cleansers.
- Vinegar cleans glass with a streak-free finish.

## NOTES AND TIPS:

- Spray this over the Bathroom Scrub to remove hard-water stains.
- This spray is safe for children over the age of two, who like to help with the chores—or are supposed to help with the chores!

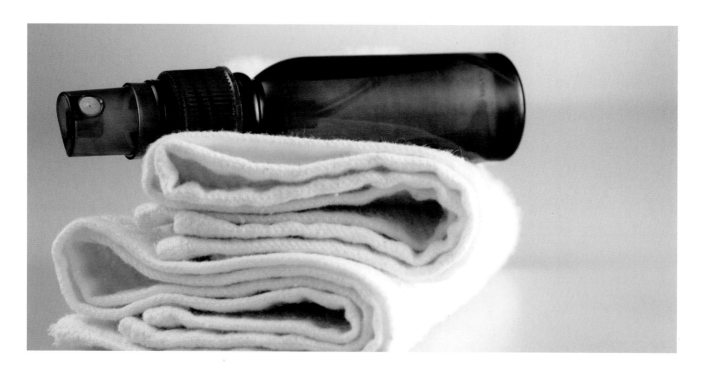

# Laundry Room

## Laundry Detergent

Making your own laundry detergent saves money and allows you to avoid the chemicals found in many commercial detergents. Dr. Bronner's bar soaps come in 5-ounce bars and Fels-Naptha bars are 5.5 ounces, so just use the whole bar—a little more or less will not make a noticeable difference in this recipe. All these ingredients can easily be purchased online.

### Ingredients:

1 (5- or 5.5-oz) bar soap (Dr. Bronner's or
    Fels-Naptha is ideal)
1 cup borax
1 cup washing soda
20 drops lavender, lemon, jasmine, or geranium
    essential oil (optional)

### Directions:

1. Grate the soap in a food processor. Then switch to the blade attachment, add borax, washing soda, and essential oil (if using) and process until it becomes a fine powder. Store in a covered container and use 1 to 2 tablespoons of detergent per load of wash.

## Reusable Dryer Sheets

Commercial dryer sheets are laden with chemicals, some of which (like alpha-terpineol and linalool) may cause nervous system disorders or are carcinogenic. So make your own reusable ones! The vinegar will help to soften the clothes and reduce static, and the essential oil will leave your laundry smelling however you want it to. Try using lavender, tea tree, or jasmine essential oil.

### Ingredients:

Cotton fabric
½ cup white vinegar, ideally organic
8 to 10 drops essential oil

### Directions:

1. Cut the fabric into four to six squares, each about 4 inches by 4 inches. Use pinking shears to help prevent fraying, or hem the edges if you're feeling ambitious. Or just don't worry about it—it's not that big a deal if your dryer sheets start to fray after a few loads. Combine the vinegar and essential oil in a glass jar with a tight-fitting lid. Place the fabric pieces inside, screw on the lid, and give the jar a shake. To use, take the squares out of the container, wring them out gently, and throw them in the dryer with your clothes. After the dryer is done, place the pieces back in the jar with the liquid until you're ready to do the next load.

## Stain Removal Cheat Sheet

While the all-purpose stain removal will work for most spots, sometimes you have something specific that you want to get out right away. Here are some of the most common stains, along with quick, natural ways to remedy them.

**Blood:** Douse with hydrogen peroxide if you catch the spot right away, then rinse thoroughly, rubbing the fabric against itself. It should disappear. If not, soak a cotton ball in hydrogen peroxide and place it on the spot for about a minute. Then rinse well to avoid bleaching the garment. Always use cold water when rinsing blood; hot water will set the stain.

**Grass:** Douse with undiluted rubbing alcohol. Let sit for 10 minutes, then wash as usual.

**Red wine:** Use white wine to quickly saturate the stain. Rinse well. Follow with seltzer water if there is still some left.

**Coffee/tea:** If the coffee or tea is black, you can use cold water and blotting to remove much of the stain. If it contained cream or sugar, you'll need to use some vinegar to help break down the proteins. Saturate the spot with vinegar, let sit for 10 minutes, then rinse with cold water.

**Ink/marker/highlighter:** Douse with undiluted rubbing alcohol. Let sit for 10 minutes, then wash as usual.

**Chocolate:** Let dry if it is solid chocolate that melted. Use a butter knife to scrape off the melted chocolate, then douse the stain with rubbing alcohol.

Ketchup/barbecue sauce: Cold water or cold seltzer water. Rinse immediately and gently rub the fabric against itself to get out any stubborn bits. Blot with vinegar if it hasn't completely come out.

**Grease/oil stains:** Rub a stick of white chalk over the stain to absorb it. Or, coat the spot liberally with cornstarch. Then hand-wash the spot with a bit of your regular shampoo (it's designed to get oil out of your hair, and it works great on clothing fibers, too).

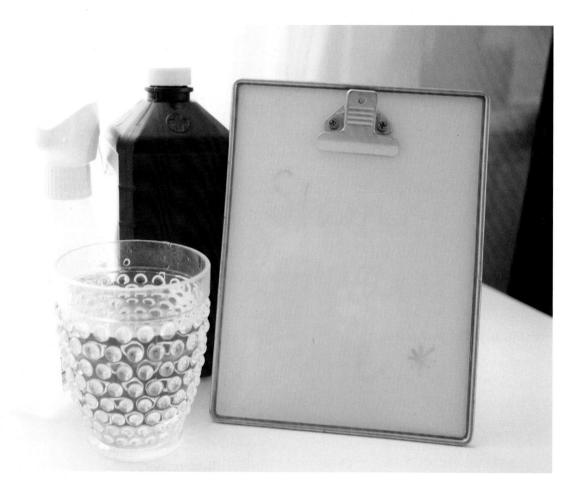

# Pet Care

## Pet Leash and Collar Wash

The grime that accumulates in pet leashes and collars, and how quickly it accumulates, is astonishing. Leashes and collars are not inexpensive, and chances are you've chosen one that suits your dog's personality, your home's color scheme, or for some other important reason (such as the kids absolutely insisted on a certain cartoon character—themed leash and you purchased it to bribe them to take the dog out more often). Keeping them clean and fresh is a simple prospect. Just be sure to do this at night when you don't need them, and that your dog is safe without a collar, or keep a backup collar on hand for cleaning the regular one. The leash should be dry enough to use by the morning.

### Ingredients:
1 teaspoon castile soap
2 tablespoons baking soda
2 cups hot water

### Directions:
1. Mix the ingredients in a basin and add the collar and leashes.
2. Let soak for 30–45 minutes to soften the grime and get into the fibers.
3. Use a clean toothbrush to scour the tough fibers and get around the buckles and hardware. Rinse well.
4. Let dry flat on a clean towel in a warm place but not in front of a heating source.

**Extra Tip**: You can give your leash and collar an extra vinegar rinse if you'd like for additional cleaning power. But you don't want to add the vinegar to the soaking mixture since it breaks down the soap and you lose that cleaning agent.

## Pretty & Peppy Puppy Pet Shampoo

Pet shampoos are expensive, and unless your pet has severe allergic reactions to skin products, this soap should work wonders. Your puppy will be pretty and peppy in no time. Not only does it lather well and get deep dirt out, it doesn't strip the natural oils of your dog's coat thanks to the glycerin. Tea tree oil soothes itchy or inflamed skin, which will help any minor irritations your dog's skin may have from scratching. Peppermint oil is cooling and refreshing, giving the peppiness to the name, along with having a pleasant scent. Use good judgment in using essential oils with your pets; most dogs respond well to them when properly diluted, but keep them away from strong doses or open bottles.

### Ingredients:
2 cups castile soap
½ cup distilled water
2 tablespoons glycerin
3 drops tea tree oil
3 drops peppermint oil

### Directions:
1. Mix all ingredients well in a 16- or 18-ounce container. Shake well to combine.
2. To Use: Use as you would regular shampoo, being sure to keep it out of your dog's eyes.

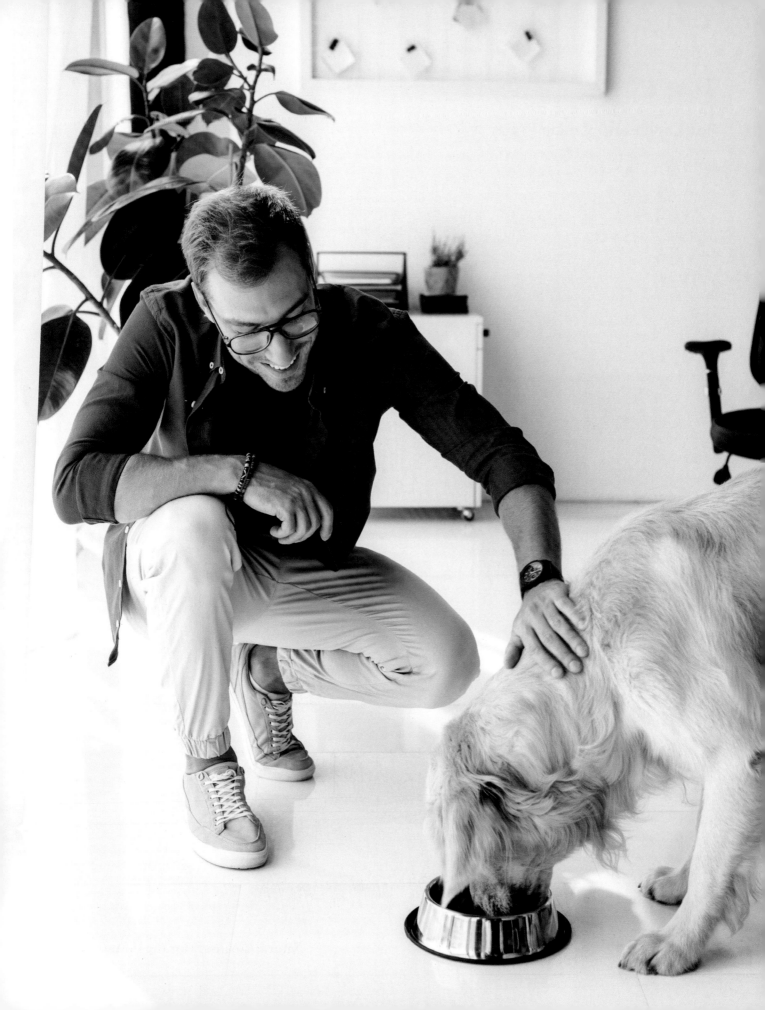

## Dog Perfume & Coat Conditioner

This might sound silly, but one of my favorite memories as a kid was when our golden retriever came back from the groomers'. He was soft, silky, fluffy . . . and he always smelled so good! We didn't know what it was until one day we asked, and found out the groomers used a special aerosol spray for dogs; basically, perfume for your dog. Laugh now, but when you spray your dog with this after they've dried from the shower and brush it in, they'll smell so wonderful you'll think I'm a genius (and our groomers were, too). Use good judgment in using essential oils with your pets; most dogs respond well to them when properly diluted, but keep them away from strong doses or open bottles. (This does not work for cats, in case you were wondering; cats are much more sensitive to essential oils and don't like citrus scents, either.)

### Ingredients:
1 cup distilled or boiled and cooled water
¼ cup jojoba oil
1 teaspoon glycerin
3 drops tangerine essential oil
3 drops geranium essential oil

### Directions:
1. Mix ingredients well in a 12-ounce spray bottle. Shake before use.
2. To Use: Spray liberally onto your dog's coat and brush in well.

## Pet Spot and Odor Remover

We've all been there, with pet spots here and there, whether they're from a new puppy, a sick cat, or a geriatric pet. This method of cleaning soaks up the odor as well as the mess and works on carpets, hardwoods, and laminate floors. However, it must be used immediately on pet stains or within 24 hours. With set accidents that have been on the carpet more than 24 hours it is nearly impossible to prevent staining. The pH level of pet urine can remove dye from carpet or, if it is white, stain it, leaving a permanent mark. Test the spray on dark-colored carpets and rugs in an inconspicuous spot first; the hydrogen peroxide may remove dyes if they aren't colorfast. The tea tree oil is naturally antibacterial, and further neutralizes odors so pets don't come back to the same spot, as they're apt to do.

If there is liquid, sprinkle it liberally with baking soda to soak up the liquid and the odor. Do not use baking soda if there is no liquid. Once it has soaked up the liquid, use a stiff brush to brush up the baking soda into a dustpan. Discard. Scoop up and discard any solids.

### Ingredients:
½ cup hydrogen peroxide
½ cup distilled or boiled and cooled water
½ teaspoon castile soap
4–5 drops tea tree oil

### Directions:
1. Mix ingredients together well in a 12- or 16-ounce spray bottle. Shake before use.
2. To Use: Shake well and spray liberally on the soiled area to fully saturate. Let sit for 2–3 minutes if your carpet is beige or white; clean immediately if it is a darker color. Use a clean rag to blot and press in the stain. Do not rub. Blot and press until it is dried and the mess is gone. Then saturate the area with plain water again and blot and press the water up for a final rinse. Dry gently with a hair dryer on warm (not hot, which may melt the glues that attach the carpet fibers) and use a clean brush to fluff the fibers as you dry the area.

## Pet Bowl Cleaner

Pet bowls tend to get a layer of buildup inside them at the water level due to hard water and lime deposits. These stick right to plastic bowls, and can even show up on metal bowls. But we know what cuts through hard-water deposits, of course . . . vinegar. The best news is vinegar is also pet-safe. We won't use any essential oils because they aren't necessary and also must be used with extreme care when used internally for dogs.

### Ingredients:
1 cup vinegar
½ cup hot water
¼ cup baking soda

### Directions:
1. Mix the three ingredients together in the food dish. Let sit for 30 minutes to 1 hour, depending on how difficult the water stains are.
2. Use a toothbrush or textured rag to work the mixture into any trouble spots. Discard the solution.
3. Wash well in hot, soapy water, and dry thoroughly.

**Extra Tip**: If the bottom of the food dish also has issues (such as mold from water getting under it), double the recipe below, and add the bowl and the solution to a basin where the entire dish can be covered.

## Litter Box Cleaner

Cleaning the litter in the litter box daily is enough of a chore it seems, but keeping the litter box itself clean is another necessary evil for kitty owners. This is a dirty job, there's no way around it. Bring the litter box outside if you can or to a basement or laundry sink. If all else fails, you can do this in the bathtub, so long as you give the bathtub a full cleaning afterward. It's important to use gloves because coming into contact with kitty poo can cause a serious illness called toxoplasmosis. This job should also be avoided if you're pregnant; pass it along to someone else! Cats can be sensitive to smells, so it's best to use the unscented castile soap here. Of course, empty the litter box completely first, and bring all of the pieces if your box has more than one component.

### Ingredients:
2 tablespoons castile soap
8 cups hot water

### Directions:
1. Mix these ingredients in a bucket and bring it outdoors to your workspace, along with your gloves and a sponge that will only be used for this purpose.
2. Fill the basin of the box with enough water to cover the line where the kitty litter usually is, and agitate with your gloved hands. Use the sponge to get it really clean, and get into all the nooks and crannies of the edge if it has a lid.
3. Let it soak while you clean the lid and ramp if your litter box has either of these pieces. Use the rest of the soap solution and the sponge to get them thoroughly cleaned.
4. Rinse well to get rid of all traces of soap and dry in the sunlight or tipped up in the sink.
5. Allow to dry thoroughly. Dump out the solution from the main box and rinse it well, too, and set it up to dry. Do not fill a damp box with kitty litter!

# Soaps

When you make your own soap, you get to choose how you want it to look, feel, and smell. Adding dyes, essential oils, texture (with oatmeal, seeds, etc.), or pouring it into molds will make your soap unique. Making soap requires time, patience, and caution, as you'll be using some caustic and potentially dangerous ingredients—especially lye (sodium hydroxide). Avoid coming into direct contact with the lye; wear goggles, rubber gloves, and long sleeves, and work in a well-ventilated area.

Be careful not to breathe in the fumes produced by the lye and water mixture. Soap is made up of three main ingredients: water, lye, and fats or oils. While lard and tallow were once used exclusively for making soaps, it is perfectly acceptable to use a combination of pure oils for the "fat" needed to make soap.

Saponification is the process in which the mixture becomes completely blended and the chemical reactions between the lye and the oils, over time, turn the mixture into a hardened bar of usable soap.

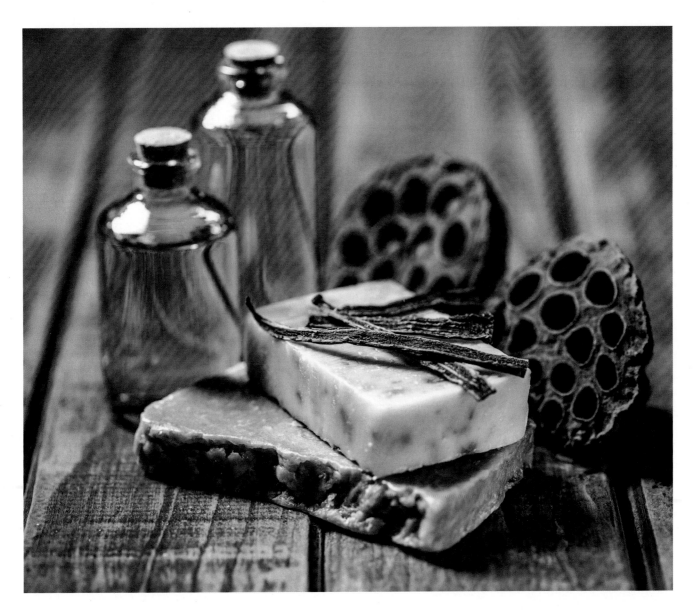

## Cold-Pressed Soap

### Ingredients and Supplies:

6.9 ounces lye (sodium hydroxide)

2 cups distilled water, cold (from the refrigerator is the best)

2 cups canola oil

2 cups coconut oil

2 cups palm oil

Goggles, gloves, and mask (optional) to wear while making the soap

Mold for the soap (a cake or bread loaf pan will work just fine; you can also find flexible plastic molds at your local arts and crafts store)

Plastic wrap or wax paper to line the molds

Glass bowl to mix the lye and water

Wooden spoon for mixing

2 thermometers (one for the lye and water mixture and one for the oil mixture)

Stainless steel or cast-iron pot for heating oils and mixing in lye mixture

Handheld stick blender (optional)

### Directions:

1. Put on the goggles and gloves and make sure you are working in a well-ventilated room.
2. Ready your mold(s) by lining with plastic wrap or wax paper. Set them aside.
3. Slowly add the lye to the cold, distilled water in a glass bowl (never add the water to the lye) and stir continually for at least a minute, or until the lye is completely dissolved. Place one thermometer into the glass bowl and allow the mixture to cool to around 110°F (the chemical reaction of the lye mixing with the water will cause it to heat up quickly at first).
4. While the lye is cooling, combine the oils in a pot on medium heat and stir well until they are melted togeth er. Place a thermometer into the pot and allow the mixture to cool to 110°F.
5. Carefully pour the lye mixture into the oil mixture in a small, consistent stream, stirring continuously to make sure the lye and oils mix properly. Continue stirring, either by hand (which can take a very long time) or with a handheld stick blender, until the mixture traces (has the consistency of thin pudding). This may take anywhere from 30 to 60 minutes or more, so be patient. It is well worth the time invested to make sure your mixture traces. If it doesn't trace all the way, it will not saponify correctly and your soap will be ruined.
6. Once your mixture has traced, pour carefully into the mold(s) and let sit for a few hours. Then, when the mixture is still soft but congealed enough not to melt back into itself, cut the soap with a table knife into bars. Let sit for a few days, then take the bars out of the mold(s) and place on brown paper (grocery bags are perfect) in a dark area. Allow the bars to cure for another 4 weeks or so before using. If you want your soap to be colored, add special soap-coloring dyes (you can find these at the local arts and crafts store) after the mixture has traced, stir them in. Or try making your own dyes using herbs, flowers, or spices.

If you are looking to have a yummy-smelling bar of soap, add a few drops of your favorite essential oils (such as lavender, lemon, or rose) after the tracing of the mixture and stir in. You can also add aloe and vitamin E at this point to make your soap softer and more moisturizing.

To add texture and exfoliating properties to your soap, you can stir some oats into the traced mixture, along with some almond essential oil or a dab of honey. This will not only give your soap a nice, pumice-like quality but it will also smell wonderful. Try adding bits of lavender, rose petals, or citrus peel to your soap for variety.

To make soap in different shapes, pour your mixture into molds instead of making them into bars. If you are looking to have round soaps, you can take a few bars of soap you've just made, place them into a resealable plastic bag, and warm them by putting the bag into hot water (120°F) for 30 minutes. Then, cut the bars up and roll them into balls. These soaps should set in about 1 hour or so.

## Soap Oils

Almost any oil can be used to make soap, but different oils have different qualities; some oils create a creamier lather, some create a bubbly lather. Oils that are high in iodine will produce a softer soap, so be sure to mix with oils that are lower in iodine. Online soap calculators are very helpful when creating your own recipes.

## Natural Dyes for Soap or Candles

| Light/Dark Brown | Cinnamon, ground cloves, allspice, nutmeg, coffee |
|---|---|
| Yellow | Turmeric, saffron, calendula petals |
| Green | Liquid chlorophyll, alfalfa, cucumber, sage, nettles |
| Red | Annatto extract, beets, grapeskin extract |
| Blue | Red cabbage |
| Purple | Alkanet root |

## Oil Qualities

| Almond Butter | Conditioning, Creamy Lather. Moderate Iodine. |
|---|---|
| Almond Oil, sweet | Conditioning, Fragrant. High Iodine. |
| Apricot Kernel Oil | Conditioning, Fragrant. High Iodine. |
| Avocado Oil | Conditioning, Creamy Lather. High Iodine. |
| Babassu Oil | Cleansing, Bubbly. Very Low Iodine. |
| Canola Oil | Conditioning. Inexpensive. High Iodine. |
| Cocoa Butter | Creamy Lather. Low Iodine. |
| Coconut Oil | Bubbly Lather, Cleansing. Low Iodine. |
| Emu Oil | Conditioning. Creamy Lather. Moderate Iodine, |
| Evening Primrose Oil | Conditioning. Very High Iodine. |
| Flax Oil, Linseed | Conditioning. Very High Iodine. |
| Ghee | Cleansing, Bubbly Lather. Very Low Iodine. |
| Grapeseed Oil | Conditioning. Very High Iodine. |
| Hemp Oil | Conditioning. Very High Iodine. |
| Lanolin Liquid Wax | Low Iodine. |
| Neem Tree Oil | Conditioning, Creamy Lather. High Iodine. |
| Olive Oil | Conditioning, Creamy Lather. High Iodine. |
| Palm Oil | Conditioning, Creamy Lather. Moderate Iodine. |
| Safflower Oil | Conditioning. Very High Iodine. |
| Sesame Oil | Conditioning. High Iodine. |
| Shea Butter | Conditioning, Creamy Lather. Moderate Iodine. |
| Ucuuba Butter | Conditioning. Creamy Lather. Low Iodine. |

# Mermaids Kisses Salty Sea Soap

This delightful soap recipe was created after a wonderful trip to the ocean. I also developed an accompanying essential oil blend that smells like the ocean breezes around the Carmel Valley that roll in with the morning mist, with swaying eucalyptus trees, refreshing lemongrass, and just a touch of rosemary—the kiss of a mermaid.

This fun soap contains sea salt and seaweed. Sea salt adds a lovely exfoliating element; it is purifying and full of nutrients essential for skin health such as potassium, calcium, and zinc. The best part about this soap is you can get all these benefits and not smell like a fish!

A note about crafting salt soaps: Salt in soap creates a quickly hardening bar accelerating the natural process of saponification created by the sodium hydroxide (lye). I cut this soap as soon as it is no longer warm to the touch. Cut it within 4 hours, otherwise it will be too hard to cut and may crumble. Alternatively, if you pour it into individual soap molds, you bypass this issue entirely.

Also, soap has a reducing effect upon bubbles. To remedy this, we use higher amounts of coconut oil, which in many cases can be far too drying. To counterbalance, I use a 20 percent super fat. This blend uses sea salt and any type of seaweed you like. I use kelp, dulse, and bladderwrack, which you can easily purchase from your local co-op or from herb stores online, but you can use just one type of seaweed if you like—or ten! There are so many to choose from! Each type of seaweed contains a varying amount of nutrients.

## Ingredients:

7 oz distilled water
2.8 oz lye
16 oz coconut oil
4 oz olive oil
½ cup sea salt
½ teaspoon powdered seaweed of your choice

## Recommended Scent Blend:

- 60 drops eucalyptus
- 30 drops lemon grass
- 30 drops rosemary

## Directions:

1. SAFETY CHECK!!
   Line your soap mold with parchment paper. Weigh your water in a heatproof nonreactive bowl and your lye in a separate container. Take these outside in a well-ventilated safe area and add your lye to your water, mixing thoroughly with a nonreactive spoon. Set in a safe spot to cool.

2. Meanwhile, weigh your oils and melt over medium heat until thoroughly melted. Remove from heat and add essential oils for scent. Check that your lye and oil temps are around 100°F to 110°F and blend your lye/water into your oil blend. Mix these thoroughly with a stick blender. Mix until you have reached trace. Now add the salt and seaweed.

3. Keep blending until the mixture has reached a pudding-like consistency; this is important so the salt will remain suspended until the soap hardens. If the mixture is too liquidy, the salt will sink to the bottom of the bar. Pour your soap into a lined soap mold.

4. At this point, spritz the tops of your soap with alcohol to keep soda ash from forming. Set aside in a safe spot to set for 4 hours, then remove your soap from the mold, peel off the freezer paper, and cut your soap. Set aside to cure for 4 to 6 weeks!
   Seaweed is incredibly beneficial for the skin. It contains a variety of minerals well known for their antiaging benefits. Seaweed draws out redness and irritations and also speeds up healing with healthy cell turnover. The iodine in seaweed helps pull out toxins in the skin. Some people say it helps the body clear out radiation.

## Goat Milk Soap

Goat milk is wonderful for sensitive, dry, and baby skin. I like to visit a local goat farmer, who allows her goats to graze and play all day in green fields before escorting them into the barn to be milked. They are the kindest little goats I've ever met; each one knows how dear to the farmer's heart they are. The goat milk itself is the sweetest, creamiest treat I get all week. I like to use this fresh milk in my soap, but store bought will work great, too!

### Ingredients:
7.6 oz goat milk
2.9 oz lye
8 oz olive oil
8 oz coconut oil
4 oz castor oil
Scent blend, if desired

### Directions:
1. SAFETY CHECK!

   Start by pouring your goat milk into ice cube trays, as goat milk is extremely high in sugar and will burn rapidly if mixed in liquid form with lye. Stick your ice cube tray in the freezer and wait until goat milk is frozen. Once the milk has frozen, remove from freezer, and place ice cubes in a heat-resistant, nonreactive mixing bowl. Next, weigh your lye in a separate container and take it plus your ice cubes to a well-ventilated, safe outdoor area. Add your lye to the goat milk ice cubes, mixing well. Set aside to cool

2. Meanwhile, weigh your oils and place over medium heat until thoroughly melted. Remove from heat, and add essential oils for scent, if you desire. Check that your lye and oil temperatures are around 100°F to 110°F and blend your lye/goat milk into your oils. Mix these thoroughly with a stick blender until you have reached trace and then mix a little longer, just to be certain. Pour your soap into a pre-lined soap mold.

3. At this point, spritz the tops of your soap with alcohol to keep soda ash from forming. Set aside in a safe and ideally a cool spot to reduce heat-related fissures and leave to sit for 12 to 24 hours. After this time, remove your soap from the mold, peel off the freezer paper, and cut your soap! Set aside to cure for 4 to 6 weeks. Enjoy!

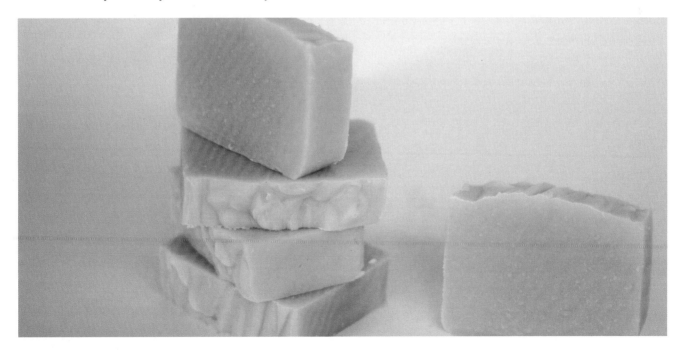

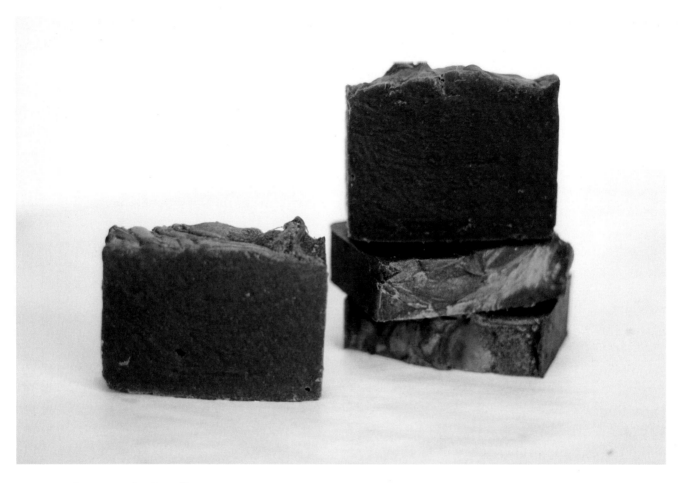

## Lavender Herbal Infusion Soap

This lovely soap contains a special herbal infusion of alkanet and olive oil that results in a deep purple hue. Lavender is very soothing and calming to the skin and mind, and it helps relieve stress and headaches. A wonderful soap to start your day with, lavender aids in the healing of burns. It can also reduce acne, heal blemishes, and calm inflammations.

### Ingredients:
7.6 oz distilled water
2.9 oz lye
2 oz alkanet-strained olive oil
6 oz olive oil
8 oz coconut oil

### Recommended Scent Blend: Lavender
- The following is based on a variety of some of my favorite lavenders on my shelves. The varieties of available lavender distillations is vast, but if you don't have a variety of lavenders and have just one, that will work great, too— just be sure to add the benzoin to "fix" the lavender or your scent will evaporate rapidly.
- 20 drops benzoin
- 40 drops *Lavender angustifolia* (Hungary)
- 40 drops *Lavender angustifolia* (Russia)
- 40 drops *Lavandin abrialis* (France)
- 40 drops *Lavandin grosso* (Oregon, USA)

### Directions:
1. SAFETY CHECK!
   Weigh your water in a heatproof, non-reactive bowl and weigh lye in a separate

container. Take these outside to a well-ventilated, safe area and add your lye to your water, mixing thoroughly with a nonreactive spoon. Set in a safe spot to cool.

2. Meanwhile, weigh your oils and keep over medium heat until thoroughly melted. Remove from heat, add essential oils for scent. Check that your lye and oil temperatures are both around 100°F and 110°F and then blend your lye/water into your oils. Mix these thoroughly with a stick blender until you have reached trace, then mix a little longer, just to be certain. Pour your soap into pre-lined soap mold.

3. At this point, spritz the tops of your soap with alcohol to keep soda ash from forming. Set aside in a safe spot to harden for 12 to 24 hours. After this time, remove your soap from the mold, peel off the freezer paper, and cut your soap! Set aside to cure for 4 to 6 weeks.

## Charcoal Soap

This is by far the most popular soap I've ever made. Thanks to the powerful healing abilities of charcoal, it's a perfect face and body soap!

### Activated Charcoal

Activated charcoal works through a process called adsorption in which it binds with toxins in the body, utilizing its negative electron charge to bond (adsorb) positive electron toxins and reducing their overall toxicity. But the magic doesn't stop there—because of the process that activated charcoal goes through to become activated, it has a massively absorbent surface area so it pulls out bacteria and grime from the skin. It also works as a wonderful complexion balancer, acne reducer, and toner.

Warning: Activated charcoal is not the same as the charcoal you use in your barbecue—that stuff is dangerous. Make sure you purchase food-grade activated charcoal for this recipe.

### Ingredients:
7.6 oz distilled water
2.9 oz lye
8 oz coconut oil
8 oz olive oil
4 oz castor oil
2 tbsp activated charcoal

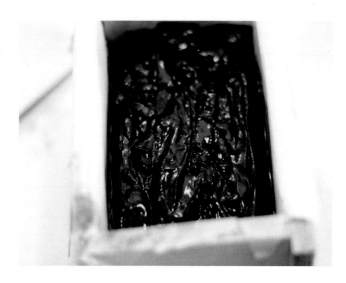

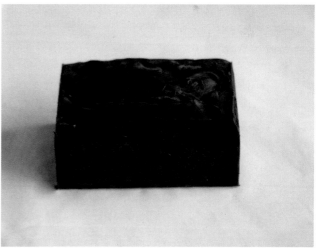

**Directions:**

1. SAFETY CHECK!

   Line your soap mold with freezer paper. Weigh your water in a heatproof, nonreactive bowl and weigh lye in a separate container. Take these outside to a well-ventilated, safe area and add your lye to your water, mixing thoroughly with a nonreactive spoon. Set in a safe spot to cool. Meanwhile, weigh your oils and place over medium heat until thoroughly melted. Remove from heat, and add essential oils for scent if you are choosing to use them.

2. Check that your lye and oil temperatures are around 100°F to 110°F and blend your lye/water into your oils. Mix these thoroughly with a stick blender until you have reached trace. Add your charcoal, stirring it in slowly before mixing or it may billow all over the place. Now, use your stick blender to mix a little longer. Pour your soap into a pre-lined soap mold.

3. At this point, spritz the tops of your soap with alcohol to keep soda ash from forming. Set aside in a safe spot for 12 to 24 hours. After this time, remove your soap from the mold, peel off the freezer paper, and cut your soap! Set aside to cure for 4 to 6 weeks. Enjoy!!

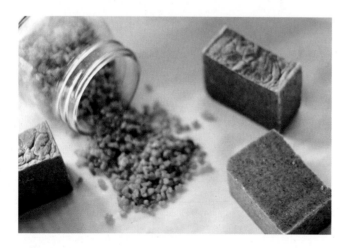

## Resin Soap Two Ways

Resin is sap from a tree. It cleanses the blood, increases circulation, moves obstructions, mends cuts, scraps, burns, bruises, and bites, etc. The following are two variations on creating soap from resin. You should choose your method based on whether you want an exfoliating effect.

One wonderful aspect of using resins in soap is the beautiful scent they naturally impart in your finished product. They being said, you can absolutely add fragrance. Personally, I like to build off the natural resin scent, creating a truly intoxicating soap aroma.

## Ingredients:

2.9 oz lye

6.6 oz distilled water

8 oz coconut oil

8 oz olive oil

4 oz castor oil

2 tbsp finely ground resin (I'm using 2 tablespoons of myrrh in the first recipe, and 2 tablespoons dragon's blood resin in the second method)

## Directions 1

This method will give you an exfoliating resin soap.

1. SAFETY CHECK!

   Weigh your lye and water, and in a well-ventilated, safe area outdoors, add your lye to your water, mixing thoroughly. Set this aside to cool. While your lye water is cooling, weigh your oils, blend these together, and set over medium heat until thoroughly melted. Remove from heat, and add essential oils for scent if you choose to do so.

2. Once your oils and lye water have both reached between 100°F and 110°F degrees, add these together. Add your resin and mix until relatively thick trace is achieved. Due to resin having a bit of density, this thickness is desirable to ensure your resin doesn't sink while setting up. Pour your soap into your pre-lined soap mold, set aside for at

least 12 to 24 hours to harden, and then cut. Set aside to cure for 4 to 6 weeks in an undisturbed area.

## Myrrh

Myrrh is wonderful for skin care—it works as an antibacterial, it's moisturizing, circulation-enhancing, and toning in nature. It cleans up acne and blemishes very well because of its blood-purifying properties. I break out for a week every month without fail and this soap is my saving grace at saving face! During summer, it helps stave off itchy issues such as bug bites and poison oak. I actually prefer using it over neem, as its smell much more pleasing in a resinous way.

## Directions 2

This method will give you a delightful resin soap without exfoliating properties.

1. SAFETY CHECK!
   To start, weigh your lye, ground resin, and distilled water. Take to a safe, outside area and add your resin to the distilled water.
2. Next add your lye, and stir well until your resin is melted. Set aside to cool.
3. While your water/lye/resin blend is cooling, weigh your oils and keep over medium heat until thoroughly melted. Gently blend in your resin powder, stirring well.
4. Take off heat and add essential oils for fragrance if you're going to do so. Once both your water and oil have reached between 120°F and 130°F, mix them together, blending until trace had been reached—this will happen very quickly.
5. Next, pour your mixture into a soap mold and set aside for 12 to 24 hours. Cut and cure for 4 to 6 weeks.

## Checkered Soap

This artistic method creates a really lovely soap, and the addition of charcoal adds some serious skin-healing abilities, although you could use anything you prefer as a colorant.

### Ingredients:

7.6 oz distilled water
2.9 oz lye
8 oz coconut oil
8 oz olive oil
4 oz castor oil
1 tbsp activated charcoal

### Additional Supplies:

- 2 large plastic bottles with a tapered screw-on top (I got mine in the tie-dye section of the craft store and cut the tip just a tiny bit.)
- 2 (4-cup) nonreactive pitchers

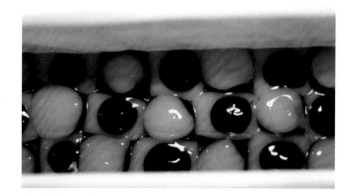

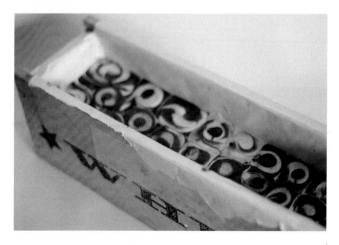

## Directions:

1. SAFETY CHECK!

   Weigh your water in a heatproof, non-reactive bowl. Weigh lye in a separate container, and then take these outside to a well-ventilated and safe area. Add your lye to your water, mixing thoroughly with a nonreactive spoon. Set in a safe spot to cool.

2. Meanwhile, weigh your oils and place over medium heat until thoroughly melted. Remove from heat, add essential oils or scent blend if you so choose. Check that your lye and oil temperatures are both around 100°F to 110°F and blend your lye/water into your oils. Mix these thoroughly with a stick blender. Mix until you have just reached trace.

3. Split your soap in half, pouring one half into one container, and pour the rest of soap into another. Add charcoal to one of your Pyrex soap pitchers and blend. Fill your plastic tapered bottles, one with white soap and one with black soap.

4. Now start with black soap in your plastic bottle with tapered lid and place dots of soap along the bottom of your soap mold. Between these dots, place white dots with white soap. The white soap will look a bit yellow but will whiten as it cures. Switch bottles and squeeze black soap into the center of the white soap. Switch bottles again and squeeze white soap into black soap centers. Keep this switching back and forth of soap colors until you have used up all the soap.

5. At this point, spritz the tops of your soap with alcohol to keep soda ash from forming. Place your soap in a safe spot to set for 12 to 24 hours. After this time, remove your soap from the mold, peel off the freezer paper, and cut your soap! Set aside to cure for 4 to 6 weeks. Enjoy!!

## Beard Wash Soap

I created this fantastic soap after spending some time around beards and finding they were rarely washed because folks simply did not want to mess with the beauty of them. They would add product and rinse them, but there was a gap in actual beard shampooing. This recipe has been formulated to enhance growth, shine, beard health, and nourishment, takes care of dander and irritation, and adds tenacity—meaning it slows down breakage and adds elasticity and strength to the follicle, caring for the beard from base to tip. I use a specially formulated herbal blend to add nutrients and quality. I cut down on super fatting by 2 percent so as to not leave greasy residue. Light oils are used to avoid weighing down the beard; I use herbal oils for their powerful beardly benefits (see beginning of recipe for instructions). An alternative would be to add straight powdered herbs, but I feel this is less desirable because it means you're putting powder in hair. But it's entirely up to you!

### Ingredients:
10 oz olive oil
0.20 oz avocado oil
0.20 oz argan oil
0.20 oz apricot kernel oil
8.60 oz coconut oil
0.60 oz cocoa butter
0.20 oz evening primrose oil
7.60 oz distilled water
2.97 oz lye

### Additional Supplies:
- Herbs, such as fo ti, nettle, bhringaraj, horsetail (½ teaspoon, powdered of each herb)*
- 2-inch PVC pipe, capped

### Recommended Scent Blend: Shakka Shakka
The following is a fun and great-smelling scent blend based on the original recipes for men's cologne.
- 20 drops vetiver

- 4 drops patchouli
- 20 drops rosewood
- 20 drops lemon
- 20 drops lime
- 20 drops lavender
- 20 drops bergamot
- 10 drops rosemary

*For this recipe, either substitute the olive oil for herbal olive oil or add them as powders.

## Directions:

1. SAFETY CHECK!

   If you you're not using powdered herbs, then you can blend all the fresh herbs into the olive oil, creating an herbal oil, and then strain. Set aside oil to use and compost your herbs. Weigh distilled water in a heatproof bowl and weigh lye in a separate container. In an outside, safe, and well-ventilated area, add your lye to the water and mix well with a non-caustic spoon. Set this blend aside in a safe and undisturbed place to cool.

2. Meanwhile, weigh your oils in a nonreactive cooking pot—this includes substituting the olive oil for your herbal olive oil if you made it. If you're planning to use powdered herbs, wait to add. Set over medium heat to melt oils. Once your oils are melted, remove from heat, and add scent now, if desired. Bring in your lye and add to oil mixture once both have reached 100°F to 110°F. Mix and add any herbs. Blend to trace. Add color, if desired, and mix until blended, and then pour into your lined mold. Set aside in a safe place for 12 to 24 hours. Remove from mold, cut, and set aside in a well-ventilated area to cure for 4 to 6 weeks. Share with your bearded friends!

## Baby's Hand-Sanitizing Spray

### Ingredients:

2 tablespoons witch hazel
2 tablespoons vegetable glycerin
2 drops geranium essential oil
2 drops melaleuca essential oil
2 drops orange essential oil

### Preparation:

1. Use a metal funnel to fill a 2-ounce blue or amber glass spray bottle with 2 tablespoons vegetable glycerin.
2. Add 2 drops each of geranium, melaleuca, and orange essential oils.
3. Swirl glycerin and essential oils together.
4. Add 2 tablespoons witch hazel.
5. Apply spray nozzle cap.
6. Shake well.

## Kid-Safe Hand-Sanitizing Spray

### Ingredients:

3 tablespoon witch hazel
1 tablespoon glycerin
3 drops geranium essential oil
3 drops melaleuca essential oil
3 drops orange essential oil
2 drops clove essential oil
1 drop lemongrass essential oil

### Preparation:

1. Use a metal funnel to fill a 2-ounce blue or amber glass spray bottle with 1 tablespoon vegetable glycerin.
2. Add 3 drops each of geranium, melaleuca, and orange essential oils, 2 drops clove essential oil, and 1 drop lemongrass essential oil.
3. Swirl glycerin and essential oils together.
4. Add 3 tablespoons witch hazel.
5. Apply spray nozzle cap.
6. Shake well.

**Benefits:**

- Geranium, orange, and clove essential oils are effective against many microbes including, but not limited to *Proteus vulgaris, Pseudomonas aeruginosa, Escherichia coli, Staphylococcus aureus, Bacillus subtilis,* and *Klebsiella pneumoniae.*
- Melaleuca has been used by Aboriginal people in Australia and New Zealand for its medicinal properties, for generations. Its antimicrobial properties make it superb for hand sanitation.
- There are a wide variety of microbes deterred by lemongrass essential oil bacteria, but it is particularly effective against phages and fungi.
- The witch hazel works as an astringent and cleanser, while the glycerin is a moisturizing carrier for the essential oils.

**NOTES AND TIPS:**

- The Baby's Hand-Sanitizing Spray is intended for babies ages six months to two years.
- The Kid-Safe Hand-Sanitizing Spray is intended for children and adults ages two and up.
- The sprays may also be used to sanitize other areas of the body, but avoid sensitive areas like the face and genitals.
- If the spray gets in the eyes, rinse with carrier oil such as coconut, almond, or olive oils.
- Some people have skin sensitivities to melaleuca. If the melaleuca irritates you or your child, replace it with lemon essential oil.

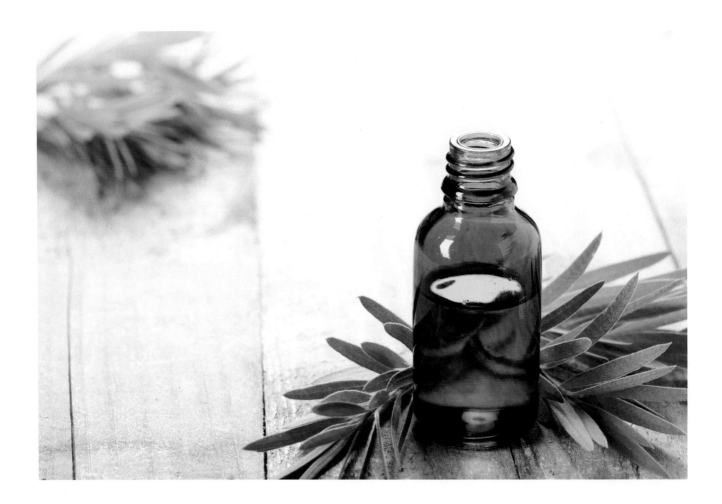

# Toothpaste and Mouthwash

## Coconut Oil Toothpaste

This recipe is incredibly simple to make, and by using it you'll avoid the fluoride, detergents, and chemicals found in many commercial toothpastes. Coconut oil is antibacterial, antifungal, and anti-microbial, and it helps to bind the other ingredients together into more of a paste than a powder. Baking soda is a cleanser, whitener, and mild abrasive. The essential oil makes the paste taste better and freshens your breath.

### Ingredients:

½ cup coconut oil
¼ cup baking soda
15 to 20 drops peppermint, cinnamon, or myrrh essential oil (or a combination)

### Directions:

1. If the coconut oil is hard, warm it slightly to soften.
2. Stir in baking soda and essential oil and store in a small mason jar or other covered dish.
3. To use, wet your toothbrush, dip it in the paste, and brush!

## Peppermint Lavender Mouthwash

Commercial mouthwash is awash in chemicals; you can tell just by looking at its atomic colors. The list of ingredients is pretty much unpronounceable, and I'm not sure why they insist on making it electric colored. There's also plenty of alcohol in there, which does no favors for your mouth's ecosystem. But mouthwash can be a helpful oral health tool when it helps balance the pH (baking soda), kills bacteria (peppermint oil and xylitol), and adds a fresh feeling (herbs and peppermint oil). Xylitol is recommended for oral health, too, and it sweetens

the mouthwash just enough to make it pleasant to swish in your mouth. Note: Keep xylitol away from dogs as it is extremely toxic to them.

### Ingredients:

1 tablespoon dried organic lavender
1 tablespoon dried organic mint
2 ½ cups distilled or boiled and cooled water
2–4 drops organic peppermint oil (or omit the lavender and use tea tree oil)
1 tablespoon baking soda
Xylitol, to taste (start with a tiny amount; a little goes a long way)

### Preparation:

1. Fill a saucepan with the 2 cups of water and the tablespoon of organic lavender and the mint. Bring to a simmer and let simmer for

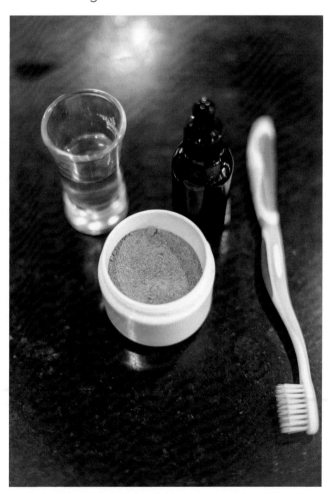

2 minutes. Turn off the heat and let cool completely. Strain the mixture and keep the liquid, composting the herbs.

2. Add the peppermint oil if you'd like (taste the mixture first to see how pepperminty it is), the baking soda, and a tiny amount of xylitol just to make the flavor appealing. Taste as you go along.

3. Pour into a 16-ounce container with a tight-fitting lid. Label well and store in the refrigerator for up to a month. Shake before using.

## Tooth and Gum Health Powder

1 part myrrh gum powder
1 part baking soda
1 part bentonite clay
½ part turmeric powder
½ part slippery elm powder
½ part chamomile powder
¼ part licorice powder
¼ part peppermint powder
¼ part clove powder

This formula is used as toothpaste. Simply dip your damp toothbrush into the powder and brush as usual. It has antibacterial healing, and soothing properties, and it leaves your mouth feeling fresh and clean.

## Tooth and Gum Health Mouthwash

**Ingredients:**
1 part comfrey
1 part echinacea
1 part sage
½ part lavender
½ part yarrow

**Directions:**
1. This formula is made as a tincture (see page 204) with the menstruum being equal parts apple cider vinegar and vodka or grain alcohol.
2. After the tincture is finished, it can be bottled in dropper bottles and used as a concentrate.
3. Add one dropper-full to a mouthful of water, and swish for at least 30 seconds.

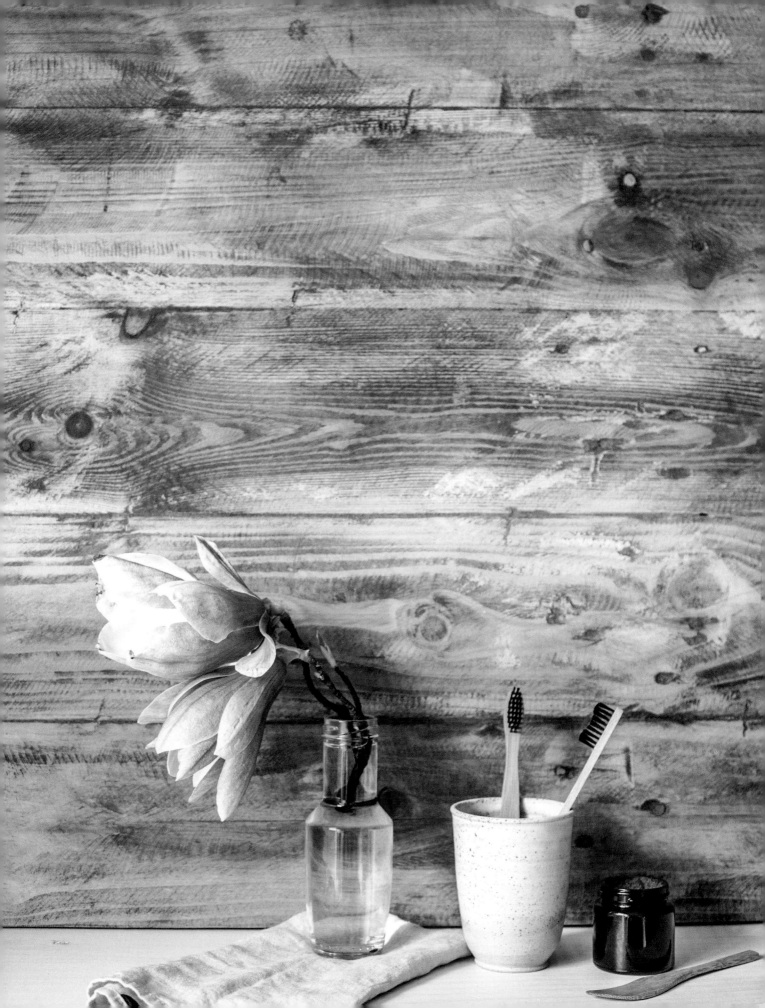

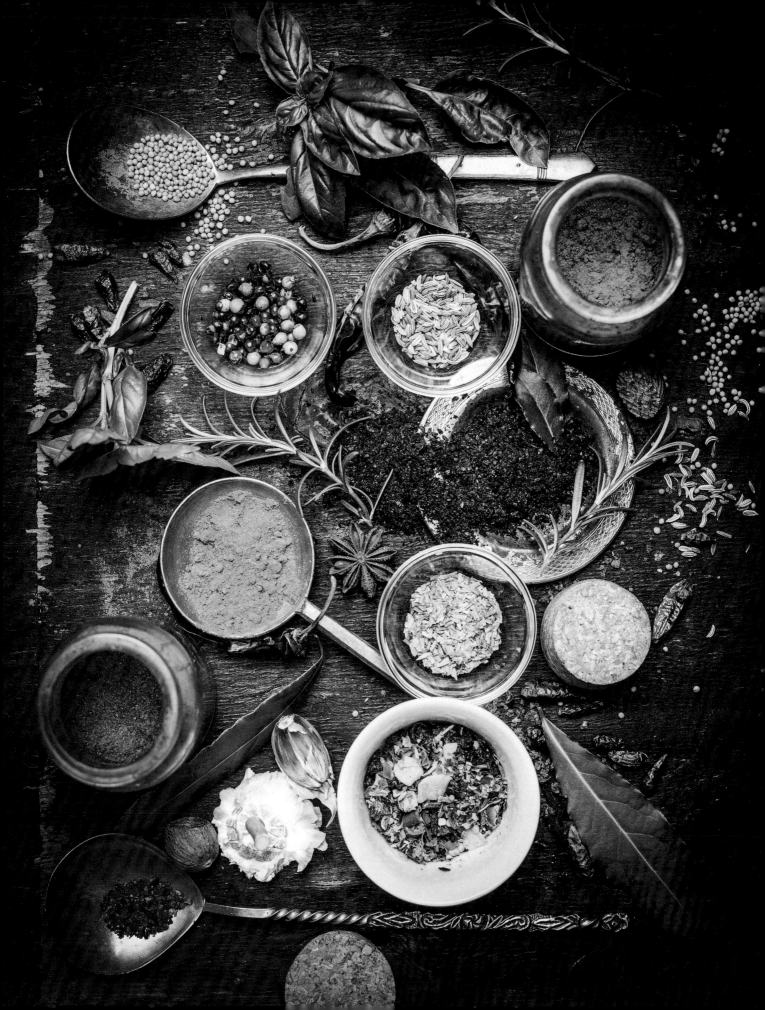

# ACKNOWLEDGMENTS

This book is a compendium of knowledge from herbalists, doctors, nutritionists, cooks, and other authors—many of whom are far more equipped to edit a book like this than I am. I have learned from each of them, and am honored to share their wisdom in these pages. Please be sure to check out their own books, which are featured at the end of this one.

Special thanks to Taylor Norton, who did the lion's share of compiling material for this tome, leaving me with the less cumbersome task of editing, arranging, and adding my own research throughout. I am not being modest when I say I could not have completed this project without her.

As always, thanks to publisher Tony Lyons for entrusting this project to me, and to production editor Chris Schultz for her skill and seemingly endless patience in making beautiful and useful books.

Alyssa Holmes, thank you for taking the time to write a thoughtful, meaningful foreword! I have so much respect for your knowledge and expertise, and it means a lot to have your stamp of approval on this book.

Last but not least, thanks to my husband Tim and my children, Anna and William, who make wellness that much more important to me.

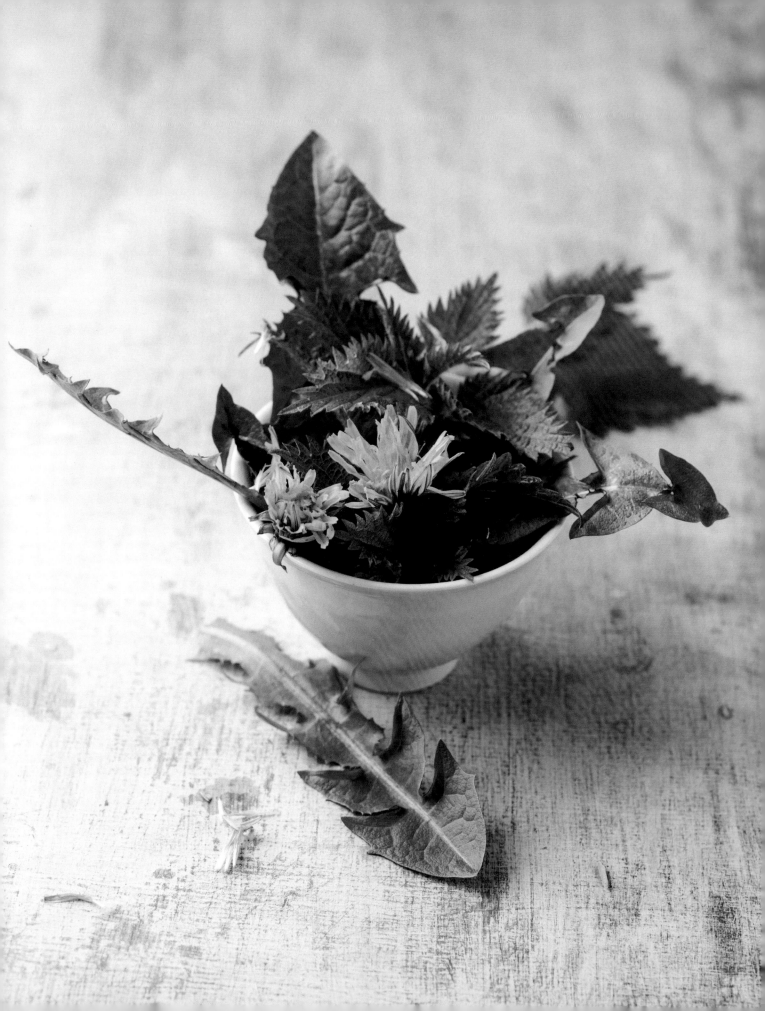

# RESOURCES

Atkinson, Alicia. *Essential Oils for Beauty, Wellness, and the Home*. New York: Skyhorse Pub., 2015. "Stress-Relieving Diffuser Blend," page 10; "Diarrhea Calming Capsule," "Diarrhea Calming Massage Blend," page 28; "Head Cold Tea," page 40; "Flu," pages 44–45; "Ingestible Hay Fever Relief," "Hay Fever Relief Diffuser Blend," page 46; "Eczema Lotion Bar," page 61; "Arthritis Joint Rub," page 78; "Menstrual Relief Massage Blend," page 94; "Warm and Woody Shaving Cream," page 107; "Comforting Diaper Cream," page 110; "Citrus Cream Deodorant," pages 284–285; "Coconut Lime Verbena Sugar Scrub," page 289; "Sweet and Subtle Sugar Scrub," page 291; "Invigorating Cellulite-Reducing Salt Scrub," page 291–292; "Orange Blossom Honey Salt Scrub," page 293; "Romantic Massage Blend," page 300; "Baby's Hand-Sanitizing Spray," page 339; "Kid-Safe Hand-Sanitizing Spray," page 339–340; "All Purpose Cleaner," page 314, "Sanitizing Counter Spray," page 315; "Citrus-Fir Dish Soap," page 317; "Gunk- and Grease-Removing Spray," page 318

Brock, Farnoosh. *The Big Book of Healing Drinks*. New York: Skyhorse Pub., 2019. "Juice Recipes," pages 177–183; "Elixirs," pages 199–200; "Tonics & Shots," pages 209–216; "Broths," page 220–224; "Beef Bone Broth in the Instant Pot," page 225; "Chicken Bone Broth in the Slow Cooker," "Vegetable Broth on the Stove," page 226

Browne, Jennifer. *The Good Living Guide to Medicinal Tea*. New York: Good Books, 2016. "Anti-Depressant Tea," page 6; "Forget-Me-Not Tea," page 8; "Tea for Migraines," page 19; "Stomach Stabilizing Tea," page 33; "Cholesterol-Lowering Tea," page 71; "Bone Up Tea," page 81; "Lactation Tea," page 90

Chase, Daniella. *Healing Smoothies*. New York: Skyhorse Pub., 2015. "Smoothies," pages 186–191

Chatagnier, Leigh Ann. *Natural Baby & Toddler Treats*. New York: Skyhorse Pub., 2019. "Natural Baby and Toddler Treats." pages 254–259

Cuadra, Morena & Escardó, Morena. *Detox Juicing*. New York: Skyhorse Pub., 2014. "The Truth About Toxins," pages 168–169; "The Power of Juicing," pages 170–173; "Detox Juicing 101," pages 174–176

Cummings, Dede & Holmes, Alyssa. *Healing Herbs*. New York: Skyhorse Pub., 2017. "Stress and Anxiety Support Syrup," page 10; "Headache Tincture," page 16; "Iron and Energy Syrup," page 70; "Healthy Moon Cycle Blend," page 95; "Herb Garden Designs," pages 122–123; "Properties and Actions of Herbs," pages 126–129; "Tea," pages 194–196; "Vitamin C Flower Power Blend," "Super Green Vitamin/Mineral Blend," "Relaxation Blend," page 196; "Wellness Blend," "Energizing Blend," "Healthy Gut/Digestion Blend," page 197; "Hormonal Balance," "High Mineral Vinegar Tincture," "Spicy Immunity Vinegar Tincture," page 204; "Beautiful Body Oil," page 266; "Skin Healing Oil," page 267; "Aphrodisiac Tea," page 300; "Tooth and Gum Health Powder," "Tooth and Gum Health Mouthwash," page 342

Dill, Linda Louisa. *Aphrodisiacs: An A-Z*. New York: Skyhorse Pub., 2015. "An Introduction to Sex Drive and Libido," page 296

Gehring, Abigail. *The Good Living Guide to Country Skills*. New York: Good Books, 2016. "Laundry Detergent," "Reusable Dryer Sheets," page 323; "Coconut Oil Toothpaste," page 341

Gehring, Abigail. *The Healthy Gluten-Free Diet*. New York: Skyhorse Pub., 2014. "Medicinal Cooking," pages 234–251

Gehring, Abigail. *The Illustrated Encyclopedia of Country Living*. New York: Skyhorse Pub., 2011. "Edible Wild Plants," pages 163–165; "Fruits and Vegetables for Your Skin" (box), page 265; "Shampoo," "Hair Conditioner," "Herbs for Your Hair" (box), page 277; "Rosemary Peppermint Foot Scrub," page 278; "Tropical Face Cleanser," page 280; "Minty Cucumber Facial Mask," page 282; "Soaps," page 329; "Cold-Pressed Soap," pages 330–331; "Soap Oils" (box), "Natural Dyes for Soap or Candles" (box), "Oil Qualities" (box), page 331

Hinchliffe, Sandra & Kerr, Stacey. *CBD Every Day*. New York: Skyhorse Pub., 2019. "Super Pain Balm," page 82; "CBD Infusion for Beverage and Broth Recipe," page 231

McGrath, Simone. *Apple Cider Vinegar for Health and Beauty*. New York: Skyhorse Pub., 2015. "Apple Cider Vinegar," page 6; "Apple Cider Vinegar," page 7; "Apple Cider Vinegar," page 24; "Apple Cider Vinegar," page 29; "Apple Cider Vinegar," page 36; "Apple Cider Vinegar," page 56; "Apple Cider Vinegar," page 60; "Apple Cider Vinegar," page 62; "Apple Cider Vinegar," page 63; "Apple Cider Vinegar Tonic," page 72; "Apple Cider Vinegar," page 78; "Apple Cider Vinegar," page 81; "Apple Cider Vinegar," page 96; "Apple Cider Vinegar," page 100; "Apple Cider Vinegar," page 111; "Apple Cider Vinegar," page 113

McGrath, Simone. *Coconut Oil for Health and Beauty*. New York: Skyhorse Pub., 2014. "Coconut Oil," page 14; "Coconut Oil," page 20; "Coconut Oil," page 24; "Coconut Oil and Crohn's Disease," page 26; "Coconut Oil," page 36; "Coconut Oil for Colds and Flu," page 40; "Coconut Oil," page 46; "Coconut Oil," page 56; "Coconut Oil," page 57; "Coconut Oil," page 58; "Coconut Oil," page 59; "Coconut Oil," page 61; "Coconut Oil," page 62; "Coconut Oil," page 64; "Coconut Oil," page 65; "Coconut Oil," page 66; "Coconut Oil," page 67; "Coconut Oil," page 72; "Coconut Oil," page 78; "Coconut Oil and Thrush," page 97; "Coconut Oil," page 98; "Coconut Oil," page 111; "Whipped Coconut Oil Body Butter," page 265; "Replenishing Conditioner Treatment for Dry Hair," "Lavender Scalp Cream," page 274; "Avocado and Coconut Oil Hydrating Face Mask," 281

McQuerry, Liz. *Natural Soap at Home*. New York: Skyhorse Pub., 2018. "Mermaids Kisses Salty Sea Soap," page 332; "Goat Milk Soap," page 333; "Lavender Herbal Infusion Soap," pages 334–335; "Charcoal Soap," pages 335–336; "Resin Soap Two Ways," pages 336–337; "Checkered Soap," pages 337–338; "Beard Wash Soap," pages 338–339

Millman, Elana. *Aromatherapy for Sensual Living*. New York: Skyhorse Pub., 2015. "Beauty Rituals," page 264; "Facial Oiling," page 270; "Facial Steams," pages 271–272; "Scrubs," 287–288

Page, Teri. *Family Homesteading*. New York: Skyhorse Pub., 2018. "Cold Care Syrup" page 38

Plimmer, Claire. *Pregnancy Made Simple*. New York: Skyhorse Pub., 2018. "Folic Acid," "Calcium and Fatty Acids," page 92; "Lifestyle Changes," page 93; "Prevention and Treatment," page 96; "What Can Men Do?," "What Should Men Avoid?," page 105; "Fertility Foods," page 105–106

Polk, Michelle. *Healing Houseplants*. New York: Skyhorse Pub., 2018. "DIY Chamomile Flower Tea," page 4; "Sleepy Time Chamomile Tincture," page 7; "Rosemary Digestive Tea," page 29; "Peppermint Oil," page 30; "Chest Congestion and

Sinus Remedy," page 38; "Aloe Vera Face Cream," page 54; "Dandelion Abscess Poultice," page 65; "Lavender Bath Salt," page 80; "Peppermint," page 90; "Calendula Tea," page 98; "Rosemary Shampoo," page 104; "Aloe Vera," pages 130–131; "Rosemary," pages 150–153; "Sage," pages 154–155; "Houseplants for Clean Air," pages 306–313

Resnick, Ariane. *The Bone Broth Miracle*. New York: Skyhorse Pub., 2015. "Basic Lamb Bone Broth," "Basic Fish Bone Broth," page 228; "Beautifier," "Inflammation Reducer," page 230

Wise, Natalie. *The Modern Organic Home*. New York: Good Books, 2018. "Bites Be Gone Anti-Itch Paste," page 63; "Calming Aromatherapy Facial Steam," page 272; "Stinky Foot Solution Soak," "Beachside Break Foot Soak," page 278; "Eye'll Be Gentle Makeup Remover," page 280; "Lemon-Honey Facial Mask," page 281; "Looking Good Enough to Eat Fruit and Veggie Cleaner," page 318; "Stain Removal Cheat Sheet," pages 323–324; "Pet Leash and Collar Wash," "Pretty & Peppy Puppy Pet Shampoo," page 325; "Dog Perfume & Coat Conditioner," "Pet Spot and Odor Remover," page 327; "Peppermint Lavender Mouthwash," page 341

Yardley, Katolen. *The Good Living Guide to Natural and Herbal Remedies*. New York: Good Books, 2016. "Beam Me Up Melissa Balm Tea," page 4; "Headache Be Gone" page 16; "Heartburn Relief," page 32; "Yarrow Rose Hip Cold and Flu Relief," page 38; "Daisy Restorative Lung Tea," "Decongestant Oregano Coconut Vapor Rub," page 42; "Bronchitis Elixir," "Sage Cherry Cough Syrup," page 48; "Sinus Relief Herbal Steam," page 50; "Cayenne Pepper," "Marigold Antiseptic Tincture," page 59; "Pineapple Weed Insect Repellent," page 63; "Poison Ivy Relief," "Anti-Itch Oatmeal Paste," page 64; "Soothe Away the Ouch Sunburn Blend," page 67; "Marigold Vein Liniment," page 74; "Mullein and Garlic Ear Oil," page 86; "Soothing Chamomile Astringent Eyewash," page 87; "Marigold," page 90; "Pain Relief Tonic," page 94; "Hair Rinse," page 104; "Soothe My Throat Gargle", page 114; "Tummy and Teething Calm Popsicle," page 116; "Herbs to Avoid During Pregnancy," page 124; "Chamomile," page 132; "Chickweed," page 134; "Daisy," page 136; "Lavender," page 138; "Lemon Balm," page 141; "Marigold," page 142–143; "Mint," page 144; "Oregano," page 146; "Parsley" page 148; "Sunflower," page 156; "Thyme," pages 158–159; "Watercress," page 160; "Tinctures," page 204; "Dry Brushing," pages 268–269; "Basil Lavender Natural Deodorant," page 285

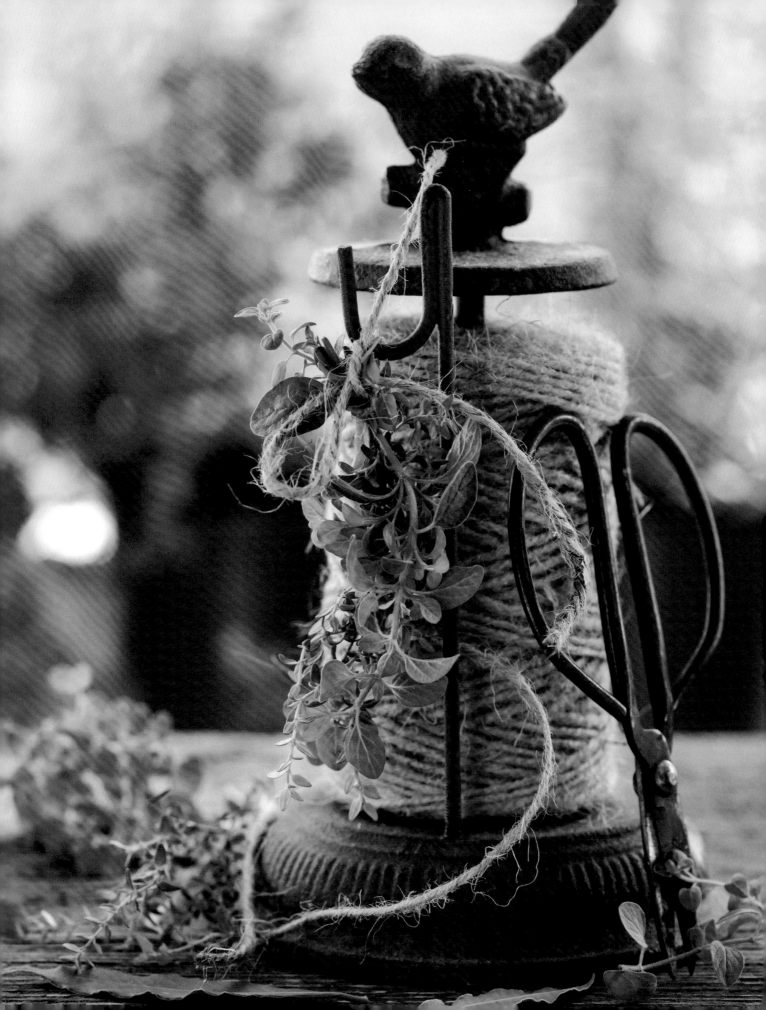

# PHOTO CREDITS

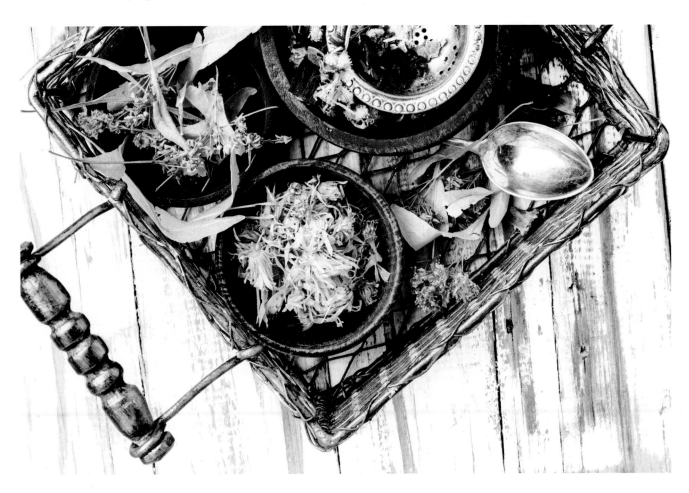

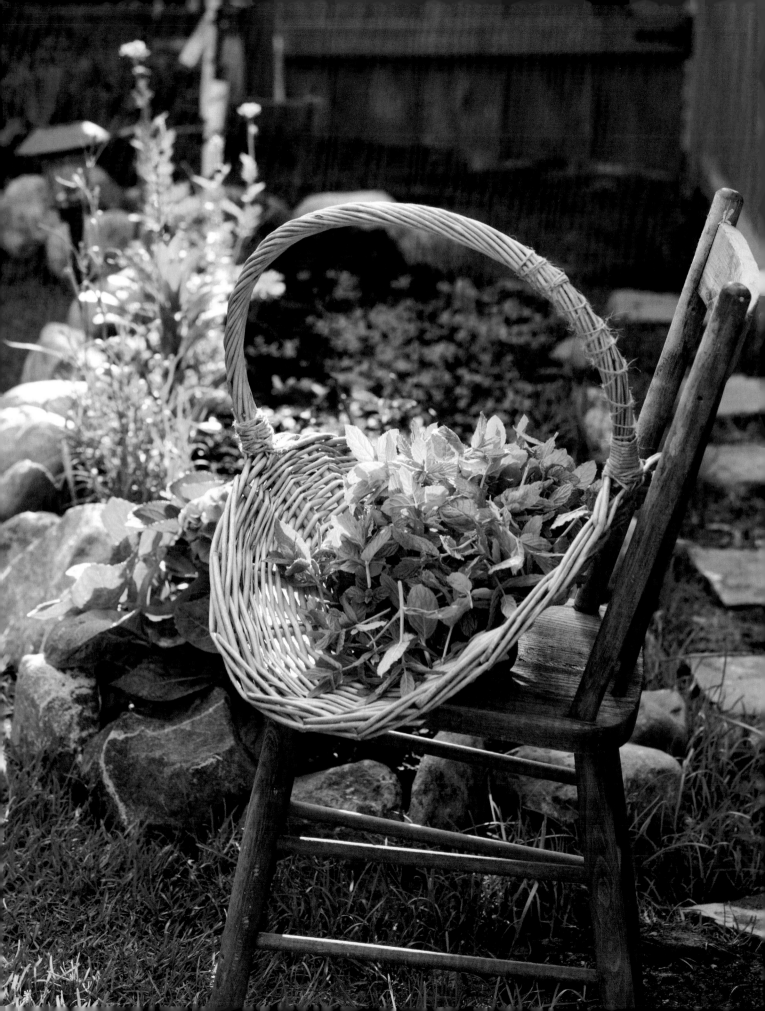

# ABOUT THE EDITOR

**Abigail R. Gehring** is the author or editor of several books on country living skills, cooking, baking, and more. A work in progress, she lives to worship Jesus wholeheartedly, and her passions include foster care and adoption, social justice, and the written word. She enjoys books, photography, gardening, experimenting in the kitchen, and spending time with loved ones. As associate publisher of Skyhorse Publishing, she has the privilege of working with authors from around the world and a wonderful team of hardworking colleagues. Abigail lives with her husband, two children, and Siberian husky in an 1800s farmstead they are restoring (another work in progress) in southern Vermont.

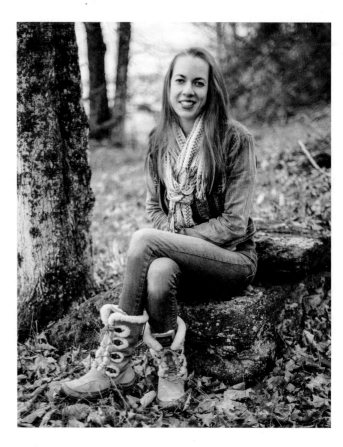

## Other books by Abigail R. Gehring:

*Back to Basics*
*Back to Basics Handbook*
*Classic Candy*
*Complete Guide to Practically Perfect Grandparenting*
*Complete Juicer*
*Country Living Handbook*
*Dangerous Jobs*
*Gluten-Free Miniature Desserts*
*Good Living Guide to Country Skills*
*Healthy Gluten-Free Diet*
*Homesteading*
*Homesteading Handbook*
*Illustrated Encyclopedia of Country Living*
*Odd Jobs*
*Quintessential Quinoa Desserts*
*Self-Sufficiency*
*Self-Sufficiency Handbook*
*Super Easy Soups & Stews*
*Tea Cocktails*
*Ultimate Guide to Old-Fashioned Country Skills*

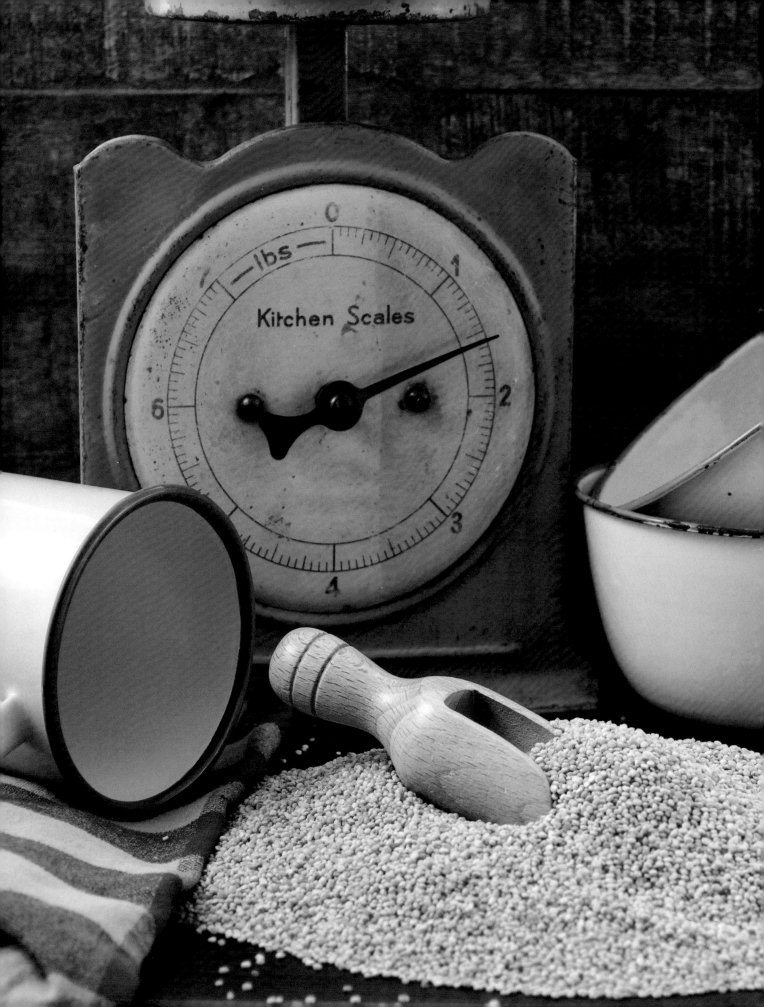

# CONVERSION CHARTS

## Metric Equivalent Measurements

| Weight (Dry Ingredients) | | |
|---|---|---|
| 1 oz | | 30 g |
| 4 oz | ¼ lb | 120 g |
| 8 oz | ½ lb | 240 g |
| 12 oz | ¾ lb | 360 g |
| 16 oz | 1 lb | 480 g |
| 32 oz | 2 lb | 960 g |

| Fahrenheit | Celcius | Gas Mark |
|---|---|---|
| 225° | 110° | ¼ |
| 250° | 120° | ½ |
| 275° | 140° | 1 |
| 300° | 150° | 2 |
| 325° | 160° | 3 |
| 350° | 180° | 4 |
| 375° | 190° | 5 |
| 400° | 200° | 6 |
| 425° | 220° | 7 |
| 450° | 230° | 8 |

| Volume (Liquid Ingredients) | | |
|---|---|---|
| ½ tsp. | | 2 ml |
| 1 tsp. | | 5 ml |
| 1 Tbsp. | ½ fl oz | 15 ml |
| 2 Tbsp. | 1 fl oz | 30 ml |
| ¼ cup | 2 fl oz | 60 ml |
| ⅓ cup | 3 fl oz | 80 ml |
| ½ cup | 4 fl oz | 120 ml |
| ⅔ cup | 5 fl oz | 160 ml |
| ¾ cup | 6 fl oz | 180 ml |
| 1 cup | 8 fl oz | 240 ml |
| 1 pt | 16 fl oz | 480 ml |
| 1 qt | 32 fl oz | 960 ml |

| Length | |
|---|---|
| ¼ in | 6 mm |
| ½ in | 13 mm |
| ¾ in | 19 mm |
| 1 in | 25 mm |
| 6 in | 15 cm |
| 12 in | 30 cm |

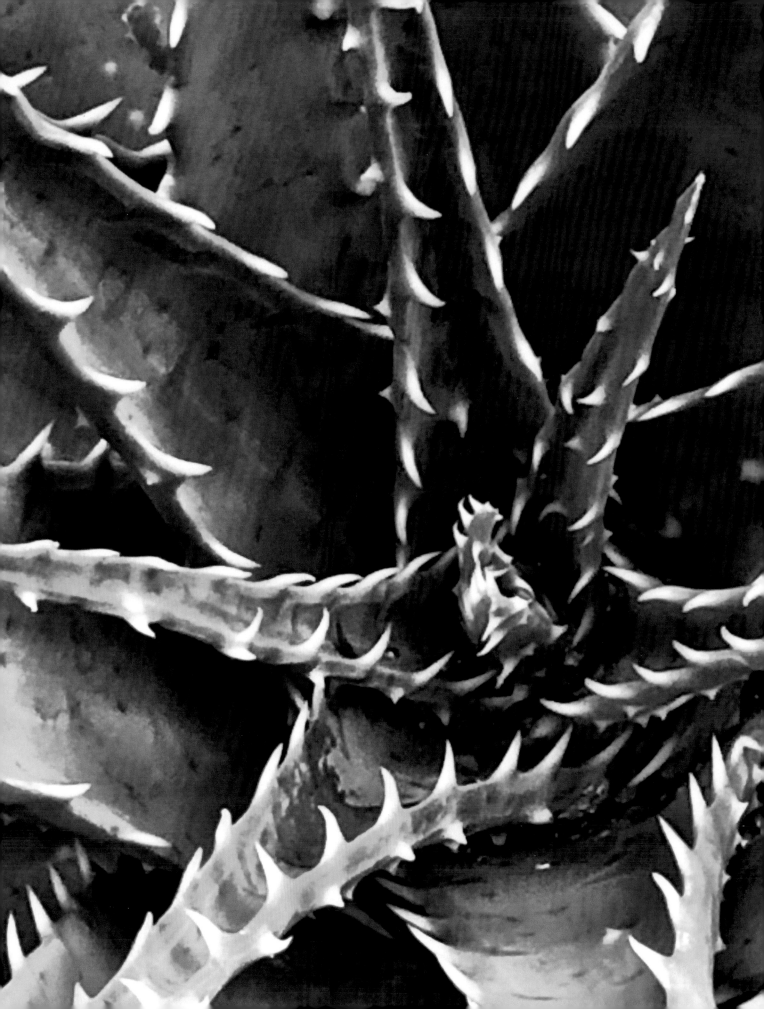

# INDEX

**A**

abortifacient, 126

acid reflux, 32

acne, 54–55

acorn squash
  Quinoa-Stuffed Acorn Squash, 242

acupuncture
  for Alzheimer's disease, 14

adaptogen, 126

air, 306–313

Air-Freshening Diffuser Blend, 321

alcohol, 93

alfalfa, 129

All-Purpose Cleaner, 314

Almond Flour Banana Bread, 240

Almond Flour Waffles, 234

almond milk
  Anti-Inflammatory Spicy Wake-Me-Up Shot, 216
  Maca Hot Chocolate, 299
  Mexican Cocoa, 191
  Trace Minerals Nightcap Shot, 216

almond oil
  Citrus Cream Deodorant, 284
  Simple Homemade Massage Oil, 267

almonds
  Amaranth Cracker Jacks, 247
  Energy Balls, 249
  Tropical Face Cleanser, 280

aloe vera, 129, 130–131, 310
  for dandruff, 60
  Soothe Away the Ouch Sunburn Blend, 67

Aloe Vera Face Cream, 54–55

alterative, 126

Alzheimer's disease, 14

amaranth
  Hot Amaranth Cereal, 236

Amaranth Cracker Jacks, 247

ammonia, 308

analgesic, 126

anemia, 70

anise seed
  Daisy Restorative Lung Tea, 42
  Lactation Tea, 90
  Starstruck Multi-Herb Elixir, 199

anodyne, 126

Anti-Anemia Cocktail, 70

antibacterial, 126

anticatarrhal, 126

antidepressant, 126

Antidepressant Tea, 6

antiemetic, 126

antifungal, 126

anti-inflammatory, 126

Anti-Inflammatory Spicy Wake-Me-Up Shot, 216

antilithic, 126

Antimicrobial Water, 44

antioxidant, 126

antiparasitic, 126

antipyretic, 126

antiseptic, 126

antispasmodic, 126

antitumor, 126

antitussive, 126

antiviral, 126

anxiety, 4

aphrodisiac, 126, 296–302

Aphrodisiac Tea, 299

apple
  Golden Berry Apple, 189
  Green Apple Glee, 178
  Green & Clean, 178
  Green Delight, 177
  Seriously Detox, 180
  Spa Day at Home, 181
  Spicy Charm, 181

apple cider vinegar
  for arthritis, 78
  for asthma, 36

for athlete's foot, 56
Chest Congestion and Sinus Remedy, 38
for constipation, 24
for dandruff, 60
for depression, 6
for diaper rash, 110
for earache, 110
for flatulence, 29
Golden Yellow Spicy Garlic Tonic, 213
Grilled Pear Salad with Green Tea Dressing, 246
for head lice, 113
for hemorrhoids, 62
Herbal Apple Cider and Honey Elixir, 200
Honey Lemon Ginger Drops, 114
for insect bites, 63
for insomnia, 7
Lemon-Honey Facial Mask, 281
for morning sickness, 96
for osteoporosis, 80
Refreshing Galangal Cider, 210
for yeast infection, 100
Apple Cider Vinegar Tonic, 72
Apple Compote, 235
apple juice
    Golden Berry Apple, 189
applesauce
    Vegan Pumpkin Brownies, 246
apricot kernel oil
    Beard Wash Soap, 338–339
apricot oil
    Tropical Face Cleanser, 280
apricots
    Cinnamon Stone Fruit Puree, 255
    Tropical Face Cleanser, 280
argan oil
    Beard Wash Soap, 338–339
arnica, 124
arrowroot
    Basil Lavender Natural Deodorant, 285
    Honey and Coconut Oil Healing Mask, 282
arthritis, 78, 126
Arthritis Joint Rub, 78
ashwagandha, 126
    for multiple sclerosis, 20
asthma, 33

astragalus, 126
    Spicy Immunity Vinegar Tincture, 204
    Stress and Anxiety Support Syrup, 10
    Wellness Blend, 197
astringent, 126
athlete's foot, 56
avocado
    Avocado and Coconut Oil Hydrating Face Mask, 281
    Replenishing Conditioner Treatment for Dry Hair, 274
    Tropical Face Cleanser, 280
Avocado and Coconut Oil Hydrating Face Mask, 281
Avocado Banana Smash, 254
avocado oil
    Beard Wash Soap, 338–339

**B**
baby food, 254–255
Baby's Hand-Sanitizing Spray, 339
Baked Frittata, 238
Baked Gluten-Free Chicken Nuggets with Homemade Ketchup, 256
baking soda
    for athlete's foot, 56
    Bites Be Gone Anti-Itch Paste, 63
    for dandruff, 60
    Poison Ivy Relief, 64
baldness, 104
bamboo palm, 310
banana
    Almond Flour Banana Bread, 240
    Avocado Banana Smash, 254
    Cocoa Pom, 189
    Mango Cream, 186
    Mexican Cocoa, 191
    Replenishing Conditioner Treatment for Dry Hair, 274
    Tropical Face Cleanser, 280
    Vanilla Bean Banana, 186
Banana Ginger Dream, 186
barberry, 124
basil, 126, 234
    Berry Good Hydrating Tonic, 213
    Starstruck Multi-Herb Elixir, 199

Basil Lavender Natural Deodorant, 285
basil oil
    Basil Lavender Natural Deodorant, 285
    Flu-Fighting Neck and Chest Rub, 44
    Lemongrass-Peppermint Toilet Drops, 320
Bathroom Scrub, 319
bath salt, 80
Beachside Break Foot Soak, 278
Beam Me Up Melissa Balm Tea, 4
beans
    black
        Vegetarian Chili, 242
    green
        Green Bean, Pear, and Tofu, 254
    red
        Vegetarian Chili, 242
Beard Wash Soap, 338–339
Beautiful Body Oil, 266
beech, 163
beef bone broth, 225
beeswax
    Basil Lavender Natural Deodorant, 285
    Eczema Lotion Bar, 61
    Super Pain Balm, 82
beet
    Red Hot Love, 177
    Rocking the Roots, 178
Beet and Sweet, 177
belladonna, 124
bell pepper
    Crown Me Queen, 178
    Peachy and Tangy, 177
    Pear and Grape Joy, 177
    Ultimate Cleanser, 181
    Vegetarian Chili, 242
bentonite
    Bites Be Gone Anti-Itch Paste, 63
    Tooth and Gum Health Powder, 342
benzene, 308
bergamot
    Stress-Relieving Diffuser Blend, 10
bergamot oil
    Beard Wash Soap, 338–339
    Citrus Cream Deodorant, 284
    Romantic Massage Blend, 301–302

Sparkling Glass Cleaner, 322
Berry Citrus Cream, 188
Berry Good Hydrating Tonic, 213
bites, insect, 63
Bites Be Gone Anti-Itch Paste, 63
bitter, 126
blackberry
    Blood Orange and Blackberry, 189
black cherry
    Sage Cherry Cough Syrup, 48
black cohosh, 124, 126
black peppercorn
    Super Pain Balm, 82
black pepper oil
    Diarrhea Calming Capsule, 28
    Flu-Fighting Neck and Chest Rub, 44
    Invigorating Cellulite-Reducing Salt Scrub, 291–
        292
blackstrap molasses
    Anti-Anemia Cocktail, 70
    Iron and Energy Syrup, 70
blessed thistle, 129
Blood Orange and Blackberry, 189
blood pressure, 72
blueberry
    Berry Good Hydrating Tonic, 213
    Golden Berry Apple, 189
blue cohosh, 124, 126
body butters, 265
body oiling, 266–267
bone broth, 220–231
boneset, 126
    Cold and Flu Tincture, 40
Bone Up Tea, 81
Boston fern, 308
brandy
    Bronchitis Elixir, 48
breastfeeding, 90
broccoli
    Crown Me Queen, 178
bronchitis, 48
Bronchitis Elixir, 48
bronchodilator, 126
brownies
    Vegan Pumpkin Brownies, 246

brushing, skin, 268–269
buchu, 124
burdock, 126, 129, 163
Butter Me Up, 183

## C

calendula, 129, 132–133
  Skin Healing Oil, 267
  Soothe My Throat Gargle, 114
  Soothing Chamomile Astringent Eyewash, 87
  for sore nipples, 90
  Topical Wash, 100
  for urinary tract infection, 98
Calendula Antiseptic Tincture, 59
Calendula Vein Liniment, 74
California poppy herb, 124
  Beam Me Up Melissa Balm Tea, 4
  Relaxation Blend, 196
calmative, 126
Calming Aromatherapy Facial Steam, 272
canola oil
  Cold-Pressed Soap, 330–331
cantaloupe
  Persimmon Cantaloupe Puree, 254
cardamom
  Sunshine Coconut, Ginger, and Turmeric Tonic, 210
  Yarrow Rose Hip Cold and Flu Relief, 38
carminative, 126
carrot, wild, 124
carrot juice
  Mango Cream, 186
carrots
  Beet and Sweet, 177
  Cherry Tasty, 180
  for eyesight, 87
  Moroccan Chickpea Slow Cooker Stew, 243
  Peachy and Tangy, 177
  Potato and Tomato Spice, 178
  Red Hot Love, 177
  Roasted Carrots with Ginger and Pumpkin, 255
  Rocking the Roots, 178
  Spa Day at Home, 181
cashew milk
  Anti-Inflammatory Spicy Wake-Me-Up Shot, 216

Trace Minerals Nightcap Shot, 216
cashews
  Amaranth Cracker Jacks, 247
castile soap
  Citrus-Fir Dish Soap, 317
  Rosemary Shampoo, 104
  Warm and Woody Shaving Cream, 107
castor oil
  Charcoal Soap, 335–336
  Checkered Soap, 337–338
  Goat Milk Soap, 333
  Resin Soap Two Ways, 336–337
cayenne, 126
  Anti-Inflammatory Spicy Wake-Me-Up Shot, 216
  Cherry Tasty, 180
  for cuts and sores, 59
  Maca Hot Chocolate, 299
  Mexican Cocoa, 191
  Potato and Tomato Spice, 178
  Sunshine Coconut, Ginger, and Turmeric Tonic, 210
CBD-infused bone broth, 231
CBD-infused murumuru butter
  Super Pain Balm, 82
cedar oil
  Pineapple Weed Insect Repellent, 63
celery
  Cherry Tasty, 180
  Mint Condition, 183
  Pear and Grape Joy, 177
  Seriously Detox, 180
  Spa Day at Home, 181
  Ultimate Cleanser, 181
Chai-Infused Coconut Milk Butternut Squash Soup, 243
chamomile, 126, 129, 134
  Calming Aromatherapy Facial Steam, 272
  DIY Chamomile Flower Tea for Anxiety and Stress, 4
  Healthy Gut/Digestion Blend, 197
  for multiple sclerosis, 20
  Relaxation Blend, 196
  Sinus Relief Herbal Steam, 50
  Sleepy Time Chamomile Tincture, 7
  Soothing Chamomile Astringent Eyewash, 87

Tooth and Gum Health Powder, 342
Topical Wash, 100
chamomile oil
    Arthritis Joint Rub, 78
    Comforting Diaper Cream, 110
    Diarrhea Calming Capsule, 28
    Diarrhea Calming Massage Blend, 28
    Eczema Lotion Bar, 61
chaparral, 124
charcoal
    Checkered Soap, 337–338
Charcoal Soap, 335–336
Checkered Soap, 337–338
cheese
    cheddar
        Baked Frittata, 238
        Spinach and Corn Quesadillas, 259
cherries
    Cherry Chocolate Bars, 297
    Dairy-Free Chocolate Cherry Popsicles, 249
    Grapefruit Rosemary, 188
cherry, black
    Sage Cherry Cough Syrup, 48
Cherry Chocolate Bars, 297
cherry juice
    Kumquat Berry Cherry, 188
Cherry Tasty, 180
Chest Congestion and Sinus Remedy, 38
chia seed
    Berry Citrus Cream, 188
    EGCG Power, 191
    Kumquat Berry Cherry, 188
    Tart Peach Cream, 191
chicken
    Baked Gluten-Free Chicken Nuggets with
        Homemade Ketchup, 256
Chickpea Chocolate Chip Cookies, 251
chickpeas
    Chickpea Chocolate Chip Cookies, 251
    Moroccan Chickpea Slow Cooker Stew, 243
chickweed, 126, 129, 136
chicory, 163–164
Chinese evergreen, 310
chocolate
    Dairy-Free Chocolate Cherry Popsicles, 249

chocolate chips
    Chickpea Chocolate Chip Cookies, 251
cholagogue, 126
choleretic, 129
cholesterol, 71
Cholesterol-Lowering Tea, 71
cilantro
    Cooling Peppermint Herb Tonic, 212
    Youth Glow, 181
cinnamon, 234
    Apple Compote, 235
    Cinnamon Stone Fruit Puree, 255
    Easy Coconut Mango Blender Sorbet, 247
    Energy Balls, 249
    Golden Yellow Spicy Garlic Tonic, 213
    Healthy Moon Cycle Blend, 95
    Hot Amaranth Cereal, 236
    Maca Hot Chocolate, 299
    Mexican Cocoa, 191
    Quinoa-Stuffed Acorn Squash, 242
    Refreshing Galangal Cider, 210
    Roasted Carrots with Ginger and Pumpkin, 255
    Roasted Vegetables, 245
    Starstruck Multi-Herb Elixir, 199
    Sweet Potato Pancakes, 236
    Yarrow Rose Hip Cold and Flu Relief, 38
cinnamon oil
    Antimicrobial Water, 44
    Flu-Fighting Gargle, 44
    Invigorating Cellulite-Reducing Salt Scrub, 291–
        292
    Menstrual Relief Massage Blend, 94
Cinnamon Stone Fruit Puree, 255
citronella oil
    Pineapple Weed Insect Repellent, 63
Citrus Cream Deodorant, 284
Citrus-Fir Dish Soap, 317
clary sage oil
    Menstrual Relief Massage Blend, 94
    Romantic Massage Blend, 301–302
clay, bentonite
    Bites Be Gone Anti-Itch Paste, 63
    Tooth and Gum Health Powder, 342
cleaning, 314–332
cleavers

Soothe My Throat Gargle, 114
clove, 126
    Cold Care Syrup, 38
    Super Pain Balm, 82
    Tooth and Gum Health Powder, 342
    Yarrow Rose Hip Cold and Flu Relief, 38
clove oil
    Flu-Fighting Gargle, 44
    Kid-Safe Hand-Sanitizing Spray, 339–340
    Menstrual Relief Massage Blend, 94
clover, red, 126
    Bone Up Tea, 81
    High Mineral Vinegar Tincture, 204
cocoa butter
    Basil Lavender Natural Deodorant, 285
    Beard Wash Soap, 338–339
Cocoa Pom, 189
cocoa powder
    Cherry Chocolate Bars, 297
coconut
    Easy Coconut Mango Blender Sorbet, 247
Coconut Lime Verbena Sugar Scrub, 289
coconut milk
    Berry Citrus Cream, 188
    Dairy-Free Chocolate Cherry Popsicles, 249
    Tart Peach Cream, 191
coconut oil
    Aloe Vera Face Cream, 54–55
    for Alzheimer's disease, 14
    for arthritis, 78
    for asthma, 36
    for athlete's foot, 56
    Avocado and Coconut Oil Hydrating Face Mask,
        281
    Basil Lavender Natural Deodorant, 285
    Beard Wash Soap, 338–339
    Beautiful Body Oil, 266
    Charcoal Soap, 335–336
    Checkered Soap, 337–338
    Cherry Chocolate Bars, 297
    Coconut Lime Verbena Sugar Scrub, 289
    for cold, 40
    Cold-Pressed Soap, 330
    for cold sores, 57
    Comforting Diaper Cream, 110

    for constipation, 24
    for corns, 58
    for dandruff, 60
    Decongestant Oregano Coconut Vapor Rub, 42
    DIY Vapor Rub, 42
    for earache, 110
    for eczema, 61
    for flu, 40
    Goat Milk Soap, 333
    for hay fever, 46
    for hemorrhoids, 62
    Honey and Coconut Oil Healing Mask, 282
    Lavender Herbal Infusion Soap, 334–335
    Lemon Pepper Anti-Dandruff Mask, 274
    Menstrual Relief Massage Blend, 94
    Mermaids Kisses Salty Sea Soap, 332
    for multiple sclerosis, 20
    for muscle sprains and pulls, 82
    Poison Ivy Relief, 64
    for psoriasis, 65
    for rashes, 66
    Replenishing Conditioner Treatment for Dry Hair,
        274
    Resin Soap Two Ways, 336–337
    Skin Healing Oil, 267
    for sunburn, 67
    Super Pain Balm, 82
    for urinary tract infection, 98
    Whipped Coconut Oil Body Butter, 265
coconut water
    Gingerly Recovery, 183
    Spicy Pomegranate and Coconut Tonic, 212
    Sunshine Coconut, Ginger, and Turmeric Tonic,
        210
coffee
    Chickpea Chocolate Chip Cookies, 251
    Invigorating Cellulite-Reducing Salt Scrub,
        291–292
cold, 38, 40, 223
Cold and Flu Tincture, 40
Cold Care Syrup, 38
Cold-Pressed Soap, 330–331
cold sores, 57
collar wash, 325
coltsfoot, 124, 126, 129

Comforting Diaper Cream, 110
comfrey, 124, 126, 129
    Skin Healing Oil, 267
    Super Green Vitamin/Mineral Blend, 196
    Tooth and Gum Health Mouthwash, 342
common cold, 38, 40, 223
constipation, 24
cookies
    Chickpea Chocolate Chip Cookies, 251
Cool as a Cucumber, 181
Cooling Peppermint Herb Tonic, 212
CoQ10
    for infertility, 105
corns, 58
    Spinach and Corn Quesadillas, 259
    Vegetarian Chili, 242
corn silk, 126
cornstarch
    Comforting Diaper Cream, 110
cough, 42, 126
cramp bark, 126
    Tummy Tamer Tea, 30
cranberry
    Amaranth Cracker Jacks, 247
    Energy Balls, 249
    for multiple sclerosis, 20
    Quinoa-Stuffed Acorn Squash, 242
cranberry juice
    Kumquat Berry Cherry, 188
    Tart Peach Cream, 191
    for urinary tract infection, 98
Creamy Mango and Yogurt, 255
Crohn's disease, 26
Crown Me Queen, 178
cucumber
    Avocado and Coconut Oil Hydrating Face Mask,
        281
    Berry Good Hydrating Tonic, 213
    Butter Me Up, 183
    Cool as a Cucumber, 181
    Crown Me Queen, 178
    Deep Kiwi Green, 181
    Gingerly Recovery, 183
    Green Apple Glee, 178
    Green Delight, 177

Kale to the Rescue, 183
    Mint Condition, 183
    Minty Cucumber Facial Mask, 282
    Pear and Grape Joy, 177
    Pine for Me, 180
    Seriously Detox, 180
    Spicy Charm, 181
    Ultimate Cleanser, 181
    Youth Glow, 181
Cucumber Pom Mint, 191
cuts, 59
cypress oil
    Flu-Fighting Neck and Chest Rub, 44

D
Dairy-Free Chocolate Cherry Popsicles, 249
daisy, 138
    Pineapple Weed Insect Repellent, 63
Daisy Restorative Lung Tea, 42
damiana, 126
    Aphrodisiac Tea, 299
dandelion, 126, 129, 164
    Digestion Tincture, 30
    Iron and Energy Syrup, 70
    for multiple sclerosis, 20
    for psoriasis, 65
    Vitamin C Flower Power Blend, 196
Dandelion Abscess Poultice, 65
dandruff, 60
dates
    Energy Balls, 249
Decongestant Oregano Coconut Vapor Rub, 42
Deep Kiwi Green, 181
demulcent, 129
deodorant, 284–285
depression, 6
DHA
    for multiple sclerosis, 20
diabetes, 155
diaper rash, 110
diaphoretic, 129
diarrhea, 28
Diarrhea Calming Capsule, 28
Diarrhea Calming Massage Blend, 28
Digestion Tincture, 30

dill
    Cool as a Cucumber, 181
    Cooling Peppermint Herb Tonic, 212
diuretic, 129
DIY Chamomile Flower Tea for Anxiety and Stress, 4
DIY Vapor Rub, 42
dog perfume, 327
dong quai, 124
    Healthy Moon Cycle Blend, 95
    Tea for Migraines, 19
dragon's blood resin
    Resin Soap Two Ways, 336–337
dry brushing, 268–269
dryer sheets, 323

**E**
earache, 110
earwax, 86
Easy Coconut Mango Blender Sorbet, 247
Easy Lentil Stew, 245
echinacea, 126, 129
    Cold and Flu Tincture, 40
    Cold Care Syrup, 38
    for multiple sclerosis, 20
    Tooth and Gum Health Mouthwash, 342
    Wellness Blend, 197
eczema, 61
Eczema Lotion Bar, 61
EGCG Power, 191
eggs
    Baked Frittata, 238
elder, 126
    Skin Healing Oil, 267
elderberries, 164
    Cold and Flu Tincture, 40
    Cold Care Syrup, 38
elder blossom
    Wellness Blend, 197
elecampene, 126, 129
eleuthero, 126
    Energizing Blend, 197
    Stress and Anxiety Support Syrup, 10
elixirs, 199–200
emetic, 129
emmenagogue, 129

emollient, 129
endive
    Deep Kiwi Green, 181
Energizing Blend, 197
Energy Balls, 249
English ivy, 308
eucalyptus oil
    Gunk and Grease-Removing Spray, 318
    Mermaids Kisses Salty Sea Soap, 332
    Sinus Relief Herbal Steam, 50
evening primrose
    Eczema Lotion Bar, 61
evening primrose oil
    Beard Wash Soap, 338–339
    Orange Blossom Honey Salt Scrub, 293
expectorant, 129
Eye'll Be Gentle Makeup Remover, 280
eye pillow, 19
eyestrain, 87

**F**
face masks, 281–282
facial oiling, 270
facial steams, 271–272
Farnoosh's Magic Potion Tonic Recipe, 214
farting, 29
*FastDiet, The* (Mosley), 169
fennel, 126, 129
    Green & Clean, 178
    Kale to the Rescue, 183
fennel oil
    Diarrhea Calming Capsule, 28
    Heartburn Relief, 32
    Menstrual Relief Massage Blend, 94
    Sage Cherry Cough Syrup, 48
fennel seed
    Healthy Gut/Digestion Blend, 197
    Healthy Moon Cycle Blend, 95
    Lavender and Orange Zest Dream Elixir, 200
    Lemongrass Ginger Thyme Elixir, 199
    Tummy and Teething Calm Popsicle, 116
fenugreek, 129
fenugreek seed
    Lactation Tea, 90
feverfew, 124

Headache Tincture, 16
Tummy and Teething Calm Popsicle, 116
fish bone broth, 228
fitness, 223–224
flamingo lily, 310
flatulence, 29
flu, 40, 44–45
Flu-Fighting Foot Rub, 45
Flu-Fighting Gargle, 44
Flu-Fighting Neck and Chest Rub, 44
folic acid
for infertility, 90, 105
foot soak, 278
foot treatments, 278
Forget-Me-Not Tea, 8
formaldehyde, 308
frankincense oil
Arthritis Joint Rub, 78
Eczema Lotion Bar, 61
free radicals, 169
fruit cleaner, 318

**G**
galactogogue, 129
galangal
Refreshing Galangal Cider, 210
gardens, herb, 122–123
garlic, 126, 129, 234
Cold and Flu Tincture, 40
Farnoosh's Magic Potion Tonic Recipe, 214
Flu-Fighting Foot Rub, 45
Golden Yellow Spicy Garlic Tonic, 213
Mullein and Garlic Ear Oil, 86
Roasted Vegetables, 245
Spicy Immunity Vinegar Tincture, 204
Vegetarian Chili, 242
geranium oil
Baby's Hand-Sanitizing Spray, 339
Bathroom Scrub, 319
Kid-Safe Hand-Sanitizing Spray, 339–340
Lemongrass-Peppermint Toilet Drops, 320
Menstrual Relief Massage Blend, 94
Orange Blossom Honey Salt Scrub, 293
Sweet and Subtle Sugar Scrub, 291
ginger, 234

Anti-Inflammatory Spicy Wake-Me-Up Shot, 216
Banana Ginger Dream, 186
Berry Good Hydrating Tonic, 213
Butter Me Up, 183
Cherry Tasty, 180
Cholesterol-Lowering Tea, 71
Cold and Flu Tincture, 40
Cool as a Cucumber, 181
Digestion Tincture, 30
Energizing Blend, 197
Farnoosh's Magic Potion Tonic Recipe, 214
Gingerly Recovery, 183
Golden Yellow Spicy Garlic Tonic, 213
Healthy Gut/Digestion Blend, 197
Honey Lemon Ginger Drops, 114
Kale to the Rescue, 183
Lemongrass Ginger Thyme Elixir, 199
Mint Condition, 183
for multiple sclerosis, 20
Pain Relief Tonic, 94
Peachy and Tangy, 177
Pine for Me, 180
Red Hot Love, 177
Rocking the Roots, 178
Sage Cherry Cough Syrup, 48
Seriously Detox, 180
Spicy Charm, 181
Spicy Immunity Vinegar Tincture, 204
Spicy Pomegranate and Coconut Tonic, 212
Stomach-Stabilizing Tea, 33
Sunshine Coconut, Ginger, and Turmeric Tonic, 210
Super Pain Balm, 82
Tummy Tamer Tea, 30
Ultimate Cleanser, 181
Yarrow Rose Hip Cold and Flu Relief, 38
Gingerly Recovery, 183
ginger oil
Arthritis Joint Rub, 78
Diarrhea Calming Massage Blend, 28
Head Cold Tea, 40
Invigorating Cellulite-Reducing Salt Scrub, 291–292
Menstrual Relief Massage Blend, 94
ginkgo

Forget-Me-Not Tea, 8
ginkgo biloba
    for multiple sclerosis, 20
ginseng, 124, 126, 129, 299
    Forget-Me-Not Tea, 8
glycerin
    Baby's Hand-Sanitizing Spray, 339
    Kid-Safe Hand-Sanitizing Spray, 339–340
    Rosemary Shampoo, 104
Goat Milk Soap, 333
Golden Berry Apple, 189
golden pothos, 308–310
goldenseal, 124, 126
    Cold and Flu Tincture, 40
Golden Yellow Spicy Garlic Tonic, 213
grapefruit
    Red Hot Love, 177
Grapefruit and Green Tea, 189
grapefruit oil
    Invigorating Cellulite-Reducing Salt Scrub,
        291–292
Grapefruit Rosemary, 188
grapefruit seed extract
    Looking Good Enough to Eat Fruit and Veggie
        Cleaner, 318
grapes, 178
    Cool as a Cucumber, 181
    Deep Kiwi Green, 181
    Gingerly Recovery, 183
    Green Apple Glee, 178
    Mint Condition, 183
    Pear and Grape Joy, 177
    Spa Day at Home, 181
    Youth Glow, 181
grape-seed oil
    Pineapple Weed Insect Repellent, 63
gravel root, 126
greater celandine, 124
Green Apple Glee, 178
Green Bean, Pear, and Tofu, 254
Green & Clean, 178
Green Delight, 177
green onion
    Head Cold Tea, 40
green tea

Banana Ginger Dream, 186
Berry Citrus Cream, 188
Blood Orange and Blackberry, 189
Cholesterol-Lowering Tea, 71
Cocoa Pom, 189
for dandruff, 60
EGCG Power, 191
Grapefruit and Green Tea, 189
Grapefruit Rosemary, 188
Grilled Pear Salad with Green Tea Dressing, 246
Kumquat Berry Cherry, 188
Mango Cream, 186
Tart Peach Cream, 191
Vanilla Bean Banana, 186
Grilled Pear Salad with Green Tea Dressing, 246
Gunk and Grease-Removing Spray, 318

**H**
hair conditioner, 277
Hair Rinse, 104
hair treatments, 274–277
hand sanitizer, 339–340
hawthorn, 129
    Antidepressant Tea, 6
hay fever, 46
Hay Fever Relief Diffuser Blend, 46
hazelnuts
    Energy Balls, 249
headache, 16, 19
Headache Be Gone, 16
Headache Tincture, 16
Head Cold Tea, 40
head lice, 113
healing, 223–224
Healthy Gut/Digestion Blend, 197
Healthy Moon Cycle Blend, 95
heartburn, 32
Heartburn Relief, 32
heart tonic, 129
hemorrhoids, 62
hemostatic, 129
hemp seed
    Blood Orange and Blackberry, 189
    Cucumber Pom Mint, 191
    Golden Berry Apple, 189

Grapefruit Rosemary, 188
Mango Cream, 186
Mexican Cocoa, 191
hepatoprotective, 129
Herbal Apple Cider and Honey Elixir, 200
herbal infusion, 194–196
herb gardens, 122–123
hibiscus
Vitamin C Flower Power Blend, 196
high blood pressure, 72
High Mineral Vinegar Tincture, 204
Homemade Crock-Pot Yogurt, 240
Honey and Coconut Oil Healing Mask, 282
Honey Lemon Ginger Drops, 114
hops, 126
hops rhizome
Pain Relief Tonic, 94
hops strobiles
Heartburn Relief, 32
horehound, 129
Hormonal Balance, 204
horseradish
Spicy Immunity Vinegar Tincture, 204
horsetail
Bone Up Tea, 81
High Mineral Vinegar Tincture, 204
Hot Amaranth Cereal, 236
houseplants, 306–313
hydrangea, 126
hypotensive, 129

I
immunomodulator, 129
infertility
in men, 105–106
in women, 90
inflammatory disorders, 220–222
influenza, 44–45
Cold and Flu Tincture, 40
infusions, 194–196
Ingestible Hay Fever Relief, 46
injury recovery, 223–224
insect bites, 63
insomnia, 7
Invigorating Cellulite-Reducing Salt Scrub, 291–292

Iron and Energy Syrup, 70
irritable bowel syndrome (IBS), 30–31
ivy, 308–310

J
jalapeño
Spicy Charm, 181
Spicy Pomegranate and Coconut Tonic, 212
Vegetarian Chili, 242
jojoba oil
Beautiful Body Oil, 266
Eye'll Be Gentle Makeup Remover, 280
Invigorating Cellulite-Reducing Salt Scrub,
291–292
Rosemary Shampoo, 104
Simple Homemade Massage Oil, 267
juices, 177–183
juicing, 170–173
juniper, 124, 126
juniper berry oil
Arthritis Joint Rub, 78

K
kale
Cool as a Cucumber, 181
Gingerly Recovery, 183
Green & Clean, 178
Green Delight, 177
Kale to the Rescue, 183
Pine for Me, 180
Quinoa-Stuffed Acorn Squash, 242
Ultimate Cleanser, 181
Kale to the Rescue, 183
kava, 126
kelp
Iron and Energy Syrup, 70
Kid-Safe Hand-Sanitizing Spray, 339–340
kiwi
Deep Kiwi Green, 181
Tropical Face Cleanser, 280
Youth Glow, 181
Kombucha, 30
Kumquat Berry Cherry, 188

## L

lactation, 90
Lactation Tea, 90
lamb bone broth, 228
laundry, 323–324
lavender, 126, 140
  Beam Me Up Melissa Balm Tea, 4
  Calming Aromatherapy Facial Steam, 272
  Headache Be Gone, 16
  Lavender and Orange Zest Dream Elixir, 200
  Lavender Bath Salt, 80
  Peppermint Lavender Mouthwash, 341
  Relaxation Blend, 196
  Stress-Relieving Diffuser Blend, 10
  Tea for Migraines, 19
  Tooth and Gum Health Mouthwash, 342
Lavender and Orange Zest Dream Elixir, 200
Lavender Bath Salt, 80
Lavender Herbal Infusion Soap, 334–335
lavender oil
  Basil Lavender Natural Deodorant, 285
  Beard Wash Soap, 338–339
  Comforting Diaper Cream, 110
  Eczema Lotion Bar, 61
  Hay Fever Relief Diffuser Blend, 46
  Ingestible Hay Fever Relief, 46
  Lavender Bath Salt, 80
  Lemon Pepper Anti-Dandruff Mask, 274
  Menstrual Relief Massage Blend, 94
  Pineapple Weed Insect Repellent, 63
  Poison Ivy Relief, 64
  Soothe Away the Ouch Sunburn Blend, 67
laxative, 129
leash wash, 325
leek
  Turnip Leek Mash, 254
lemon
  Beet and Sweet, 177
  Butter Me Up, 183
  Cherry Tasty, 180
  Chest Congestion and Sinus Remedy, 38
  for dandruff, 60
  Deep Kiwi Green, 181
  Farnoosh's Magic Potion Tonic Recipe, 214
  Gingerly Recovery, 183

  Golden Yellow Spicy Garlic Tonic, 213
  Honey Lemon Ginger Drops, 114
  Kale to the Rescue, 183
  Lemon Pepper Anti-Dandruff Mask, 274
  Pine for Me, 180
  Potato and Tomato Spice, 178
  Rocking the Roots, 178
  Seriously Detox, 180
  Spicy Pomegranate and Coconut Tonic, 212
  Ultimate Cleanser, 181
lemon balm, 126, 143
  Antidepressant Tea, 6
  Beam Me Up Melissa Balm Tea, 4
  Headache Tincture, 16
  Stress and Anxiety Support Syrup, 10
  Tummy Tamer Tea, 30
  Vitamin C Flower Power Blend, 196
lemongrass
  Cooling Peppermint Herb Tonic, 212
  Energizing Blend, 197
  Herbal Apple Cider and Honey Elixir, 200
  Sunshine Coconut, Ginger, and Turmeric Tonic, 210
Lemongrass Ginger Thyme Elixir, 199
lemongrass oil
  Air-Freshening Diffuser Blend, 321
  All-Purpose Cleaner, 314
  Antimicrobial Water, 44
  Bathroom Scrub, 319
  Citrus-Fir Dish Soap, 317
  Kid-Safe Hand-Sanitizing Spray, 339–340
  Lemongrass-Peppermint Toilet Drops, 320
  Mermaids Kisses Salty Sea Soap, 332
  Sanitizing Counter Spray, 315
Lemongrass-Peppermint Toilet Drops, 320
Lemon-Honey Facial Mask, 281
lemon oil
  Air-Freshening Diffuser Blend, 321
  All-Purpose Cleaner, 314
  Antimicrobial Water, 44
  Bathroom Scrub, 319
  Beard Wash Soap, 338–339
  Citrus Cream Deodorant, 284
  Citrus-Fir Dish Soap, 317
  Decongestant Oregano Coconut Vapor Rub, 42

Flu-Fighting Gargle, 44
Gunk and Grease-Removing Spray, 318
Hay Fever Relief Diffuser Blend, 46
Ingestible Hay Fever Relief, 46
Sparkling Glass Cleaner, 322
Stress-Relieving Diffuser Blend, 10
Lemon Pepper Anti-Dandruff Mask, 274
lemon verbena
Coconut Lime Verbena Sugar Scrub, 289
lentils
Easy Lentil Stew, 245
lettuce
Butter Me Up, 183
lice, 113
licorice, 124
Tooth and Gum Health Powder, 342
Yarrow Rose Hip Cold and Flu Relief, 38
lime
Anti-Anemia Cocktail, 70
Blood Orange and Blackberry, 189
Cherry Tasty, 180
Crown Me Queen, 178
Cucumber Pom Mint, 191
Green Apple Glee, 178
Mint Condition, 183
Spa Day at Home, 181
Sunshine Coconut, Ginger, and Turmeric Tonic, 210
Ultimate Cleanser, 181
Youth Glow, 181
lime oil
Air-Freshening Diffuser Blend, 321
All-Purpose Cleaner, 314
Beard Wash Soap, 338–339
Citrus Cream Deodorant, 284
Citrus-Fir Dish Soap, 317
Coconut Lime Verbena Sugar Scrub, 289
litter box cleaner, 328
liver, 168
Looking Good Enough to Eat Fruit and Veggie Cleaner, 318
lye
Beard Wash Soap, 338–339
Charcoal Soap, 335–336
Checkered Soap, 337–338

Cold-Pressed Soap, 330–331
Goat Milk Soap, 333
Lavender Herbal Infusion Soap, 334–335
Mermaids Kisses Salty Sea Soap, 332
Resin Soap Two Ways, 336–337
lymphagogue, 129

**M**
Maca Hot Chocolate, 299
makeup remover, 280
mandala garden, 122
mango
Creamy Mango and Yogurt, 255
Easy Coconut Mango Blender Sorbet, 247
Mango Cream, 186
Mango Cream, 186
Maple Citrus-Glazed Salmon, 241
maple syrup
Cooling Peppermint Herb Tonic, 212
Lavender and Orange Zest Dream Elixir, 200
marjoram oil
Comforting Diaper Cream, 110
Menstrual Relief Massage Blend, 94
masks, 281–282
massage oil
Simple Homemade Massage Oil, 267
mayonnaise
Replenishing Conditioner Treatment for Dry Hair, 274
medicine wheel garden, 123
melaleuca oil
Air-Freshening Diffuser Blend, 321
All-Purpose Cleaner, 314
Baby's Hand-Sanitizing Spray, 339
Citrus Cream Deodorant, 284
Flu-Fighting Gargle, 44
Flu-Fighting Neck and Chest Rub, 44
Kid-Safe Hand-Sanitizing Spray, 339–340
memory loss, 8, 154
menopause, 155
men's health, 104–107
Menstrual Relief Massage Blend, 94
menstruation, 94–95
menstruum
Digestion Tincture, 30

Headache Tincture, 16
Hormonal Balance, 204
Mermaids Kisses Salty Sea Soap, 332
Mexican Cocoa, 191
migraine, 19
mint, 144
Cucumber Pom Mint, 191
DIY Chamomile Flower Tea for Anxiety and Stress, 4
Herbal Apple Cider and Honey Elixir, 200
Kale to the Rescue, 183
Lemongrass Ginger Thyme Elixir, 199
Mint Condition, 183
Minty Cucumber Facial Mask, 282
Peppermint Lavender Mouthwash, 341
Refreshing Galangal Cider, 210
Spicy Pomegranate and Coconut Tonic, 212
Ultimate Cleanser, 181
Mint Condition, 183
Minty Cucumber Facial Mask, 282
mistletoe, 124
molasses
Anti-Anemia Cocktail, 70
Baked Gluten-Free Chicken Nuggets with
Homemade Ketchup, 256
Iron and Energy Syrup, 70
moon garden, 122
morning sickness, 96
Moroccan Chickpea Slow Cooker Stew, 243
Mosley, Michael, 169
motherwort, 126, 129
mouthwash, 341–342
muffins
Oatmeal Pumpkin Muffins, 238
mugwort, 126
mu huang, 124
mullein, 126, 129
Mullein and Garlic Ear Oil, 86
mullein leaf
Bronchitis Elixir, 48
Sage Cherry Cough Syrup, 48
Mullein Tea, 36
multiple sclerosis, 20
murumuru butter
Super Pain Balm, 82

muscle sprains and pulls, 82
mushrooms
Baked Frittata, 238
Quinoa Risotto with Shiitake Mushrooms and
Arugula, 241
mustard, 299
myrrh, 124, 337
Resin Soap Two Ways, 336–337
Tooth and Gum Health Powder, 342
myrrh oil
Arthritis Joint Rub, 78

N
nausea, 33
nervine, 129
nettle, 126, 129, 164
Healthy Moon Cycle Blend, 95
High Mineral Vinegar Tincture, 204
Iron and Energy Syrup, 70
Lactation Tea, 90
Super Green Vitamin/Mineral Blend, 196
nipples, sore, 90
nutritive, 129

O
oatmeal
for poison ivy, 64
Oatmeal Pumpkin Muffins, 238
oat tops, 126, 129
Relaxation Blend, 196
Stress and Anxiety Support Syrup, 10
olive oil
Beard Wash Soap, 338–339
Charcoal Soap, 335–336
Checkered Soap, 337–338
Flu-Fighting Foot Rub, 45
Goat Milk Soap, 333
Gunk and Grease-Removing Spray, 318
Lavender Herbal Infusion Soap, 334–335
Mermaids Kisses Salty Sea Soap, 332
Mullein and Garlic Ear Oil, 86
Resin Soap Two Ways, 336–337
Skin Healing Oil, 267
Sweet and Subtle Sugar Scrub, 291
omega-3 fatty acids

for Alzheimer's disease, 14
for infertility, 105
for multiple sclerosis, 20
for sore nipples, 90
omega-6 fatty acids, 90
for multiple sclerosis, 20
omega-9 fatty acids, 90
onion
Spicy Immunity Vinegar Tincture, 204
onion, green
Head Cold Tea, 40
orange
Beet and Sweet, 177
blood
Blood Orange and Blackberry, 189
Refreshing Galangal Cider, 210
Cocoa Pom, 189
Cool as a Cucumber, 181
Cooling Peppermint Herb Tonic, 212
Golden Yellow Spicy Garlic Tonic, 213
Lavender and Orange Zest Dream Elixir, 200
Starstruck Multi-Herb Elixir, 199
Orange Blossom Honey Salt Scrub, 293
orange juice
Banana Ginger Dream, 186
Berry Citrus Cream, 188
Grapefruit Rosemary, 188
Vanilla Bean Banana, 186
orange oil
Baby's Hand-Sanitizing Spray, 339
Bathroom Scrub, 319
Citrus Cream Deodorant, 284
Diarrhea Calming Massage Blend, 28
Invigorating Cellulite-Reducing Salt Scrub, 291–292
Kid-Safe Hand-Sanitizing Spray, 339–340
Orange Blossom Honey Salt Scrub, 293
Sparkling Glass Cleaner, 322
orange peel
Aphrodisiac Tea, 299
Healthy Gut/Digestion Blend, 197
Heartburn Relief, 32
oregano, 146
Spicy Pomegranate and Coconut Tonic, 212
Starstruck Multi-Herb Elixir, 199

oregano oil
Decongestant Oregano Coconut Vapor Rub, 42
Flu-Fighting Foot Rub, 45
Flu-Fighting Gargle, 44
Sanitizing Counter Spray, 315
osha, 126
osteoporosis, 80
overeating, 168–169

P
pain, general, 80
Pain Relief Tonic, 94
palm oil
Cold-Pressed Soap, 330
papaya
Tropical Face Cleanser, 280
parsley, 124, 148
Butter Me Up, 183
Forget-Me-Not Tea, 8
Gingerly Recovery, 183
Green Delight, 177
Healthy Moon Cycle Blend, 95
Kale to the Rescue, 183
Pine for Me, 180
Seriously Detox, 180
Spa Day at Home, 181
Spicy Charm, 181
Spicy Immunity Vinegar Tincture, 204
parsnip
Cherry Tasty, 180
Spa Day at Home, 181
passion flower
Relaxation Blend, 196
patchouli
Beard Wash Soap, 338–339
peace lily, 310
peach
Banana Ginger Dream, 186
Grapefruit and Green Tea, 189
Mint Condition, 183
Tart Peach Cream, 191
Tropical Face Cleanser, 280
Peachy and Tangy, 177
peanut butter
Chickpea Chocolate Chip Cookies, 251

pear
    Crown Me Queen, 178
    Deep Kiwi Green, 181
    Green & Clean, 178
    Pear and Grape Joy, 177
Pear and Grape Joy, 177
pennyroyal, 124, 126
peppermint, 126
    Calming Aromatherapy Facial Steam, 272
    Energizing Blend, 197
    Headache Be Gone, 16
    Healthy Gut/Digestion Blend, 197
    for multiple sclerosis, 20
    for sore nipples, 90
    Stomach-Stabilizing Tea, 33
    Super Green Vitamin/Mineral Blend, 196
    Tea for Migraines, 19
    Tooth and Gum Health Powder, 342
Peppermint Lavender Mouthwash, 341
peppermint oil
    Cooling Peppermint Herb Tonic, 212
    Diarrhea Calming Capsule, 28
    Hay Fever Relief Diffuser Blend, 46
    Ingestible Hay Fever Relief, 46
    for irritable bowel syndrome, 30
    Lemongrass-Peppermint Toilet Drops, 320
    Lice Repellent, 113
    Peppermint Lavender Mouthwash, 341
    Poison Ivy Relief, 64
    Rosemary Peppermint Foot Scrub, 278
    Rosemary Shampoo, 104
Persimmon Cantaloupe Puree, 254
pet care, 325
pillow, eye, 19
pineapple
    EGCG Power, 191
    Pine for Me, 180
    Vanilla Bean Banana, 186
pineapple weed
    Beam Me Up Melissa Balm Tea, 4
    Heartburn Relief, 32
    Pineapple Weed Insect Repellent, 63
Pineapple Weed Insect Repellent, 63
Pine for Me, 180
plantain leaf, 126, 129

    Sage Cherry Cough Syrup, 48
plums
    Cinnamon Stone Fruit Puree, 255
pneumonia, 48
poison ivy, 64
Poison Ivy Relief, 64
pokeweed, 124
pomegranate juice
    Cocoa Pom, 189
    Cucumber Pom Mint, 191
    EGCG Power, 191
pomegranate seeds
    Spicy Pomegranate and Coconut Tonic, 212
poppy, 126
popsicle
    Dairy-Free Chocolate Cherry Popsicles, 249
    Tummy and Teething Calm Popsicle, 116
potato
    Easy Lentil Stew, 245
    Roasted Vegetables, 245
potato, sweet
    Potato and Tomato Spice, 178
    Roasted Vegetables, 245
    Rocking the Roots, 178
Potato and Tomato Spice, 178
pregnancy, 96, 124
prunes
    Energy Balls, 249
psoriasis, 65
pumpkin
    Oatmeal Pumpkin Muffins, 238
    Roasted Carrots with Ginger and Pumpkin, 255
    Vegan Pumpkin Brownies, 246

Q
quesadillas
    Spinach and Corn Quesadillas, 259
quinoa
    Cherry Chocolate Bars, 297
Quinoa Risotto with Shiitake Mushrooms and
    Arugula, 241
Quinoa-Stuffed Acorn Squash, 242

R
rashes, 66

raspberry leaf, 126
    Healthy Moon Cycle Blend, 95
    High Mineral Vinegar Tincture, 204
    Hormonal Balance, 204
    Pain Relief Tonic, 94
    Soothing Chamomile Astringent Eyewash, 87
    Super Green Vitamin/Mineral Blend, 196
red clover, 126
    Bone Up Tea, 81
    High Mineral Vinegar Tincture, 204
Red Hot Love, 177
red raspberry leaf, 126
    High Mineral Vinegar Tincture, 204
    Hormonal Balance, 204
    Pain Relief Tonic, 94
    Soothing Chamomile Astringent Eyewash, 87
Refreshing Galangal Cider, 210
Relaxation Blend, 196
Replenishing Conditioner Treatment for Dry Hair,
    274
Resin Soap Two Ways, 336–337
Roasted Carrots with Ginger and Pumpkin, 255
Roasted Vegetables, 245
Rocking the Roots, 178
Roman chamomile
    Eczema Lotion Bar, 61
Roman chamomile oil
    Arthritis Joint Rub, 78
    Comforting Diaper Cream, 110
Romantic Massage Blend, 301–302
rosebuds
    Calming Aromatherapy Facial Steam, 272
rose geranium oil
    Basil Lavender Natural Deodorant, 285
rose hips
    Vitamin C Flower Power Blend, 196
    Wellness Blend, 197
rosemary, 150–153, 234
    Grapefruit Rosemary, 188
    Hair Rinse, 104
    Headache Be Gone, 16
    Headache Tincture, 16
    Herbal Apple Cider and Honey Elixir, 200
    Kumquat Berry Cherry, 188
    Roasted Vegetables, 245

Rosemary Digestive Tea, 29
    Rosemary Peppermint Foot Scrub, 278
    Sinus Relief Herbal Steam, 50
    Soothe My Throat Gargle, 114
    Starstruck Multi-Herb Elixir, 199
Rosemary Digestive Tea, 29
rosemary oil, 153
    Beard Wash Soap, 338–339
    Flu-Fighting Gargle, 44
    Invigorating Cellulite-Reducing Salt Scrub,
        291–292
    Mermaids Kisses Salty Sea Soap, 332
    Rosemary Peppermint Foot Scrub, 278
    Rosemary Shampoo, 104
Rosemary Peppermint Foot Scrub, 278
Rosemary Shampoo, 104
rose petals
    Aphrodisiac Tea, 299
roses
    Vitamin C Flower Power Blend, 196
rosewood
    Beard Wash Soap, 338–339
rue, 124

S
safflower oil
    Lavender Bath Salt, 80
sage, 124, 126, 154–155
    Berry Good Hydrating Tonic, 213
    for multiple sclerosis, 20
    Sage Cherry Cough Syrup, 48
    Tooth and Gum Health Mouthwash, 342
Sage Cherry Cough Syrup, 48
salmon
    Maple Citrus-Glazed Salmon, 241
sandalwood oil
    Romantic Massage Blend, 301–302
    Sweet and Subtle Sugar Scrub, 291
    Warm and Woody Shaving Cream, 107
Sanitizing Counter Spray, 315
sassafras, 124
Scotch broom, 124
scrubs, 287–293
seaweed
    Mermaids Kisses Salty Sea Soap, 332

sedative, 129
selenium
    for infertility, 105
self-heal, 165
    Calendula Vein Liniment, 74
    Mullein and Garlic Ear Oil, 86
Seriously Detox, 180
sesame oil
    Arthritis Joint Rub, 78
shampoo, 277
    pet, 325
shatavari
    Aphrodisiac Tea, 299
shaving (men), 107
shea butter
    Basil Lavender Natural Deodorant, 285
    Bites Be Gone Anti-Itch Paste, 63
    DIY Vapor Rub, 42
    Eczema Lotion Bar, 61
    Warm and Woody Shaving Cream, 107
Simple Homemade Massage Oil, 267
sinusitis, 50
Sinus Relief Herbal Steam, 50
skin brushing, 268–269
Skin Healing Oil, 267
skullcap, 126, 129
sleep, 223
Sleepy Time Chamomile Tincture, 7
slippery elm, 129
    Honey Lemon Ginger Drops, 114
    Tooth and Gum Health Powder, 342
smoking, 93
smoothies, 170–172, 186–191
snake plant, 310
soaps, 329–340
Soothe Away the Ouch Sunburn Blend, 67
Soothe My Throat Gargle, 114
Soothing Chamomile Astringent Eyewash, 87
sores, 59
sore throat, 114
Soup Enhancer, 45
Spa Day at Home, 181
Sparkling Glass Cleaner, 322
spearmint
    Heartburn Relief, 32

Sinus Relief Herbal Steam, 50
    Soothe Away the Ouch Sunburn Blend, 67
    Tummy and Teething Calm Popsicle, 116
    Yarrow Rose Hip Cold and Flu Relief, 38
Spicy Charm, 181
Spicy Immunity Vinegar Tincture, 204
Spicy Pomegranate and Coconut Tonic, 212
spider plant, 310
spinach
    Gingerly Recovery, 183
    Mint Condition, 183
    Pine for Me, 180
    Seriously Detox, 180
    Spicy Charm, 181
    Youth Glow, 181
Spinach and Corn Quesadillas, 259
sprains, 82
squash
    Chai-Infused Coconut Milk Butternut Squash
        Soup, 243
    Moroccan Chickpea Slow Cooker Stew, 243
    Quinoa-Stuffed Acorn Squash, 242
stain remover, 323
star anise
    Starstruck Multi-Herb Elixir, 199
Starstruck Multi-Herb Elixir, 199
stimulant, 129
stimulation, 296–302
Stinky Foot Solution Soak, 278
St. John's wort, 126
    Antidepressant Tea, 6
    for multiple sclerosis, 20
stomachic, 129
Stomach-Stabilizing Tea, 33
strawberries
    Berry Citrus Cream, 188
    Berry Good Hydrating Tonic, 213
    Kale to the Rescue, 183
    Kumquat Berry Cherry, 188
    Tropical Face Cleanser, 280
stress, 10, 31
Stress and Anxiety Support Syrup, 10
Stress-Relieving Diffuser Blend, 10
sunburn, 67
sunflower, 156

sunflower lecithin
    Super Pain Balm, 82
sunflower seeds
    Bronchitis Elixir, 48
Sunshine Coconut, Ginger, and Turmeric Tonic, 210
Super Green Vitamin/Mineral Blend, 196
Super Pain Balm, 82
sweet almond oil
    Beautiful Body Oil, 266
    Diarrhea Calming Massage Blend, 28
    Flu-Fighting Neck and Chest Rub, 44
    Orange Blossom Honey Salt Scrub, 293
    Romantic Massage Blend, 301–302
    Rosemary Peppermint Foot Scrub, 278
    Warm and Woody Shaving Cream, 107
Sweet and Subtle Sugar Scrub, 291
sweet potato
    Moroccan Chickpea Slow Cooker Stew, 243
    Potato and Tomato Spice, 178
    Roasted Vegetables, 245
    Rocking the Roots, 178
Sweet Potato Pancakes, 236
sweet violet
    Daisy Restorative Lung Tea, 42
Swiss chard
    Deep Kiwi Green, 181

T
Tart Peach Cream, 191
tea, 194–197
    Antidepressant Tea, 6
    Aphrodisiac Tea, 299
    Bone Up Tea, 81
    Cholesterol-Lowering Tea, 71
    Daisy Restorative Lung Tea, 42
    DIY Chamomile Flower Tea for Anxiety and Stress, 4
    green
        Banana Ginger Dream, 186
        Berry Citrus Cream, 188
        Blood Orange and Blackberry, 189
        Cholesterol-Lowering Tea, 71
        Cocoa Pom, 189
        for dandruff, 60
        EGCG Power, 191
        Grapefruit and Green Tea, 189
        Grapefruit Rosemary, 188
        Grilled Pear Salad with Green Tea Dressing, 246
        Kumquat Berry Cherry, 188
        Mango Cream, 186
        Tart Peach Cream, 191
        Vanilla Bean Banana, 186
    Head Cold Tea, 40
    Kombucha, 30
    Rosemary Digestive Tea, 29
    Tummy Tamer Tea, 30
Tea for Migraines, 19
tea tree oil, 126
    for athlete's foot, 56
    Bites Be Gone Anti-Itch Paste, 63
    for dandruff, 60
    Lice Repellent, 113
    Mullein and Garlic Ear Oil, 86
teething, 116
thistle, 165
throat, sore, 114
thyme, 126, 158–159
    Cold and Flu Tincture, 40
    Cooling Peppermint Herb Tonic, 212
    Daisy Restorative Lung Tea, 42
    Herbal Apple Cider and Honey Elixir, 200
    Lemongrass Ginger Thyme Elixir, 199
    Refreshing Galangal Cider, 210
    Roasted Vegetables, 245
    Soothe My Throat Gargle, 114
    Starstruck Multi-Herb Elixir, 199
    Topical Wash, 100
tincture, 204
    Calendula Antiseptic Tincture, 59
    Cold and Flu Tincture, 40
    Digestion Tincture, 30
    Sleepy Time Chamomile Tincture, 7
tofu
    Green Bean, Pear, and Tofu, 254
tomato
    Baked Gluten-Free Chicken Nuggets with
        Homemade Ketchup, 256
    Butter Me Up, 183
    Cherry Tasty, 180

Moroccan Chickpea Slow Cooker Stew, 243
Potato and Tomato Spice, 178
Ultimate Cleanser, 181
Vegetarian Chili, 242
tonic, 129, 210–214
Tooth and Gum Health Mouthwash, 342
Tooth and Gum Health Powder, 342
toothpaste, 341–342
Topical Wash, 100
tortillas
Spinach and Corn Quesadillas, 259
toxins, 168–169
Trace Minerals Nightcap Shot, 216
trichloroethylene, 308
Tropical Face Cleanser, 280
Tummy and Teething Calm Popsicle, 116
Tummy Tamer Tea, 30
turmeric, 126, 129, 234
Anti-Inflammatory Spicy Wake-Me-Up Shot, 216
Cooling Peppermint Herb Tonic, 212
Farnoosh's Magic Potion Tonic Recipe, 214
Maca Hot Chocolate, 299
for multiple sclerosis, 20
Pine for Me, 180
Rocking the Roots, 178
Seriously Detox, 180
Spicy Charm, 181
Sunshine Coconut, Ginger, and Turmeric Tonic, 210
Super Pain Balm, 82
Tooth and Gum Health Powder, 342
Ultimate Cleanser, 181
Turnip Leek Mash, 254

## U

Ultimate Cleanser, 181
urinary tract infection, 98

## V

valerian, 126, 129
Vanilla Bean Banana, 186
varicose veins, 74
Vegan Pumpkin Brownies, 246
vegetable broth, 226
Quinoa Risotto with Shiitake Mushrooms and
Arugula, 241

vegetable cleaner, 318
vegetable glycerin
Rosemary Shampoo, 104
Vegetarian Chili, 242
vitamin B1
for multiple sclerosis, 20
vitamin C
for infertility, 105
Vitamin C Flower Power Blend, 196
vitamin E
Basil Lavender Natural Deodorant, 285
Eye'll Be Gentle Makeup Remover, 280
for infertility, 105
Lavender Bath Salt, 80
Pineapple Weed Insect Repellent, 63
vitex
Healthy Moon Cycle Blend, 95
Hormonal Balance, 204
vodka
Sleepy Time Chamomile Tincture, 7
vomiting, 33
vulnerary, 129

## W

waffles, 234
walnuts
Energy Balls, 249
Warm and Woody Shaving Cream, 107
watercress, 160
Green Apple Glee, 178
watermelon
EGCG Power, 191
Watermelon Raspberry Cooler, 188
Wellness Blend, 197
Whipped Coconut Oil Body Butter, 265
white fir oil
All-Purpose Cleaner, 314
Citrus-Fir Dish Soap, 317
witch hazel
Baby's Hand-Sanitizing Spray, 339
Bathroom Scrub, 319
Calendula Vein Liniment, 74
Eye'll Be Gentle Makeup Remover, 280
Kid-Safe Hand-Sanitizing Spray, 339–340
Soothe Away the Ouch Sunburn Blend, 67

women's health, 90–100
wormwood, 124, 126

## X
xylene, 308

## Y
yam
    Hormonal Balance, 204
yarrow
    Calendula Vein Liniment, 74
    Hair Rinse, 104
    Pain Relief Tonic, 94
    Tooth and Gum Health Mouthwash, 342
    Wellness Blend, 197
Yarrow Rose Hip Cold and Flu Relief, 38
yeast infection, 100
yellow dock, 129
    Iron and Energy Syrup, 70

Super Green Vitamin/Mineral Blend, 196
ylang-ylang oil
    Romantic Massage Blend, 301–302
    Sweet and Subtle Sugar Scrub, 291
yogurt
    Baked Frittata, 238
    Creamy Mango and Yogurt, 255
    Homemade Crock-Pot Yogurt, 240
    Honey and Coconut Oil Healing Mask, 282
    Lemon-Honey Facial Mask, 281
    Minty Cucumber Facial Mask, 282
    Tropical Face Cleanser, 280
Youth Glow, 181

## Z
zinc
    for infertility, 105

# NOTES

# NOTES

# NOTES

# NOTES

# Also Available

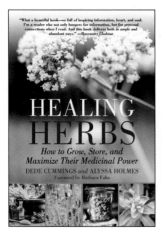

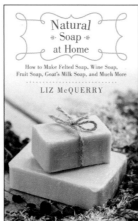

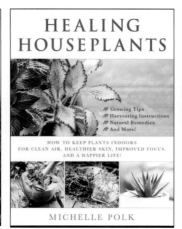

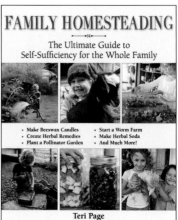

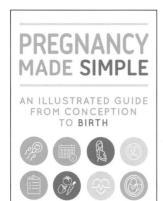

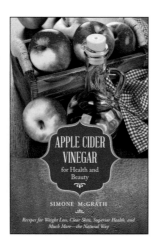

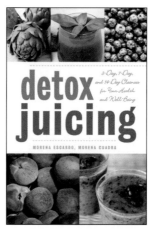

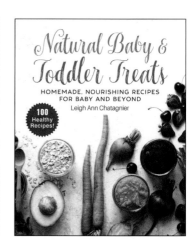

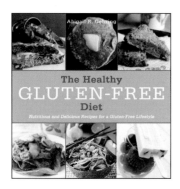

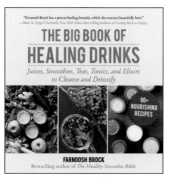

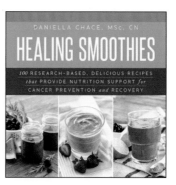

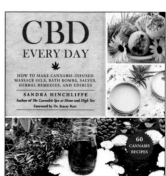

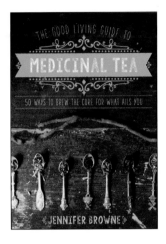

THE GOOD LIVING GUIDE TO
**MEDICINAL TEA**
50 WAYS TO BREW THE CURE FOR WHAT AILS YOU
JENNIFER BROWNE

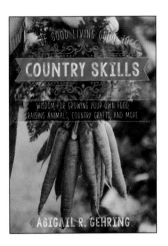

THE GOOD LIVING GUIDE TO
**COUNTRY SKILLS**
WISDOM FOR GROWING YOUR OWN FOOD, RAISING ANIMALS, COUNTRY CRAFTS, AND MORE
ABIGAIL R. GEHRING

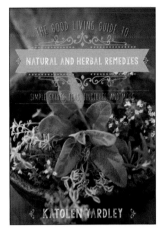

THE GOOD LIVING GUIDE TO
**NATURAL AND HERBAL REMEDIES**
SIMPLE SALVES, TEAS, TINCTURES, AND MORE
KATOLEN YARDLEY

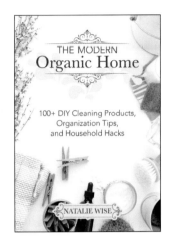

THE MODERN
**Organic Home**
100+ DIY Cleaning Products, Organization Tips, and Household Hacks
NATALIE WISE

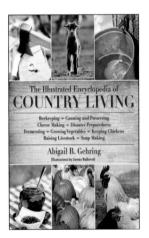

The Illustrated Encyclopedia of
**COUNTRY LIVING**
Beekeeping • Canning and Preserving
Cheese Making • Disaster Preparedness
Fermenting • Growing Vegetables • Keeping Chickens
Raising Livestock • Soap Making
Abigail R. Gehring
Illustrations by James Balkovek

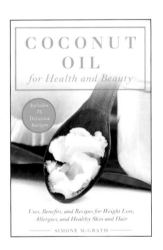

**COCONUT OIL**
*for Health and Beauty*
Includes 75 Delicious Recipes
Uses, Benefits, and Recipes for Weight Loss, Allergies, and Healthy Skin and Hair
SIMONE MCGRATH

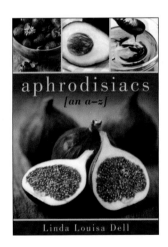

**aphrodisiacs**
[an a–z]
Linda Louisa Dell

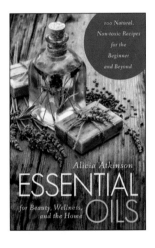

100 Natural, Non-toxic Recipes for the Beginner and Beyond
Alicia Atkinson
**ESSENTIAL OILS**
for Beauty, Wellness, and the Home

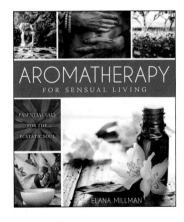

**AROMATHERAPY**
FOR SENSUAL LIVING
ESSENTIAL OILS FOR THE ECSTATIC SOUL
ELANA MILLMAN

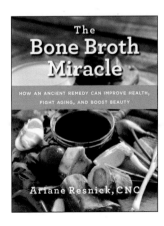

The
**Bone Broth Miracle**
HOW AN ANCIENT REMEDY CAN IMPROVE HEALTH, FIGHT AGING, AND BOOST BEAUTY
Ariane Resnick, CNC